Comparative Neuropsychology

Comparative Neuropsychology

Edited by

A. David Milner
School of Psychology
University of St Andrews

Oxford New York Tokyo
OXFORD UNIVERSITY PRESS
1998

Oxford University Press, Great Clarendon Street, Oxford OX2 6DP

Oxford New York
Athens Auckland Bangkok Bogota Bombay
Buenos Aires Calcutta Cape Town Dar es Salaam
Delhi Florence Hong Kong Istanbul Karachi
Kuala Lumpur Madras Madrid Melbourne
Mexico City Nairobi Paris Singapore
Taipei Tokyo Toronto Warsaw
and associated companies in
Berlin Ibadan

Oxford is a trade mark of Oxford University Press

Published in the United States
by Oxford University Press Inc., New York

A catalogue record for this book is available from the British Library

Library of Congress Cataloging in Publication Data
Comparative neuropsychology / edited by A. David Milner.
"A tribute to the memory of George Ettlinger" – Foreword.
Includes bibliographical references and index.
1. Neuropsychology. 2. Comparative neurobiology. 3. Ettlinger, E. G. (E. George) I. Milner, A. D. (A. David)
[DNLM: 1. Neuropsychology. 2. Brain–physiology. 3. Cognition–physiology. 4. Evolution. WL 103.5 C737 1998]
QP360.C65 1998 612.8'2–dc21 97-41989
ISBN 0 19 852411 0 (Hbk)

Typeset by Downdell, Oxford
Printed in Great Britain by
Biddles Ltd, Guildford & King's Lynn

In memory of George Ettlinger (1927–1993)

Foreword

ENNIO DE RENZI

In this book, distinguished neuroscientists pay a tribute to the memory of George Ettlinger, one of the leading figures in neuropsychological research in the course of the past 40 years. I first met George Ettlinger in 1963 at one of the earliest International Neuropsychology Symposia. At that time they were organized every year by Henry Hécaen, who used to gather people—mostly neurologists, and mostly from around Europe—who were interested in the effects of brain damage on higher nervous functions. The atmosphere was relaxed, and presentations were mostly given in the speaker's own language, which a few participants, conversant in foreign languages, would translate in a low voice for their near neighbours. Communications tended to be in a typical clinical style, being based on data and beliefs drawn from long clinical experience and anecdotal evidence. So, it was rather surprising to hear George starting his presentation, which concerned the then new issue of the relationship of memory disorders to temporal lobe damage, with the following words: 'I will only concern myself with findings that have been validated at a probability level of $p < 0.05$. If anybody wishes to know the reasons for this selection, I am ready to give them.' I am not sure that the audience of mostly greying clinicians was altogether familiar with the subtlety of statistical methodology or wholly convinced of the need to meet its requirements before accepting a statement. Be that as it may, nobody asked questions and George went on with his critical review of recent research. His covert polemic foreshadowed the way that neuropsychology was to change in the following years, as experimental psychologists entered the field in greater numbers.

George was lucky to have been trained by Oliver Zangwill, one of the few scientists that in the 1950s were to rekindle interest in the study of cognitive disorders and to fight against the disheartening feeling of impotence that, between the two World Wars, had followed the controversy between localizationists and anti-localizationists. Along with Henry Hécaen, Hans-Lucas Teuber, Arthur Benton, and a few others, Zangwill was convinced that the study of brain-damaged patients had much to teach people interested in the relation of brain to mind, and had instilled his enthusiasm into a group of young scientists he gathered at Queen Square in London. Among them was George Ettlinger, who soon proved his talent in two papers that remain landmarks in the history of clinical neuropsychology. He was the first author in one of these early studies to provide evidence of the specific role played by the right hemisphere in visuo-spatial tasks. In the other, he made a substantial contribution to settling an old issue that had plagued the interpretation of agnosia for many years. He succeeded in providing quantitative evidence from a group study—a methodological novelty in those days—that visual agnosia could not be accounted for by concomitant sensory deficits, since their severity was not commensurate with the recognition impairment, a conclusion that has been recently borne out (see Chapter 2).

After having devoted his early years to human neuropsychology, Ettlinger turned to monkey research, convinced, as he said, that progress in the understanding of the relation of brain to behaviour could only be achieved by bridging the gulf dividing clinical from experimental work and elucidating discontinuities as well as commonalities between human and non-human primates. It would be impossible, and outside the realm of my specific competence, to summarize here the contributions he made to providing animal models for the interpretation of neurological disorders originally delineated in a clinical setting. I would like, however, to recall two particular areas in which I found his research enlightening when I addressed the same topics from the perspective of human neuropsychology:

(1) the disruption of spatial behaviour following parietal ablation (see Chapter 5); and
(2) the unexpected finding that unilateral lesions of the second somatosensory area brought about a bilateral impairment of tactile discrimination and learning.

The energy and time George devoted to animal experiments and the important results he obtained did not divert his attention from clinical issues, and indeed he was, in a sense, unique among people pursuing the investigation of brain and behaviour for his enduring interest in both sides of the discipline. I cannot think of any other neuropsychologist, with the exception of Denny-Brown, who remained so active in the two areas, plundering the knowledge acquired in either one or the other to gain a better perspective in both. A good exemplar of this cross-fertilization would be his research on the callosal syndrome, which he investigated both in the commissurotomized monkey and in patients with callosal agenesis (see Chapters 8 and 9).

George had an unobtrusive and selfless personality that I came to appreciate in the course of the exchanges we had in the editorship of *Cortex*. I knew that I could always rely on his thoughtful and well-balanced opinion and that his advice was both open-minded and rigorous. George never made a issue of prestige, nor tried to be flamboyant 'on stage', but once you had gained his confidence, you could rely on his loyal friendship. He also had a wry sense of humour. When he came to Italy for the San Geminiano meeting of the INS in 1964, he lodged at an inexpensive hotel, which did not provide warm water from the taps, in spite of the fact that one of them bore an F (*freddo* for cold) and the other a C (*caldo* for hot). He did not complain of this to me, but merely commented that Italian hotel-keepers know English remarkably well and were even kind enough to provide the guest with information both in Italian and English. Obviously, he surmised, they used F for *freddo* and C for cold!

The legacy of George Ettlinger as a researcher is inherited by the community of neuroscientists; that of him as a man lives in the memory of those who had the privilege to become acquainted with his sensibility and discretion. Both will miss him.

Preface

This book grew out of discussions I had with Dr Alick Elithorn and then with Dr Dick Passingham during the summer of 1995. Alick was the first to propose the idea of publishing a book in honour of George Ettlinger, who met an untimely death at the age of 66 in December 1993. Dick and I were the beneficiaries of George's wisdom and enthusiasm as contemporaneous doctoral students with him in the late 1960s. During the period I spent in his laboratory (1966–1970), George was perhaps at his most productive, and I have vivid memories of his many collaborators, including the late Cyril Rashbass, Bert Morton, George Fenton, Donald Scott, Colin B. Blakemore, John Wilson, Rosalind Ridley, Martin Jarvis, and (especially) the late Adrienne Moffett, as well as several visiting researchers, including Denyse Gautrin, Tullio Manzoni, and Arthur Schwartz. George was the most important scientific influence in my life: he taught me both how to be a scientist, and how to communicate science in writing.

But this book is not simply a salute to George Ettlinger, it is also intended as a stock-taking exercise for a scientific movement in which George was a major player. Comparative neuropsychology began to gather momentum during the 1950s, and it soon came to provide a major component in the contents of the first journal to be devoted to neuropsychology (*Neuropsychologia*, founded in 1963). The journal took as its main aim the advancement of our understanding of human brain function, but it saw the road towards this goal as needing inputs from animal research as well as from clinical research and research with normal human subjects. The first editorial of *Neuropsychologia*, for example, defined neuropsychology as an area of neurology 'of common interest to neurologists, psychiatrists, psychologists and neurophysiologists', and it went on 'information of great value to human pathology is to be obtained from animal experiment, which may be expected to throw valuable light on the basic mechanisms of cerebral organisation.' (*Neuropsychologia*, **1**, 1–2). George Ettlinger joined the Board of Associate Editors of *Neuropsychologia* during its first year.

However, despite the exciting work done during the 1950s and 1960s, neuropsychology remained a minority interest until the early 1970s, at which point it finally matured as a recognized sub-discipline within experimental psychology. That increased popularity owed much to the fact that cognitive psychologists began to realize that studies of human brain damage could cast powerful light on models of normal cognition. Much of the credit for launching what became known as 'cognitive' neuropsychology must be given to Elizabeth Warrington, by virtue of her pioneering studies of amnesia and acquired dyslexia during the late 1960s and early 1970s. But some cognitive neuropsychologists (of whom Warrington was not one) have regarded the brain as a 'black box' that does not need to be studied in its own right: for them brain-damaged patients have provided merely a convenient test bed for cognitive theories.

Comparative neuropsychologists reject that view absolutely: for them the brain is all-important. In particular, they acknowledge the need for the detailed neuroanatomy and neurophysiology that only animal research can provide. And they believe that it is only through a knowledge of the brain that we can fully investigate continuities (and discontinuities) in the evolution of behaviour. For these reasons, while comparative neuropsychology provided the launch pad for cognitive neuropsychology, it still remains most decidedly alive and well in its own right in the closing years of the 1990s. Indeed, it continues to flourish as an indispensable part of current neuroscience, paradoxically in large part within the ambit of 'cognitive' neuroscience.

This book is intended as a testament to that bill of health. It includes chapters by several ex-colleagues and students of George Ettlinger and by others who knew him well or corresponded with him over matters of mutual interest. Most of all it is intended to cover the areas of Ettlinger's active research interests, which encompassed almost the entire breadth of neuropsychology. I am most grateful for the encouragement and help of Madeline Ettlinger in bringing the book to fruition.

University of St Andrews A.D.M.
November 1997

Contents

List of contributors xv

1 Introduction: comparative neuropsychology 1
A. David Milner

2 Sensory factors in human visual agnosia 15
Andrew W. Young

3 Ettlinger at Bay: can visual agnosia be explained by low-level visual impairments? 30
Alan Cowey, Paul Dean, and Larry Weiskrantz

4 Cross-modal associations, intramodal associations, and object identification in macaque monkeys 51
Elisabeth A. Murray, Ludise Malkova, and Sonia Goulet

5 Visual processing in the primate parietal lobe 70
A. David Milner and H. Chris Dijkerman

6 Memory and the human temporal lobes 95
John M. Oxbury and Susan M. Oxbury

7 Memory systems in primates: episodic, semantic, and perceptual learning 109
Amanda Parker and David Gaffan

8 Interhemispheric transfer following partial commissurotomy in humans and monkeys 127
Madeline J. Eacott

9 Visual integration in callosal agenesis 143
Malcolm A. Jeeves

10 Towards a unified view of cerebral hemispheric specializations in vertebrates 167
Peter F. MacNeilage

11 Brain mechanisms of apraxia 184
Ulrike Halsband

12 Perspectives on visuospatial neglect 213
Monika Harvey

13 Cognition in great apes 228
Richard W. Byrne

14 Mental representation in human and monkey neuropsychology 245
Rosalind M. Ridley and Harry F. Baker

15 The specializations of the human neocortex 271
Richard E. Passingham

Index 299

Contributors

Harry F. Baker

Department of Experimental Psychology, University of Cambridge, Innes Building, School of Clinical Veterinary Medicine, Madingley Road, Cambridge CB3 0ES, UK

Richard W. Byrne

School of Psychology, University of St Andrews, St Andrews KY16 9JU, Scotland, UK

Alan Cowey

Department of Experimental Psychology, University of Oxford, South Parks Road, Oxford OX1 3UD, UK

Paul Dean

Department of Psychology, University of Sheffield, Sheffield S10 2TN, UK

Ennio De Renzi

Clinica Neurologica dell'Università, via del Pozzo 71, 41000 Modena, Italy

H. Chris Dijkerman

School of Psychology, University of St Andrews, St Andrews KY16 9JU, Scotland, UK

Madeline J. Eacott

Department of Psychology, University of Durham, South Road, Durham DH1 3LE, UK

David Gaffan

Department of Experimental Psychology, University of Oxford, South Parks Road, Oxford OX1 3UD, UK

Sonia Goulet

Laboratory of Neuropsychology, National Institute of Mental Health, Bldg 49, Room 1B80, Bethesda, MD 20892, USA

Ulrike Halsband

Eberhard-Karls-Universität Tübingen, Institute for Medical Psychology and Behavioural Neurobiology, Gartenstrasse 29, D-72074 Tübingen, Germany

Monika Harvey

Department of Psychology, University of Bristol, Bristol BS8 1TN, UK

Malcolm A. Jeeves

School of Psychology, University of St Andrews, St Andrews KY16 9JU, Scotland, UK

Peter F. MacNeilage

Department of Psychology, University of Texas, Austin TX 78712, USA

Ludise Malkova

Laboratory of Neuropsychology, National Institute of Mental Health, Bldg 49, Room 1B80, Bethesda, MD 20892, USA

A. David Milner

School of Psychology, University of St Andrews, St Andrews KY16 9JU, Scotland UK

Elisabeth A. Murray

Laboratory of Neuropsychology, National Institute of Mental Health, Bldg 49, Room 1B80, Bethesda, MD 20892, USA

John M. Oxbury

Department of Neurology, Radcliffe Infirmary, Oxford OX2 6HE, UK

Susan M. Oxbury

Department of Clinical Neuropsychology, Radcliffe Infirmary, Oxford OX2 6HE, UK

Amanda Parker

Department of Experimental Psychology, University of Oxford, South Parks Road, Oxford OX1 3UD, UK

Richard E. Passingham

Department of Experimental Psychology, University of Oxford, South Parks Road, Oxford OX1 3UD, UK

Rosalind M. Ridley

Department of Experimental Psychology, University of Cambridge, Innes Building, School of Clinical Veterinary Medicine, Madingley Road, Cambridge CB3 0ES, UK

Larry Weiskrantz

Department of Experimental Psychology, University of Oxford, South Parks Road, Oxford OX1 3UD, UK

Andrew W. Young

Department of Psychology, University of York, Heslington, York YO1 5DD, UK

1

Introduction: comparative neuropsychology

A. DAVID MILNER

1.1 A potted history

What is comparative neuropsychology? For present purposes, it is quite simply *the study of human brain and behaviour from a biological perspective*. Neuropsychology has grown out of a wedding between the traditions of clinical neurology and those of experimental psychology. Neurologists began to develop their own systematic investigative procedures for examining damaged brain function during the years during and after the First World War, notably exemplified by the work of Holmes and Horrax (1919) and Poppelreuter (1917) with brain-injured war veterans. Even at that early stage, the influence of experimental psychologists (notably those of the *Gestalt* school) was becoming apparent in Germany (e.g. Goldstein and Gelb 1918). In effect this cross-fertilization signalled the birth of neuropsychology, although the term was not coined until 1949, by Donald Hebb, a student of Karl Lashley's (Hebb 1949). In America, the Behaviorist school was all-powerful in psychology during the inter-war years, but with the migration of German scientists during those years, the new interest in combining neurology with experimental psychology spread across the Atlantic. When Lashley arrived at the University of Chicago in 1927, he was already combining the behavioural techniques of animal learning theorists with investigations of brain anatomy in rodents. It was natural in this intellectual climate for Heinrich Klüver, trained in the German tradition, to begin his classic behavioural studies of cortical lesions in monkeys when he joined Lashley the following year. Between the two of them, they set the scene for a true comparative neuropsychology to be born (e.g. Klüver and Bucy 1938; Klüver 1942; Beach *et al.* 1960).

But it took another World War for neuropsychology truly to come into its own. There were important reports by Oliver Zangwill and his colleagues in the UK (e.g. Paterson and Zangwill 1944) and, subsequently, the highly influential series of papers by Hans-Lucas Teuber and his group (see Teuber *et al.* 1960). One of Teuber's group, Josephine Semmes, provided a link with the comparative tradition, through her work with Karl Pribram, a neurosurgeon who had been trained in experimental neuropsychology by Lashley. Pribram set up a laboratory at the Institute of Living in Hartford, Connecticut, and it was within this environment that a number of post-doctoral researchers, including Mort Mishkin, Larry Weiskrantz, Martha Wilson, Bill Wilson, and George Ettlinger, as well as Semmes, acquired their research training prior to setting up their own primate laboratories elsewhere. Also in the 1950s, important independent developments were beginning in California and in Canada. It was at this time that Roger Sperry and Ronald Myers began their pioneering research on callosal transection in cats and primates at the California Institute of Technology, which subsequently led in the 1960s to the first neuropsychological studies of total cerebral commissurotomy in humans. And at the same time, Brenda Milner, who had recently emigrated from England, began her highly influential experimental studies of the effects of unilateral and bilateral temporal-lobe surgery on memory and perception at the Montréal Neurological Institute.

While not all of the researchers active at this time combined both human and animal research, they all took it for granted that a full understanding of human brain function would require considerable input from studies of the neuroanatomy, neurophysiology, and behaviour of animals, particularly our primate relatives. In this way the blossoming of neuropsychology in the 1950s and 1960s was a truly comparative enterprise. George Ettlinger was in the thick of this post-war development. He had received his postgraduate training and Ph.D. supervision from Zangwill at the Institute of Neurology in London, graduating in 1955. His thesis research appeared as a highly influential paper arguing against a sensory basis for visual agnosia (Ettlinger 1956*a*). He then spent a formative year (1956–57) in Pribram's laboratory. His earliest work with monkeys included a study comparing the effects of frontal and posterior parietal lesions (Ettlinger and Wegener 1958) and one on visual pattern discrimination following combined lesions of the optic tract, inferior temporal cortex, and corpus callosum (Ettlinger 1959*a*). George Ettlinger was one of the few who actively combined human and animal research, and he did so consistently throughout his scientific career. He thus embodied the biological study of brain and behaviour with a commitment matched by few others. He also made a point of looking at behaviour *directly*, in the true biological tradition, not only through formal techniques such as discrimination training (see Ettlinger 1968).

1.2 This book

In this volume, I have tried to assemble authoritative essays by current experts in a number of the areas that interested George Ettlinger during his career, though because of the sheer breadth of those interests, this aim has not been wholly achieved. His earliest concerns, relating to the nature of visual agnosia and the brain systems underlying visual recognition, are addressed in the chapters by Andrew Young (Chapter 2) and by Alan Cowey and colleagues (Chapter 3). Cross-modal recognition was a capacity that Ettlinger first began to look for in monkeys in 1960 (Burton and Ettlinger 1960), and recent developments are described in the essay by Betsy Murray and her colleagues (Chapter 4). Issues of parietal lobe function in vision, another of his long-running preoccupations, are addressed by Chris Dijkerman and myself (Chapter 5). Ettlinger studied the role of temporal lobe systems in memory and learning in work done with patients and animals with focal epilepsy, as well as by use of ablation and electrophysiological techniques (Blakemore *et al.* 1966; Ettlinger and Gautrin 1971; Ridley and Ettlinger 1973). These topics are addressed in the essays by John and Susan Oxbury (Chapter 6) and Amanda Parker and David Gaffan (Chapter 7).

Ettlinger began to study the effects of callosal section in monkeys at an early stage of his career (Ettlinger 1959*a*), and subsequently carried out studies also in humans, though in this case testing individuals with *congenital* absence of the corpus callosum. These research areas are addressed in the chapters by Madeline Eacott (Chapter 8) and Malcolm Jeeves (Chapter 9). Lateral preferences in monkeys and their implications for human laterality was another of his long-standing interests, dating back to 1961 (Ettlinger 1961*a*): this topic is discussed by Peter MacNeilage (Chapter 10). Ettlinger's interest in laterality in animals arose of course from the hope that it would help us understand human brain asymmetries, as manifest in such neurological conditions as unilateral neglect and apraxia. He published theoretical and experimental papers on both of these conditions, which are addressed in the chapters by Ulrike Halsband (Chapter 11) and Monika Harvey (Chapter 12). Both of these authors worked with Ettlinger in Germany during the last phase of his career, in the 1980s.

During the 1970s and 1980s, Ettlinger took his interest in comparative neuropsychology one step further, by embarking on studies of the cognitive and linguistic capacities of chimpanzees. The essay by Dick Byrne (Chapter 13) provides an update on current research in ape and monkey cognition. Finally, the last two chapters of this book discuss critically questions basic to the whole comparative enterprise: whether and how we can validly transplant concepts derived from human cognitive psychology to monkey neuropsychology, and whether there are evolutionary discontinuities in cortical brain structures among the higher primate species, including humans. These basic comparative questions concerned George Ettlinger for many years, as first exemplified in the paper by Drewe *et al.* (1970); they are discussed here by Rosalind Ridley and Harry Baker (Chapter 14), and Dick Passingham (Chapter 15).

1.3 Publications of George Ettlinger (1927–1993)

1955

Ettlinger, G. and Jackson, C. V. Organic factors in developmental dyslexia. *Proceedings of the Royal Society of Medicine*, **48**, 998–1000.

Ettlinger, G., Jackson, C. V., and Zangwill, O. L. Dysphasia following right temporal lobectomy in a right-handed man. *Journal of Neurology, Neurosurgery and Psychiatry*, **18**, 214–17.

1956

Ettlinger, G. Sensory deficits in visual agnosia. *Journal of Neurology, Neurosurgery and Psychiatry*, **19**, 297–307.

Ettlinger, G. The fusion frequency of flicker in the central and peripheral field with photopic levels of surround luminance. *Quarterly Journal of Experimental Psychology*, **8**, 172–81.

Ettlinger, G., Jackson, C. V., and Zangwill, O. L. Cerebral dominance in sinistrals. *Brain*, **79**, 569–88.

1957

Ettlinger, G. Visual discrimination following successive unilateral temporal excisions in monkeys. *Journal of Physiology*, **140**, 38–39P.

Ettlinger, G., Warrington, E., and Zangwill, O. L. A further study of visual–spatial agnosia. *Brain*, **80**, 335–61.

1958

Ettlinger, G. and Wegener, J. Somaesthetic alternation, discrimination and orientation after frontal and parietal lesions in monkeys. *Quarterly Journal of Experimental Psychology*, **10**, 177–86.

1959

Ettlinger, G. Visual discrimination following successive temporal ablations in monkeys. *Brain*, **82**, 232–50.

Ettlinger, G. Visual discrimination with a single manipulandum following temporal ablations in the monkey. *Quarterly Journal of Experimental Psychology*, **11**, 164–74.

1960

Bates, J. A. V. and Ettlinger, G. Posterior biparietal ablations in the monkeychanges to neurological and behavioral testing. *Archives of Neurology*, **3**, 177–92.

Burton, D. and Ettlinger, G. Cross-modal transfer of training in monkeys. *Nature*, **186**, 1071–2.

Casey, T. and Ettlinger, G. The occasional 'independence' of dyslexia and dysgraphia from dysphasia. *Journal of Neurology, Neurosurgery and Psychiatry*, **12**, 228–36.

Ettlinger, G. Cross-modal transfer of training in monkeys. *Behaviour*, **16**, 56–65.

Ettlinger, G. Discrimination learning theory: excitatory vs. inhibitory tendencies in monkeys. *Quarterly Journal of Experimental Psychology*, **12**, 41–4.

Ettlinger, G. The description and interpretation of pictures in cases of brain lesion. *Journal of Mental Science*, **106**, 1337–46.

1961

Cole, M., Chorover, S. L., and Ettlinger, G. Cross-modal transfer in man. *Nature*, **191**, 1225–6.

Ettlinger, G. Lateral preferences in monkeys. *Behaviour*, **17**, 275–87.

Ettlinger, G. Learning in two sense-modalities. *Nature*, **191**, 308.

Ettlinger, G. and Kalsbeck, J. E. The effect of successive posterior parietal lobe ablations on tactile shape discrimination in the monkey. *Journal of Physiology*, **156**, 34–35P.

Ettlinger, G. and Wyke, M. Defects in identifying objects visually in a patient with cerebrovascular disease. *Journal of Neurology, Neurosurgery and Psychiatry*, **24**, 254–59.

Wyke, M. and Ettlinger, G. Efficiency of recognition in the left and right visual fields. *Archives of Neurology*, **5**, 659–65.

1962

Ettlinger, G. Interhemispheric integration in the somatic sensory system. In *Interhemispheric relations and cerebral dominance*, (ed. V. B. Mountcastle), Ch. 5. Johns Hopkins University Press, Baltimore.

Ettlinger, G. Relationship between test difficulty and the visual impairment in monkeys with ablations of temporal cortex. *Nature*, **196**, 911–12.

Ettlinger, G. and Elithorn, A. Transfer between the hands of a mirror-image tactile shape discrimination. *Nature*, **194**, 1101–2.

Ettlinger, G. and Hurwitz, L. Dyslexia and its associated disturbances. *Neurology*, **12**, 477–80.

Ettlinger, G. and Kalsbeck, J. E. Changes in tactile discrimination and in visual reaching after successive and simultaneous bilateral posterior parietal ablations in the monkey. *Journal of Neurology, Neurosurgery and Psychiatry*, **25**, 256–68.

1963

Curzon, G., Ettlinger, G., Cole, M., and Walsh, J. The biochemical, behavioral, and neurologic effects of high l-tryptophan intake in the Rhesus monkey. *Neurology*, **13**, 431–8.

Ettlinger, G. High dietary tryptophan intake: methods used to investigate possible behaviour changes in the monkey. *Proceedings of the International Conference on Psychopharmacology, Prague, 1961.*

Ettlinger, G. Defective identification of fingers. *Neuropsychologia*, **1**, 39–45.

Ettlinger, G. and Morton, H. B. Callosal section: its effect on performance of a bimanual skill. *Science*, **139**, 485–6.

1964

Ettlinger, G. and Moffett, A. Lateral preferences in the monkey. *Nature*, **204**, 606.

1965

Ettlinger, G., de Reuck, A. V. S., and Porter, R. (ed.) *Functions of the corpus callosum.* Churchill, London.

Scott, D. F., Moffett, A., Mathews, A., and Ettlinger, G. Non-verbal learning and retention in epileptic subjects. *Proceedings of the 8th International Congress of Neurology, Vienna.*

1966

Blakemore, C. B., Ettlinger, G., and Falconer, M. A. Cognitive abilities in relation to frequency of seizures and neuropathology of the temporal lobes in man. *Journal of Neurology, Neurosurgery and Psychiatry*, **29**, 268–72.

Ettlinger, G. and Blakemore, C. B. Cross-modal transfer of conditional discrimination training in monkeys. *Nature*, **210**, 117–18.

Ettlinger, G. and Morton, H. B. Tactile discrimination performance in the monkey: transfer of training between the hands after commissural section. *Cortex*, **2**, 30–49.

Ettlinger, G., Morton, H. B., and Moffett, A. Tactile discrimination performance in the monkey: the effect of bilateral posterior parietal and lateral frontal ablations, and of callosal section. *Cortex*, **2**, 5–29.

Moffett, A. and Ettlinger, G. Opposite responding in two sense modalities. *Science*, **153**, 205–6.

1967

Cobb, W. A., Ettlinger, G., and Morton, H. B. Visual evoked potentials in binocular rivalry. *Electroencephalography and Clinical Neurophysiology—evoked potentials* (Suppl. 26), 100–7.

Cobb, W. A., Morton, H. B., and Ettlinger, G. Cerebral potentials evoked by pattern reversal and their suppression in visual rivalry. *Nature*, **216**, 1123–5.

Ettlinger, G. Visual alexia. In *Models for the perception of speech and visual form*, (ed. W. Wathen-Dunn). MIT Press, Cambridge, MA.

Ettlinger, G. Analysis of cross-modal effects and their relationship to language. In *Brain mechanisms underlying speech and language*, (ed. C. H. Millikan and F. L. Darley). Grune and Stratton, New York.

Ettlinger, G. and Blakemore, C. B. Cross-modal matching in the monkey. *Neuropsychologia*, **5**, 147–54.

Moffett, A. and Ettlinger, G. Opposite responding to position in the light and dark. *Neuropsychologia*, **5**, 59–62.

Moffett, A., Ettlinger, G., Morton, H. B., and Piercy, M. F. Tactile discrimination performance in the monkey: the effect of ablation of various subdivisions of posterior parietal cortex. *Cortex*, **3**, 59–96.

Scott, D. F., Moffett, A., Mathews, A., and Ettlinger, G. The effect of epileptic discharges on learning and memory in patients. *Epilepsia*, **8**, 188–94.

1968

Blakemore, C. B. and Ettlinger, G. The independence of visual and tactile learning in the monkey. *Journal of Physiology*, **196**, 127P.

Cobb, W. A., Ettlinger, G., and Morton, H. B. Cerebral potentials evoked in man by pattern reversal and their suppression in visual rivalry. *Journal of Physiology*, **195**, 33–34P.

Ettlinger, G. The neurological examination of animals. In *Analysis of behavioural change*, (ed. L. Weiskrantz), Ch. 12. Harper and Row, London.

Ettlinger, G. and Blakemore, C. B. Cross-modal transfer set in the monkey. *Neuropsychologia*, **7**, 41–7.

Ettlinger, G., Blakemore, C. B., and Milner, A. D. Opposite hand preferences in two sense-modalities. *Nature*, **218**, 1276.

Ettlinger, G., Iwai, E., Mishkin, M., and Rosvold, R. E. Visual discrimination in the monkey following serial ablation of interotemporal and preoccipital cortex. *Journal of Comparative and Physiological Psychology*, **65**, 110–17.

Driver, M., Ettlinger, G., Moffett, A. M., and St. John-Loe, P. Epileptogenic lesions in the monkey. *Journal of Physiology*, **196**, 93–94P.

Milner, A. D., Ettlinger, G., Morton, H. B., and Moffett, A. M. The evidence for perseveration on a delayed alternation task. *Cortex*, **4**, 138–43.

1969

Ettlinger, G. Apraxia considered as a disorder of movements that are language dependent: evidence from cases of brain bi-section. *Cortex*, **5**, 285–9.

Ettlinger, G. and Blakemore, C. B. The behavioral effects of commissural section. In *Contributions to clinical neuropsychology* (ed. A. L. Benton), Ch. 2. Aldine, Chicago.

Ettlinger, G. and Dawson, R. F. Hand preferences in the monkey: the effect of unilateral cortical removals. *Neuropsychologia*, **7**, 161–6.

1970

Drewe, E. A., Ettlinger, G., Milner, A. D., and Passingham, R. E. A comparative review of the results of neuropsychological research on man and monkey. *Cortex*, **6**, 129–63.

Ettlinger, G. Man, chimpanzee and monkey: a neuropsychological comparison. *Brain Research*, **24**, 555.

Ettlinger, G. Training monkeys by Linc-8 computer. *Cortex*, **6**, 410–16.

Ettlinger, G. and Moffett, A. M. Learning in dysphasia. *Neuropsychologia*, **8**, 465–74.

Gautrin, D. and Ettlinger, G. Lateral preferences in the monkey. *Cortex*, **6**, 287–92.

Milner, A. D. and Ettlinger, G. Cross-modal transfer of serial reversal learning in the monkey. *Neuropsychologia*, **8**, 251–8.

Moffett, A. M. and Ettlinger, G. Tactile discrimination performance in the monkey: the effect of unilateral posterior parietal ablations. *Cortex*, **6**, 47–67.

Moffett, A. M., Driver, M. V., St. John-Loe, P., and Ettlinger, G. Tactile discrimination performance in the monkey: the effect of unilateral posterior parietal discharging lesions. *Cortex*, **6**, 68–86.

1971

Ettlinger, G. Unterschiede und Übereinstimmungen zwischen der Organisation des Menschen- und Affengehirns im Licht neuropsychologischer Erkenntnise. *Klinische Wochenschrift*, **49**, 786–90.

Ettlinger, G. and Gautrin, D. Visual discrimination performance in the monkey: the effect of unilateral removals of temporal cortex. *Cortex*, **7**, 317–31.

Gautrin, D., Fenton, G., and Ettlinger, G. Aluminium hydroxide implants on the infero-temporal cortex of the monkey: their mode of influencing visual discrimination performance. *Experimental Neurology*, **33**, 459–74.

Manzoni, T. and Ettlinger, G. Impairment of tactile discrimination performance in monkeys with tectal damage. *Neuropsychologia*, **9**, 289–92.

1972

Ettlinger, G. Brain bi-section; some unsolved problems. In *Cerebral interhemispheric relations*, (ed J. Cernacek and F. Podivinsky), Ch. 24. Slovak Academy of Sciences, Bratislava.

Ettlinger, G., Blakemore, C. B., Milner, A. D., and Wilson, J. Agenesis of the corpus callosum: a behavioural investigation. *Brain*, **95**, 327–46.

Cooper, J. D., Ettlinger, G., and Goldsmith, F. H. A method of recording unit activity from ventral temporal cortex in the undrugged and lightly restrained monkey. *Journal of Physiology*, **222**, 133–134P.

Milner, A. D. and Ettlinger, G. Response latencies in go, no-go discrimination performance by monkeys. *Neuropsychologia*, **10**, 375–8.

Passingham, R. E. and Ettlinger, G. Tactile discrimination learning after selective prefrontal ablations in monkeys (*Macaca mulatta*). *Neuropsychologia*, **10**, 17–26.

1973

Ettlinger, G. The transfer of information between sense-modalities: a neuropsychological review. In *Memory and transfer of information*, (ed. H. P. Zippel), pp. 42–64. Plenum Press, New York.

Ettlinger, G., Ridley, R. M., and Hester, N. S. Successive visual discrimination performance in the monkey with brief stimuli. *Neuropsychologia*, **11**, 477–80.

Frampton, G. G., Milner, A. D., and Ettlinger, G. Cross-modal transfer between vision and touch of go, no-go discrimination learning in the monkey. *Neuropsychologia*, **11**, 231–3.

Hartje, W. and Ettlinger, G. Reaching in light and dark after unilateral posterior parietal ablations in the monkey. *Cortex*, **9**, 344–54.

Manzoni, T., Hunter, M., Maccabe, J. J., and Ettlinger, G. Tactile discrimination performance in the monkey: the effect of commissure section on transfer of training between the hands. *Cortex*, **9**, 40–55.

Nie, V, Upton, A., and Ettlinger, G. Behavioral impairment in the monkey following implantation of aluminum hydroxide on the temporal cortex: the role of cortical destruction. *Experimental Neurology*, **40**, 632–51.

Ridley, R. M. and Ettlinger, G. Visual discrimination performance in the monkey: the activity of single cells in infero-temporal cortex. *Brain Research*, **55**, 179–82.

1974

Ettlinger, G., Blakemore, C. B., Milner, A. D., and Wilson, J. Agenesis of the corpus callosum: a further behavioural investigation. *Brain*, **97**, 225–34.

Ettlinger, G., Hester, H., and Ridley, R. M. Recording from single-cells in inferotemporal cortex of the monkey during discrimination performance. *Journal of Physiology*, **237**, 6–8P.

Nie, V. and Ettlinger, G. Ablation of the primary inferotemporal epileptogenic focus in rhesus monkeys with independent secondary spike discharges. *Brain Research*, **69**, 149–52.

Nie, V., Maccabe, J. J., Ettlinger, G., and Driver, M. V. The development of secondary epileptic discharges in the rhesus monkey after commissure section. *Electroencephalography and Clinical Neurophysiology*, **37**, 473–81.

Passingham, R. E. and Ettlinger, G. A comparison of cortical functions in man and the other primates. *International Review of Neurobiology*, **16**, 233–99.

1975

Ettlinger, G. and Ridley, R. M. Visual discrimination in the monkey: distinguishing the incorrect response. *Neuropsychologia*, **13**, 111–13.

Ettlinger, G., Teuber, H.-L., and Milner, B. The seventeenth international symposium of neuropsychology. *Neuropsychologia*, **13**, 125–33.

Hunter, M., Ettlinger, G., and Maccabe, J. J. Intermanual transfer in the monkey as a function of amount of callosal sparing. *Brain Research*, **93**, 223–40.

Jarvis, M. J. and Ettlinger, G. Transfer of spatial alternation between responding in the light and in the dark. *Neuropsychologia*, **13**, 115–16.

Ridley, R. M. and Ettlinger, G. Tactile and visuo-spatial discrimination performance in the monkey: the effect of total and partial posterior parietal removals. *Neuropsychologia*, **13**, 191–206.

1976

Elliott, R. C., Ettlinger, G., Maccabe, J. J., and Richardson, N. Bi-manual motor performance in the monkey: successive division of the forebrain and cerebellum. *Experimental Neurology*, **50**, 48–59.

Ettlinger, G. and Jarvis, M. J. Cross-modal transfer in the chimpanzee. *Nature*, 259, 44–5.

Ettlinger, G. and Lowrie, M. B. An immunological factor in epilepsy. *Lancet*, **i**, 1386.

Ettlinger, G. and Rashbass, C. Adjusting the amount of overtraining to the difficulty of discrimination learning. *Neuropsychologia*, **14**, 257–60.

Hunter, M., Maccabe, J. J., and Ettlinger, G. Transfer of training between the hands in a split-brain monkey with chronic parietal discharges. *Cortex*, **12**, 27–30.

Hunter, M., Maccabe, J. J., and Ettlinger, G. Intermanual transfer of tactile training in the monkey: the effect of bilateral parieto-prestriate ablations. *Neuropsychologia*, **14**, 385–9.

Ridley, R. M. and Ettlinger, G. Impaired tactile learning and retention after removals of the second somatic sensory projection cortex (SII) in the monkey. *Brain Research*, **107**, 656–60.

1977

Elliott, R. C., Norris, E., Ettlinger, G., and Mishkin, M. Some factors influencing non-matching to sample in the monkey. *Bulletin of the Psychonomic Society*, **9**, 395–6.

Ettlinger, G. Interactions between sensory modalities in nonhuman primates. In *Behavioral primatology: advances in research and theory* (ed. A. M. Schrier), Ch. 3, pp. 71–104. Erlbaum, Hillsdale NJ.

Ettlinger, G. Parietal cortex in visual orientation. In *Physiological aspects of clinical neurology*, (ed. F. C. Rose), Ch. 6, pp. 93–100. Blackwell, Oxford.

Ettlinger, G. Agenesis of the corpus callosum. In *Handbook of Clinical Neurology*, Part 1, Vol. 30, *Congenital malformations of the brain and skull*, (ed. P. J. Vinken and G. W. Bruyn), pp. 285–97. North–Holland, Amsterdam.

Ettlinger, G., Holmes, O., and Nie, V. Unitary activity in temporal epileptic foci of the monkey. *Journal of Physiology*, **270**, 49–50P.

Hunter, M., Lowrie, M. B., Ettlinger, G., and Maccabe, J. J. The effect of prolonged pre-operative transfer testing on intermanual transfer of training in the monkey. *Cortex*, **13**, 215–16.

Jarvis, M. J. and Ettlinger, G. Cross-modal recognition in chimpanzees and monkeys. *Neuropsychologia*, **15**, 499–506.

Lowrie, M. B. and Ettlinger, G. Tactile discrimination performance in split-brain monkeys with secondary posterior parietal discharges. *Psychological Research*, **39**, 389–92.

Ratcliff, G., Ridley, R. M., and Ettlinger, G. Spatial disorientation in the monkey. *Cortex*, **13**, 62–5.

Ridley, R. M., Hester, N. S., and Ettlinger, G. Stimulus- and response-dependent units from the occipital and temporal lobes of the unanaesthetized monkey performing learnt visual tasks. *Experimental Brain Research*, **27**, 539–52.

1978

Brown, D. P. F., Lenneberg, E. H., and Ettlinger, G. Ability of chimpanzees to respond to symbols of quantity in comparison with that of children and of monkeys. *Journal of Comparative and Physiological Psychology*, **92**, 815–20.

Ettlinger, G. Language and its origins, a synthesis. In *Recent advances in primatology*, Vol. 1, *Behaviour*, (ed. D. J. Chivers and J. Herbert), pp. 933–7. Academic Press, London.

Ettlinger, G. The second somatosensory projection arearecent behavioural observations. *Trends in Neurosciences*, **1**, 144–6.

Ettlinger, G. Have we forgotten the infant? Comment on 'On the biological basis of human laterality' (by M. C. Corballis and M. J. Morgan). *Behavioral and Brain Sciences*, **2**, 294.

Ettlinger, G., Brown, J. V., and Davenport, R. K. The relevance of object categorization to cross-modal performance by chimpanzees. *Neuropsychologia*, **16**, 539–43.

Garcha, H. S. and Ettlinger, G. Sorting of objects by the chimpanzee and the monkey. In *Recent advances in primatology*, Vol. 1, *Behaviour*, (ed. D. J. Chivers and J. Herbert), pp. 957–9. Academic Press, London.

Garcha, H. S. and Ettlinger, G. The effects of unilateral or bilateral removals of the second somatosensory cortex (area SII): a profound tactile disorder in monkeys. *Cortex*, **14**, 319–26.

Hewett, T. D. and Ettlinger, G. Cross-modal performance: the absence of transfer in non-human primates capable of recognition. *Neuropsychologia*, **16**, 361–6.

Jarvis, M. J. and Ettlinger, G. Cross-modal performance in monkeys and apes: is there a substantial difference? In *Recent advances in primatology*, Vol. 1, *Behaviour* (ed. D. J. Chivers and J. Herbert), pp. 953–6. Academic Press, London.

Lowrie, M. B., Maccabe, J. J., and Ettlinger, G. The effects of ablations on primary and secondary epileptic discharges in commissure-sectioned rhesus monkeys. *Electroencephalography and Clinical Neurophysiology*, **44**, 23–36.

Norris, E. and Ettlinger, G. Cross-modal performance in the monkey: non-matching to sample with edible shapes. *Neuropsychologia*, **16**, 99–102.

Ridley, R. M. and Ettlinger, G. Further evidence of impaired tactile learning after removals of the second somatic sensory projection cortex (SII) in the monkey. *Experimental Brain Research*, **31**, 475–88.

Sugishita, M., Ettlinger, G., and Ridley, R. M. Disturbance of cage-finding in the monkey. *Cortex*, **14**, 431–8.

1979

Ettlinger, G. Interhemispheric transmission of learning and of abnormal discharges: why should there be differences? In *Structure and function of cerebral commissures*, (ed. I. S. Russell, M. W. van Hof, and G. Berlucchi), pp. 385–9. Macmillan, London.

Ettlinger, G. Experimental epilepsy in monkeys. In *Psychiatry, genetics and pathography: a tribute to Elliot Slater*, (ed. M. Roth and V. Cowie), pp. 147–60. Gaskell, London.

Ettlinger, G. Does development tell us about evolution? Comment on 'A developmental model of the evolution of language and intelligence in early hominids' (by S. T. Parker and K. R. Gibson). *Behavioral and Brain Sciences*, **2**, 384.

Ettlinger, G. and Hester, N. S. Learnt significance of stimuli in the monkey. *Journal of Physiology*, **296**, 50–51P.

Garcha, H. S. and Ettlinger, G. Object sorting by chimpanzees and monkeys. *Cortex*, **15**, 213–24.

Garcha, H. S., Malone, D., and Ettlinger, G. Susceptibility of vervet monkeys to anesthetic. *Laboratory Primate Newsletter*, **18**, 4–5.

Hewett, T. D. and Ettlinger, G. Cross-modal performance: the nature of the failure at 'transfer' in non-human primates capable of 'recognition'. *Neuropsychologia*, **17**, 511–14.

Winner, E. and Ettlinger, G. Do chimpanzees recognize photographs as representations of objects? *Neuropsychologia*, **17**, 413–20.

1980

Baltz, M. L., Ettlinger, G., Parrish, K., Pepys, M. B., and Rogers, S. Epileptic discharges produced in monkeys by injection of spleen cells from rabbits immunised with monkey brain. *Journal of Neurological Science*, **49**, 335–40.

Ettlinger, G. How can we resolve the enigma of parietal cortex? Comment on 'The functional organization of posterior parietal cortex' (by J. C. Lynch). *Behavioral and Brain Sciences*, **3**, 502.

Ettlinger, G. The development of secondary foci in the monkey: the role of the commissures. In *Advances in epileptology: the Xth Epilepsy International Symposium*, (ed. J. A. Wada and J. K. Penry), p. 492. Raven Press, New York.

Ettlinger, G. The development of secondary foci in the monkey: the evidence from microelectrode recordings. In *Advances in epileptology: Xth Epilepsy International Symposium*, (ed. J. A. Wada and J. K. Penry), p. 492. Raven Press, New York.

Ettlinger, G. and Garcha, H. S. Cross-modal recognition by the monkey: the effects of cortical removals. *Neuropsychologia*, **18**, 685–92.

Garcha, H. S. and Ettlinger, G. Tactile discrimination learning in the monkey: the effects of unilateral or bilateral removals of the second somatosensory cortex (area SII). *Cortex*, **16**, 397–412.

Holmes, O., Ettlinger, G., and Nie, V. Unitary activity recorded concurrently in primary and secondary temporal epileptic foci of the monkey. *Experimental Neurology*, **69**, 599–616.

Holmes, O., Ettlinger, G., and Nie, V. Time-locking of unitary activity with ictal and interictal epileptic spikes in the monkey. *Electroencephalography and Clinical Neurophysiology*, **49**, 97P.

Lowrie, M. B. and Ettlinger, G. The development of independent secondary ('mirror') discharges in the monkey: failure to replicate earlier findings. *Epilepsia*, **21**, 25–30.

1981

Ettlinger, G. Cerebral predominance in the monkey? Comment on 'Hemispheric laterality in animals and the effects of early experience' (by V. H. Denenberg). *Behavioral and Brain Sciences*, **4**, 25–6.

Holmes, O. and Ettlinger, G. Neuronal activity associated with vertex spikes in Macaca mulatta. *Electroencephalography and Clinical Neurophysiology*, **52**, 102P.

Muncer, S. J. and Ettlinger, G. Communication by a chimpanzee: first-trial mastery of word order that is critical for meaning, but failure to negate conjunctions. *Neuropsychologia*, **19**, 73–8.

1982

Brown, J. V., Ettlinger, G., and Garcha, H. S. Visually guided reaching and tactile discrimination performance in the monkey: the effects of removals of parietal cortex soon after birth. *International Journal of Primatology*, **3**, 266.

Ettlinger, G. An appreciation of the late Cyril Rashbass. *Perception*, **11**, 245–6.

Garcha, H. S., Ettlinger, G, and Maccabe, J. J. Unilateral removal of the second somatosensory projection cortex in the monkey: evidence for cerebral predominance? *Brain*, **105**, 787–810.

McNally, C., Ettlinger, G., and Smith, A. M. R. Cross-modal performance in patients with cerebral lesions. *Cortex*, **18**, 91–104.

Muncer, S. J., Malone, D., and Ettlinger, G. Language in a monkey? *Perceptual and Motor Skills*, **55**, 159–62.

1983

Brown, J. V. and Ettlinger, G. Intermanual transfer of mirror-image discrimination by monkeys. *Quarterly Journal of Experimental Psychology*, **35B**, 119–24.

Brown, J. V., Ettlinger, G., and Garcha, H. S. Visually guided reaching and tactile discrimination performance in the monkey: the effects of removals of parietal cortex soon after birth. *Brain Research*, **267**, 67–79.

Ettlinger, G. A comparative evaluation of the cognitive skills of the chimpanzee and monkey. *International Journal of Neuroscience*, **22**, 7–20.

Rivers, A., Bartecki, U., Brown, J. V., and Ettlinger, G. An unexpected 'epidemic' of a rare stereotypy: unidentified stress or imitation? *Laboratory Primate Newsletter*, **22**, 5–7.

1984

Ettlinger, G. Subcortical neglect. *Neurology*, **34**, 261.

Ettlinger, G. Neue Ansätze zu einer Theorie des Traumschlafs. *Nervenarzt*, **55**, 613.

Ettlinger, G. Humans, apes and monkeys: the changing neuropsychological viewpoint. *Neuropsychologia*, **22**, 685–96.

1985

Ettlinger, G. Somatotopic map of the flying fox. *Nature*, **315**, 285.

Fehn, U., Streicher, M., Ettlinger, G., and Brown, J. V. Confusion of laterally inverted mirror-images: a relationship to brain anatomy? *Cortex*, **21**, 91–110.

Halsband, U., Gruhn, S., and Ettlinger, G. Unilateral spatial neglect and defective performance in one half of space. *International Journal of Neuroscience*, **28**, 173–95.

Hörster, W. and Ettlinger, G. An association between hand preference and tactile discrimination performance in the rhesus monkey. *Neuropsychologia*, **23**, 411–13.

Niemann, H., Boenick, H. E., Schmidt, R. C., and Ettlinger, G. Cognitive development in epilepsy. The relative influence of epileptic activity and of brain damage. *European Archives of Psychiatry and Neurological Science*, **234**, 399–403.

1986

Brown, J. V. and Ettlinger, G. West German Universities. *Nature*, **320**, 390.

Holmes, O. and Ettlinger, G. Tracing the generators of EEG transients in monkeys. In *The Proceedings of the Third International Conference on Measurement in Clinical Medicine*, pp. 89–94. Institute of Measurement and Control, London.

Römer, G., Gresch, H., Ettlinger, G., and Brown, J. V. Tactile recognition of laterally inverted mirror images by children: intermanual transfer and rotation of the palm. *Perception*, **15**, 303–12.

Streicher, M. and Ettlinger, G. Cross-modal recognition by the monkey: can the experience in the first modality be reduced to a single trial? *Neuropsychologia*, **24**, 255–9.

1987

Blaschke, M. and Ettlinger, G. Pointing as an act of social communication by monkeys. *Animal Behaviour*, **35**, 1520–3.

Brown, J. V., Sepehr, M. M., Ettlinger, G., and Skreczek, W. Differential accuracy of aimed movements to visual and somatic targets in young children. *Cortex*, **23**, 381–98.

Ettlinger, G. Primate handedness: how nice if it were really so. *Behavioral and Brain Sciences*, **10**, 271–3.

Ettlinger, G. Cross-modal sensory integration. In *The Oxford companion to the mind*, (ed. R. L. Gregory), pp. 173–4. Oxford University Press, Oxford.

Hörster, W. and Ettlinger, G. Unilateral removal of the posterior insula or of area SII: inconsistent effects on tactile, visual and auditory performance in the monkey. *Behavioural Brain Research*, **26**, 1–17.

Streicher, M. and Ettlinger, G. Cross-modal recognition of familiar and unfamiliar objects by the monkey: the effect of ablation of poly-sensory neocortex or of the amygdaloid complex. *Behavioural Brain Research*, **23**, 95–107.

1988

Ettlinger, G. Hand preference, ability and hemispheric specialization: in how far are these factors related in the monkey? *Cortex*, **24**, 389–98.

Heath, B., Ettlinger, G., and Brown, J. V. Tactile recognition of mirror images by children: intermanual transfer and rotation of the palm. *Perception*, **17**, 535–47.

Sepehr, M. M., Brown, J. V., Ettlinger, G., and Skreczek, W. The relationship between metaphoric and crossmodal abilities during development. *International Journal of Neuroscience*, **38**, 53–67.

1989

Brechmann, M., Ettlinger, G., and Skreczek, W. Guidance of visual reaching with the aid of a TV monitor: the effects of monitor position and of left/right and up/down reversals of the image in relation to age. *Neuropsychologia*, **27**, 1383–97.

Brown, J. V., Schumacher, U., Rohlmann, A., Ettlinger, G., Schmidt, R. C., and Skreczek, W. Aimed movements to visual targets in hemiplegic and normal children: is the 'good' hand of children with infantile hemiplegia also normal? *Neuropsychologia*, **27**, 283–302.

Hörster, W., Rivers, A., Schuster, B., Ettlinger, G., Skreczek, W., and Hesse, W. The neural structures involved in cross-modal recognition and tactile discrimination performance: an investigation using 2-DG. *Behavioural Brain Research*, **33**, 209–27.

1990

Ettlinger, G. 'Object vision' and 'spatial vision': the neuropsychological evidence for the distinction. *Cortex*, **26**, 319–41.

Ettlinger, G. and Wilson, W. A. Cross-modal performance: behavioural processes, phylogenetic considerations and neural mechanisms. *Behavioural Brain Research*, **40**, 169–92.

Niediek, T., Franke, H. G., Degen, R., and Ettlinger, G. The development of independent foci in epileptic patients. *Archives of Neurology*, **47**, 406–11.

1991

Ettlinger, G. Microsoft Word for Windows, Version 1.1—double glazing for word-smiths? *The Psychologist*, **14**, 224.

1992

Bulla-Helwig, M., Ettlinger, G., Dommasch, D., Ebel, E., and Skreczek, W. Impaired visual perceptual categorization in right brain-damaged patients: failure to replicate. *Cortex*, **28**, 261–72.

1993

Bulla-Helwig, M., Ettlinger, G., Dommasch, D., Ebel, E., and Skreczek, W. Perceptual categorization is associated with sensory performance in patients with unilateral cerebral lesions. *International Journal of Neuroscience*, **69**, 73–84.

Other cited references

Beach, F. A., Hebb, D. O., and Morgan, C. T. (1960). *The neuropsychology of Lashley*. McGraw-Hill, New York.

Goldstein, K. and Gelb, A. (1918). Psychologische Grundlagen hirnpathologischer Fälle auf Grund von Untersuchungen Hirnverletzter. *Zeitschrift für die gesamte Neurologie und Psychiatrie*, **41**, 1–142.

Hebb, D. O. (1949). *The organization of behavior: A neuropsychological theory*. Wiley, New York.

Holmes, G. and Horrax, G. (1919). Disturbances of spatial orientation and visual attention with loss of stereoscopic vision. *Archives of Neurology and Psychiatry*, **1**, 385–407.

Klüver, H. (1942). Functional significance of the geniculo-striate system. *Biological Symposia*, **7**, 253–99.

Klüver, H. and Bucy, P. C. (1938). An analysis of certain effects of bilateral temporal lobectomy in the rhesus monkey, with special reference to 'psychic blindness'. *Journal of Psychology*, **5**, 33–54.

Paterson, A. and Zangwill, O. L. (1944). Disorders of visual space perception associated with lesions of the right cerebral hemisphere. *Brain*, **67**, 331–58.

Poppelreuter, W. (1917). Die psychische Schädigungen durch Kopfschuss im Kriege 1914/16. Band 1: Die Störungen der niederen und höheren Sehleistungen durch Verletzungen des Okzipitalhirns. L. Voss, Leipzig. (Translated into English as *Disturbances of lower and higher visual capacities caused by occipital damage*, by J. Zihl and L. Weiskrantz. Oxford University Press, Oxford, 1990.)

Teuber, H.-L., Battersby, W., and Bender, M. B. (1960). *Visual field defects after penetrating missile wounds of the brain*. MIT Press, Cambridge, MA.

2

Sensory factors in human visual agnosia

ANDREW W. YOUNG

2.1 Background

The classic report of visual agnosia was by Lissauer (1890; Shallice and Jackson 1988), who described case G.L., an 80-year-old man who had suffered a head injury when a storm blew him against a fence. G.L. could still see; he had near-normal visual acuity for his age, and he could draw accurate copies of seen objects. Yet he no longer recognized the things about him. Instead, he looked around in a perplexed manner, as if everything was unfamiliar. He thought that pictures in his room were boxes, and tried to search in them for things he could not find. He mistook his jacket for a pair of trousers, and at mealtimes he could not recognize the pieces of cutlery on the table.

Other investigations showed that G.L. had not lost his knowledge of objects; he referred to them appropriately in conversation, and he could recognize them immediately if he handled them, or from characteristic sounds. When shown a whistle, for example, he had no idea what it was, yet he recognized it straight away when it was blown.

Lissauer called this *Seelenblindheit*—psychic blindness or mind-blindness—but 'agnosia' is now preferred. The term agnosia is derived from the Ancient Greek, roughly translating as 'not-knowing'; it is credited to Freud (1891; 1953). Use of the term agnosia is usually taken to imply that the recognition disorder is not a consequence of general intellectual deterioration, language impairment, or basic sensory dysfunction; the person with a visual agnosia can still see things, and has not forgotten what they are, yet fails to recognize them.

Modern studies indicate several different causes of visual object agnosia (Humphreys and Riddoch 1987). Lissauer (1890) himself realized this; he proposed that visual recognition can be separated into apperceptive and associative stages, and that each when impaired had its own characteristic agnosia. The apperceptive stage would correspond to the final stage of purely perceptual processing; it was considered to be intact if a brain-injured person could accurately copy items they could not recognize. The associative stage would give the percept meaning by linking it to previous experience; leading to the widely adopted description of associative agnosia as corresponding to a normal percept 'stripped of its meaning'.

2.1.1 Bay's critique

Although Lissauer's (1890) investigation of G.L. was thorough and in many respects remarkably astute (Shallice and Jackson 1988), the concept of visual agnosia did not go unchallenged. In particular, there was resistance to the idea that a higher-order functional impairment of visual recognition might occur independently of frank visual perceptual deficits. Convincing cases of visual agnosia were (and remain) rare, leading to the suspicion that there might be some uninvestigated or unemphasized aspects of putative cases which could account for their problems in recognizing seen objects.

Bay (1950, 1953) was a strong proponent of this view, maintaining that significant visual disabilities were present in all putative cases of agnosia where there was no obvious intellectual deterioration or language disorder. He examined local adaptation times to visual stimuli in different regions of the visual field, and found abnormalities in eight out of nine people with brain injuries he tested. Importantly, he pointed out that such abnormalities were present even for people with good overall visual acuity and normal visual fields on conventional perimetric testing. Since these tests were usually used to establish adequate vision, there was thus a clear possibility that they were failing to pick up significant visual problems.

These contentions were not well received when discussed at a meeting of leading German neurologists in 1951 (see Ettlinger 1956). For example, only one of Bay's cases had been diagnosed as agnosic, which brought into question the importance of these abnormalities in local adaptation rates, since on these data alone they did not seem sufficient in themselves to cause visual agnosia. In addition, Bay's method for assessing adaptation deficits by simply subtracting performance from a control mean gave no adequate indication as to whether performance actually fell outside the normal range.

Despite these logical and technical deficiencies, Bay's conclusions were widely cited. Even though his own data were not very persuasive, he had managed to convince people that it might be insufficient to rely only on acuity and standard perimetric testing to demonstrate fully normal vision. Similar concerns have since been reiterated from time to time (Bender and Feldman 1972; Campion 1987).

2.1.2 Ettlinger's study

The seminal paper by Ettlinger (1956) represented the first attempt to explore the issues Bay (1950, 1953) had raised, in a careful, systematic manner. What Bay had succeeded in doing was to open up the possibility that agnosia-like disturbances, which had previously been taken to indicate higher-order perceptual impairment, might reflect more basic perceptual problems. Ettlinger (1956) was concerned to find out whether this was actually the case. To this end, he carried out a thorough investigation of basic visual functions for 30 people who had suffered brain injuries, comparing their performance to that of a control group of 48 neurologically normal individuals. The brain-injured group was subdivided on the basis of visual field defects and evidence of higher perceptual disorder; 12 people had no visual field defects or clinical signs of higher perceptual disorder, 10 people had field defects but no other obvious perceptual disorder, and eight people had both field defects and various types of perceptual disorder. Everyone was tested for brightness discrimination, flicker fusion, acuity for small objects, local adaptation, tachistoscopic acuity, and apparent movement perception. These measurements were taken systematically for several different locations in the visual field, using a specially constructed apparatus which allowed factors unrelated to those being assessed to be held constant. All in all, it was an impressive technical achievement.

Ettlinger's results (1956) showed significant impairment of performance in the group of people with brain injuries and no visual field defects. This was exactly as Bay (1950, 1953) had found, confirming his point that full visual fields are not in themselves an indication of completely normal vision. However, these impairments were mostly of moderate severity, and much more pronounced problems were noted for the group with brain injury and visual field defects. It was therefore apparent that, although the absence of visual field defects cannot be taken as a guarantee of fully intact vision, it is not usually accompanied by visual deficits of the severity found for people with field defects.

The more important question Ettlinger (1956) wanted to address concerned the relation between the visual deficits revealed by his tests and clinical signs of higher perceptual disorder. His results showed that, although his group of people with field defects and various types of clinically recognizable perceptual disorder also performed below normal levels on his tests, they did no worse overall than the people with visual field defects and no clinical signs of higher perceptual disorder. This, Ettlinger reasoned, gave no grounds for thinking that the low-level perceptual deficits he had observed were causing the higher-order problems directly, since he could identify individuals with or without higher-order problems yet with equally severe low-level perceptual deficits. Indeed, pushing this logic further, he could actually find some individuals with relatively severe lower-order deficits who did not have any clinically apparent higher-order problems. He concluded (Ettlinger 1956, p.306) that:

> We are thus able to confirm Bay's finding that bilateral visual discrimination defects may follow unilateral cerebral lesions. We cannot, however, find confirmation of his view that such deficits play an appreciable part in the genesis of the visual agnosias.

2.2 Face processing and contrast sensitivity

Although clearly a landmark study, which strongly supported the view that the classical distinction of lower-order from higher-order visual perceptual impairment had much to commend it, Ettlinger's paper of 1956 did not leave the matter completely closed. Instead, two caveats concerning his work have from time to time been expressed. The first caveat concerns the particular tests Ettlinger used, and the second the nature of the higher-order deficits in the cases he investigated. These issues were raised most strongly by Campion (1987), who argued that Ettlinger's conclusions were misleading, and that he had not refuted the theory that visual agnosia is due to sensory loss. While we recognized the force of Ettlinger's (1956) position, and his major contribution to the area, my colleagues and I thus thought the matter worthy of further investigation.

First, the tests Ettlinger used. Although they were state of the art in 1956, knowledge of visual functions has moved on since then, leading to different ideas about which types of test might be most revealing. A particularly important change has been the introduction of testing based on the spatial contrast sensitivity function, pioneered by Campbell and his colleagues (Campbell 1983). The principle underlying the spatial contrast sensitivity function is that all visual stimuli can be decomposed mathematically into signals varying between high spatial frequencies (fine detail, changing rapidly across small areas of the scene) and low spatial frequencies (coarse detail, relatively unchanging across broad areas). The spatial contrast sensitivity function charts this by measuring the lowest contrast at which signals of different spatial frequencies can be detected.

The spatial contrast sensitivity function provides a more useful description of what a person can see than standard tests of acuity because the human visual system is normally more sensitive to some spatial frequencies than others, being maximally sensitive to intermediate rather than high or low spatial frequencies. Furthermore, in two influential review papers, Sergent (1983, 1984) argued that the right cerebral hemisphere is differentially sensitive to information carried by low spatial frequencies and the left cerebral hemisphere to high spatial frequencies. From this it follows that people with impaired perception of particular spatial frequencies might show problems in tasks which depend critically on information carried by these frequencies. This would have obvious implications for the recognition of visual stimuli such as objects and faces.

Newcombe *et al.* (1989) examined this for face-processing tasks. They studied a group of ex-servicemen with long-standing unilateral brain lesions, mostly sustained from shrapnel injuries during the D-day landings and the subsequent Normandy campaign. Newcombe and her colleagues (Newcombe and Russell 1969; Newcombe *et al.* 1987) had already shown double dissociations between impairments of face perception and visually guided maze learning for these ex-servicemen; they interpreted these as reflecting different forms of higher-order perceptual impairment. To investigate the alternative possibility derived from Sergent's (1983, 1984) theory, that people with face processing impairments have a basic perceptual difficulty which interferes with their ability to see faces properly, Newcombe *et al.* (1989) measured the spatial contrast sensitivity functions of neurologically normal controls and groups of ex-servicemen with unilateral brain lesions affecting the left or right cerebral hemispheres, and examined their performance of face-perception and face-recognition tasks.

Figure 2.1 shows mean spatial contrast sensitivity functions for ex-servicemen with unilateral injuries of the left or right cerebral hemispheres, and neurologically normal control subjects matched for age and intelligence (Newcombe *et al.* 1989). The characteristic inverted U-shaped function, with maximum sensitivity to intermediate spatial frequencies, is clearly seen in the control data. The ex-servicemen performed more poorly than controls, but the impairment was constant across all spatial frequencies and did not differ between left or right hemisphere injured groups. In sum, the data are inconsistent with Sergent's (1983, 1984) position; although people with unilateral brain injuries do have somewhat impaired vision, there is no hint of any differential deficit between those with left or with right hemisphere injuries.

This pattern makes an interesting contrast with problems in face perception measured for the same subject groups. To do this, Newcombe *et al.* (1989) used a 'face decision' task, in which people were asked to decide as quickly as possible whether or not a line drawing was of a properly organized or slightly scrambled face: examples of the stimuli are shown in Fig. 2.2, and mean reaction times are presented in Fig. 2.3. The ex-servicemen with right hemisphere lesions show the longest reaction times, indicating that they had problems in carrying out this simple task. The interesting point of the contrast between the data presented in Figs 2.1 and 2.3 is that although both groups of ex-servicemen showed equally impaired vision (Fig. 2.1), the group with right hemisphere injuries were more severely impaired at perceiving faces (Fig. 2.3). This suggests that the right hemisphere contributes something to face perception over and above its involvement in more basic visual abilities.

The same conclusion is apparent from individual data. Table 2.1 summarizes details concerning three ex-servicemen with unilateral missile-wound injuries from the series studied by Newcombe *et al.* (1989). Spatial contrast sensitivity functions have been tabulated for each person, alongside performance on the face-perception task (reaction time to decide whether or not a stimulus is a properly organized face). Cases T.C. and B.S. (both with left hemisphere lesions) showed impaired contrast sensitivity without a corresponding impairment of face perception, whereas P.G. (who had a right hemisphere lesion) performed very poorly on the face perception task and yet had unimpaired contrast sensitivity for all spatial frequencies that were tested.

The likely reason for these essentially negative findings concerning spatial contrast sensitivity is that higher-order representations that can pool information derived from a range of spatial frequencies are involved in face perception. However, it is not claimed that there is no relation at all between

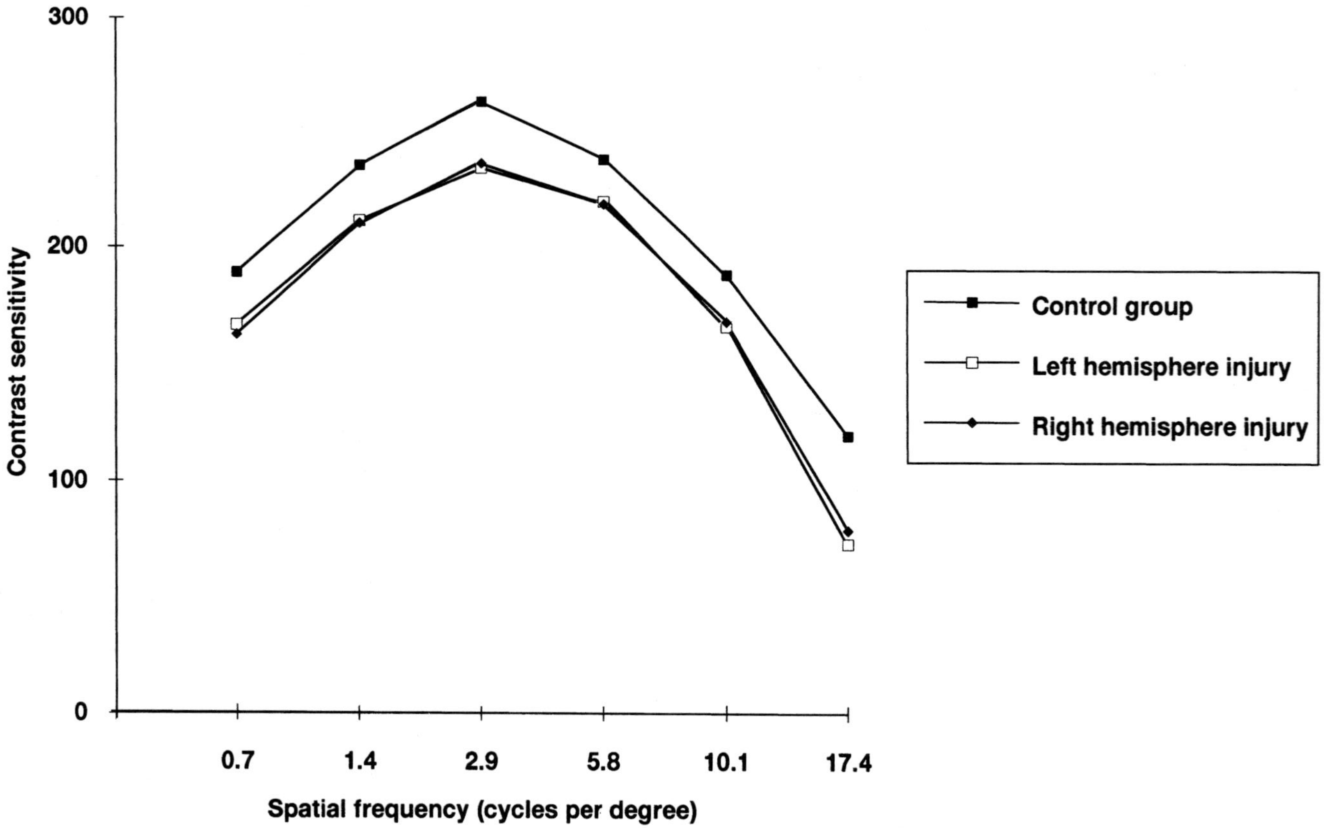

Fig. 2.1 Mean spatial contrast sensitivity functions for ex-servicemen with unilateral injuries of the left or right cerebral hemispheres, and a neurologically normal control group (from Newcombe *et al.* 1989).

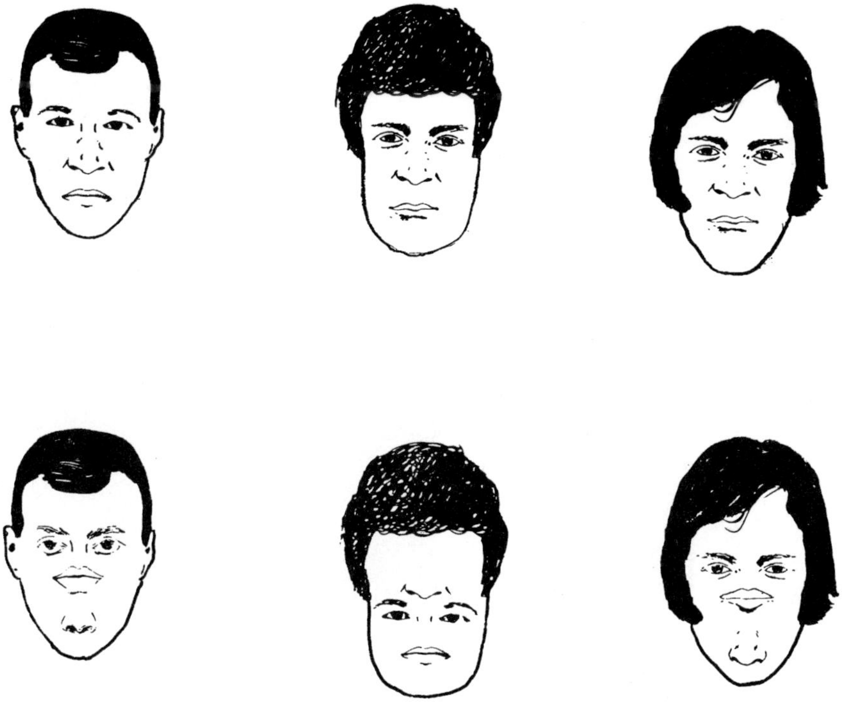

Fig. 2.2 Examples of stimuli from the face-decision task used by Newcombe *et al.* (1989). The task involves deciding as quickly as possible whether each is a properly organized or scrambled face.

'basic' and 'higher-order' visual impairments. For example, T.C. (Table 2.1) had very poor contrast sensitivity for all spatial frequencies and although his performance of the face-perception task was not significantly impaired, it did seem to be compromised to some degree. This is as one might expect if basic visual abilities 'feed' higher-order representations. Yet cases like B.S. (Table 2.1), who had a less severe contrast sensitivity impairment and could perform the face-perception task with ease, show that this is only a loose linkage.

Of course, one might argue that the reaction time data shown in Fig. 2.3 might not reflect a problem in face perception per se for the people with right hemisphere injuries. The most obvious possibility is that they are simply slower at performing any speeded task. To rule this out, Newcombe *et al.* (1989) carried out a further experiment which involved (1) deciding whether photographs showed familiar (famous) or unfamiliar faces, and (2) deciding whether printed names belonged to familiar or unfamiliar people. Mean

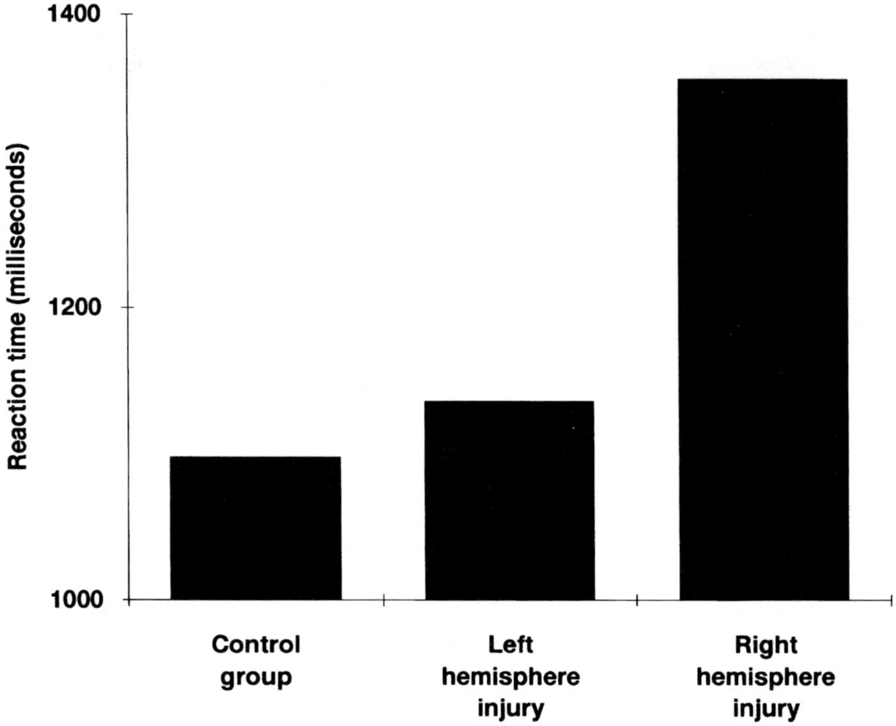

Fig. 2.3 Mean reaction times for correct responses in the face-decision task for neurologically normal control subjects and ex-servicemen with unilateral injuries of the left or right cerebral hemispheres (from Newcombe *et al.* 1989).

reaction times are shown in Fig. 2.4. Again, the ex-servicemen with right hemisphere injuries performed most poorly when faces were used as stimuli, but when names were used it was the group with left hemisphere injuries who were now slowest. Hence it is evident that the perceptual problems of the right hemisphere injured group reflect something which is needed for the analysis of faces and not needed for words.

In fact, the neuropsychological literature has often linked word recognition to the left cerebral hemisphere and face recognition to the right hemisphere, both for people with brain injuries and in studies of the neurologically normal brain (Ellis 1983; Young 1987). In addition, the face-perception tasks used by Newcombe *et al.* (1989) were chosen on the basis that they were already known to be associated with right hemisphere superiority in normal perceivers (Young *et al.* 1985a,b). There is thus an impressive convergence of findings in normal and brain-injured groups.

Table 2.1 *Cases drawn from the study of Newcombe* et al. *(1989), demonstrating dissociable impairments of face perception and contrast sensitivity. The table shows reaction times (in milliseconds) for the face-perception task (see Fig. 2.2), and contrast sensitivity (2-log$_{10}$ contrast) for sinusoidal gratings with spatial frequencies ranging from 0.72 to 17.40 cycles per degree (cpd)*

	RT (milliseconds) for face perception task	Contrast sensitivity (2-log$_{10}$ contrast)					
		0.72 cpd	1.43 cpd	2.88 cpd	5.80 cpd	10.10 cpd	17.40 cpd
Unilateral brain injury							
T.C.	1443	158.6**	187.6***	185.5***	159.7***	100.3**	000.0***
B.S.	854	151.7***	192.1***	217.2*	208.5	120.0*	031.5**
P.G.	2220***	191.6	255.1	287.6	278.9	225.0	150.6
Controls ($n = 20$)							
Mean	1098	189.5	236.0	263.8	238.5	188.5	119.5
SD	210	11.3	13.7	20.5	19.4	31.5	33.7

Longer reaction times and lower contrast sensitivities indicate poorer performance. Asterisked scores differ significantly from the control mean: *, $p < 0.05$; **, $p < 0.01$; ***, $p < 0.001$.

2.3 Sensory status and visual agnosia

The findings of Newcombe *et al.* (1989) showed with more modern testing procedures that Ettlinger's (1956) conclusion remains valid: dissociations are still evident between basic and higher-order visual deficits.

However, a second caveat concerns the forms of higher-order deficit present in the people Ettlinger (1956) investigated. Unfortunately, none of these constituted a case of visual object agnosia. Instead, they showed a range of deficits, including alexia, unilateral neglect, simultanagnosia, visual constructive defects, and prosopagnosia. It was thus possible that more severe visual impairments would be present in cases of genuine object agnosia. Ettlinger (1956) was aware of this, but noted that prosopagnosia can be considered a restricted form of visual agnosia, and that his prosopagnosic patient showed less severe sensory impairment than three other people who were free from problems in face recognition. Comparable findings have since been reported for contrast sensitivity testing in cases of prosopagnosia, which may show little impairment (Rizzo *et al.* 1986) or impairments that are no greater than for matched controls with poor vision but no problems in face recognition (Young and Ellis 1989).

Even so, the possibility of a contribution of defective vision to impaired recognition of seen objects could not be ruled out. On the contrary, Campion (1987) maintained it should be ruled in, since it was clearly so for apperceptive

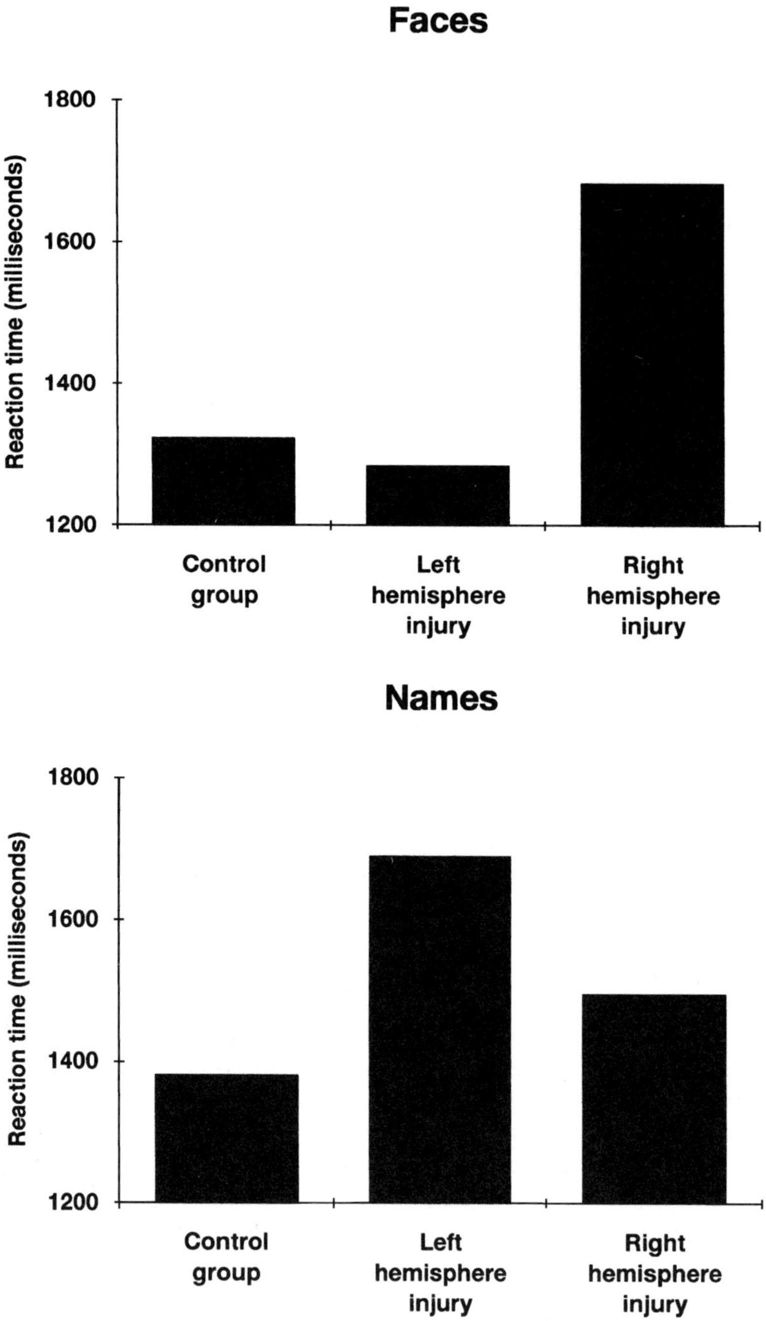

Fig. 2.4 Mean reaction times for correct responses in deciding whether faces or names are familiar, for neurologically normal control subjects and ex-servicemen with unilateral injuries of the left or right cerebral hemispheres (from Newcombe *et al.* 1989).

agnosias. However, this argument is unconvincing because the crucial issue relates to putative cases of associative (rather than apperceptive) agnosia, where the theoretical claim is that visual abnormalities do not account for observed difficulties in visual recognition.

A further study was therefore carried out by de Haan *et al.* (1995). This included an assessment of sensory status across a range of visual parameters for three people with impaired visual recognition of objects and faces, five ex-servicemen with unilateral brain injuries, and groups of control subjects. Ability to recognize seen objects and faces was formally tested for these participants, rather than relying on clinical judgement as to what is or is not normal or impaired. The group of five ex-servicemen were selected from the series investigated by Newcombe's group, using the criteria that they showed severe impairment on one or more of the sensory perception tasks and no problems in recognition of faces or objects.

Table 2.2 shows data for face-recognition and object-naming tasks (de Haan *et al.* 1995). The face recognition task involved 20 famous faces, to which subjects had to give identifying information (name, or details of occupation). The object-naming test was that devised by Oldfield and Wingfield, and comprises 36 line drawings of objects of differing degrees of familiarity (Newcombe *et al.* 1971). Case descriptions for the three agnosic people have been given in previous reports (Ratcliff and Newcombe 1982; de Haan *et al.* 1987, 1992); M.S. and N.R. are both clinically agnosic for objects and faces, whereas P.H. shows more obvious clinical problems for face than for object recognition. The formal test data presented in Table 2.2, however, reveal a complete inability to recognize familiar faces, and severely impaired object recognition for all three agnosics, with M.S.'s object-recognition problems being the worst, and those of N.R. and (especially) P.H. somewhat less. In contrast, none of the ex-servicemen with unilateral brain injuries showed any problems in recognizing objects or faces—but of course this was one of the selection criteria.

Sensory status was evaluated with an oddity paradigm involving three vertically aligned stimuli: either the top stimulus or the bottom stimulus was identical to a central reference stimulus, and subjects were asked to respond manually by touching the odd one out. Fifty trials were used, during which a discrimination threshold was established by increasing task difficulty whenever three consecutive correct choices were made, and decreasing difficulty whenever there was an error. The stimuli were chosen so that the choice had to be based on variation in the shape of a rectangle, location of a dot in a circle, colour, greyness, shape from movement, correlated movement of elements in the display, texture density, or line orientation, with each of these being assessed in separate blocks of 50 trials. Results are shown in Table 2.3.

None of the three agnosic people had fully intact vision. However, there was no relation between their sensory status and the severity of the agnosia, with M.S. showing the best overall visual performance despite having the most severe object recognition deficit. When compared to age-matched controls,

Table 2.2 *Performance of three agnosic people, five ex-servicemen with unilateral brain injuries, and 25 controls on face- and object-naming tasks (de Haan* et al. *1995)*

	Familiar face recognition (max. = 20)	Object recognition (max. = 36)
Agnosic		
P.H.	0***	20***
N.R.	0***	13***
M.S.	0***	8***
Unilateral brain injury		
A.T.	19	33
E.H.	18	34
S.J.	18	34
R.R.	18	34
J.O.	17	34
Controls		
Mean	17.9	34.1
SD	1.6	1.8

Lower scores indicate poorer performance. Asterisked scores differ significantly from the control mean: *, $p < 0.05$; **, $p < 0.01$; ***, $p < 0.001$.

M.S.'s scores were only significantly impaired for colour vision, which could not be tested because of his achromatopsia. Yet he was impaired at recognizing line drawings of objects, to which colour makes no contribution.

This pattern in itself gives a strong indication that visual recognition deficits do not relate directly to sensory status. Even more important, though, is the double dissociation between the performance of the three agnosic people and the five ex-servicemen with unilateral brain injuries. Visual recognition was severely compromised for the agnosic people but normal (in terms of accuracy) for the people with unilateral brain injuries, whereas visual sensation was much more severely impaired in the unilateral brain-injury group. People such as A.T. were performing worse than any of the agnosics on nearly all of the sensory measures, yet showing good visual recognition accuracies for objects and for faces.

2.4 Conclusions

The results summarized here point unequivocally to the conclusion that Ettlinger (1956) got it right. We have not been able to find any consistent relationship between visual sensory deficits and visual recognition problems.

Table 2.3 *Performance of visual-sensory tasks by three agnosic people, five people with unilateral brain injuries, and three separate age-matched control groups (de Haan* et al. *1995). The table shows discrimination thresholds for shape (S, mm), location (L, mm), colour (C, in arbitrary units), greys (G, candelas), shape from movement (SM, mm) correlated movement (CM, % correct), texture (T, % difference), and line orientation (LO, degrees)*

	S	L	C	G	SM	CM	T	LO
Agnosic								
P.H.	1.1	2.8***	1.0	0.9	1.8**	5.0	1.7*	2.7
N.R.	2.5***	4.1***	1.0	0.95	10.9***	5.0	2.3***	2.0
M.S.	1.4	2.1	A	1.21	1.2	5.0	3.0	2.7
Unilateral brain injury								
A.T.	5.4***	5.8***	A	2.0*	24.0***	41.7***	6.3***	2.7
E.H.	2.9***	4.9***	4.3***	3.4***	3.8	15.0	2.3	2.7
S.J.	1.8	12.5***	1.7*	2.6***	9.3***	NT	6.3***	5.7***
R.R.	2.3**	5.3***	1.0	1.5	4.0**	NT	3.0*	3.7
J.O.	2.1*	3.4**	1.3	1.1	3.4*	NT	1.0	6.7***
Young controls (for P.H. and N.R.; $n = 6$)								
Mean	0.74	0.99	1.00	1.10	1.06	5.00	1.14	1.60
SD	0.36	0.49	–	0.36	0.25	–	0.31	0.89
Middle-aged controls (for M.S.; $n = 6$)								
Mean	1.28	2.64	1.00	1.03	1.84	7.50	2.33	1.83
SD	0.78	2.44	–	0.68	0.93	5.59	1.63	1.17
Elderly controls (for unilateral brain injury cases; $n = 25$)								
Mean	1.12	1.53	1.10	1.09	1.66	7.53	1.48	2.30
SD	0.44	0.80	0.30	0.54	0.85	5.44	0.66	0.95

Higher scores indicate poorer performance. Asterisked scores differ significantly from the appropriate control mean: *, $p < 0.05$; **, $p < 0.01$; ***, $p < 0.001$.
NT, Not tested; A, achromatopsic.

It is true that detailed testing of people with visual agnosias does tend to uncover sensory problems, but these seem to be coincidental. The idea that they are causing the visual recognition deficits is undermined by the fact that much more severe sensory problems can be found in people who do not seem to have any consequent problems affecting visual recognition.

Of course, it is a truism in experimental psychology that one can never prove the null hypothesis. It remains possible that some other (as yet unthought of, or untried) measure might in future show that visual agnosias are indeed a consequence of sensory loss. But we can state with confidence that the weight of the evidence deriving from Ettlinger's (1956) work and follow-up studies makes this unlikely.

References

Bay, E. (1950). Agnosie und Funktionswandel. *Monographien aus dem Gesamtgebiet der Neurologie und Psychiatrie*, **73**, 1–94.

Bay, E. (1953). Disturbances of visual perception and their examination. *Brain*, **76**, 515–50.

Bender, M. B. and Feldman, M. (1972). The so-called 'visual agnosias'. *Brain*, **95**, 173–86.

Campbell, F. W. (1983). Why do we measure contrast sensitivity? *Behavioural Brain Research*, **10**, 87–97.

Campion, J. (1987). Apperceptive agnosia: the specification and description of constructs. In *Visual object processing: a cognitive neuropsychological approach*, (ed. G. W. Humphreys and M. J. Riddoch), pp. 197–232. Lawrence Erlbaum, London.

de Haan, E. H. F., Young, A., and Newcombe, F. (1987). Face recognition without awareness. *Cognitive Neuropsychology*, **4**, 385–415.

de Haan, E. H. F., Young, A. W., and Newcombe, F. (1992). Neuropsychological impairment of face recognition units. *Quarterly Journal of Experimental Psychology*, **44A**, 141–75.

de Haan, E. H. F., Heywood, C. A., Young, A. W., Edelstyn, N., and Newcombe, F. (1995). Ettlinger revisited: the relationship between agnosia and sensory impairment. *Journal of Neurology, Neurosurgery, and Psychiatry*, **58**, 350–6.

Ellis, H. D. (1983). The role of the right hemisphere in face perception. In *Functions of the right cerebral hemisphere*, (ed. A. W. Young), pp. 33–64. Academic Press, London.

Ettlinger, G. (1956). Sensory deficits in visual agnosia. *Journal of Neurology, Neurosurgery, and Psychiatry*, **19**, 297–307.

Freud, S. (1891). *Zur Auflasung der Aphasien. Eine Kritische Studie*. Deuticke, Leipzig.

Freud, S. (1953). *On aphasia: a critical study*. International University Press, London.

Humphreys, G. W. and Riddoch, M. J. (1987). The fractionation of visual agnosia. In *Visual object processing: a cognitive neuropsychological approach*, (ed. G. W. Humphreys and M. J. Riddoch), pp. 281–306. Lawrence Erlbaum, London.

Lissauer, H. (1890). Ein Fall von Seelenblindheit nebst einem Beitrage zur Theorie derselben. *Archiv für Psychiatrie und Nervenkrankheiten*, **21**, 222–70.

Newcombe, F. and Russell, W. R. (1969). Dissociated visual perceptual and spatial deficits in focal lesions of the right hemisphere. *Journal of Neurology, Neurosurgery, and Psychiatry*, **32**, 73–81.

Newcombe, F., Oldfield, R. C., Ratcliff, G. G., and Wingfield, A. (1971). Recognition and naming of object-drawings by men with focal brain wounds. *Journal of Neurology, Neurosurgery, and Psychiatry*, **34**, 329–40.

Newcombe, F., Ratcliff, G., and Damasio, H. (1987). Dissociable visual and spatial impairments following right posterior cerebral lesions: clinical, neuropsychological and anatomical evidence. *Neuropsychologia*, **25**, 149–61.

Newcombe, F., de Haan, E. H. F., Ross, J., and Young, A. W. (1989). Face processing, laterality, and contrast sensitivity. *Neuropsychologia*, **27**, 523–38.

Ratcliff, G. and Newcombe, F. (1982). Object recognition: some deductions from the clinical evidence. In *Normality and pathology in cognitive functions*, (ed. A. W. Ellis), pp. 147–71. Academic Press, London.

Rizzo, M., Corbett, J. J., Thompson, S., and Damasio, A. R. (1986). Spatial contrast sensitivity in facial recognition. *Neurology*, **36**, 1254–6.

Sergent, J. (1983). Role of the input in visual hemispheric asymmetries. *Psychological Bulletin*, **93**, 481–512.

Sergent, J. (1984). Inferences from unilateral brain damage about normal hemispheric functions in visual pattern recognition. *Psychological Bulletin*, **96**, 99–115.

Shallice, T. and Jackson, M. (1988). Lissauer on agnosia. *Cognitive Neuropsychology*, **5**, 153–92.

Young, A. W. (1987). Cerebral hemisphere differences and reading. In *Cognitive approaches to reading*, (ed. J. Beech and A. Colley), pp. 139–68. Wiley, Chichester.

Young, A. W. and Ellis, H. D. (1989). Childhood prosopagnosia. *Brain and Cognition*, **9**, 16–47.

Young, A. W., Hay, D. C., and McWeeny, K. H. (1985*a*). Right cerebral hemisphere superiority for constructing facial representations. *Neuropsychologia*, **23**, 195–202.

Young, A. W., Hay, D. C., McWeeny, K. H., Ellis, A. W., and Barry, C. (1985*b*). Familiarity decisions for faces presented to the left and right cerebral hemispheres. *Brain and Cognition*, **4**, 439–50.

3

Ettlinger at Bay: can visual agnosia be explained by low-level visual impairments?

ALAN COWEY, PAUL DEAN, AND LARRY WEISKRANTZ

3.1 Introduction

In the mid-1950s George Ettlinger seemed to some of his contemporaries to be ploughing a lonely furrow in arguing against Bay's theory (Bay 1953) that visual object agnosia was little more than the result of some combination of visual sensory impairment, dulled intellect, and language disorder. His demonstration (1956), the first of its kind, that the visual sensory status of patients with and without associative agnosia did not differ and could therefore not explain visual agnosia, was a rare milestone in the development of neuropsychology. Since Lissauer (1889), visual agnosia had been subdivided into apperceptive (roughly, an impoverished ability to create effective percepts) and associative (where perceptual registration is *apparently* normal but the meaning of visual percepts is impoverished). Ettlinger was studying patients with associative agnosia in his evaluation of Bay's theory, but in our own experiments with monkeys we had in mind that two different groups of monkeys with cortical lesions known to impair visual learning and retention might mimic patients with apperceptive or associative agnosia, and that measurements of a variety of visual thresholds might shed light on their possible contrasting disorders.

Ettlinger had another feather in his cap: the belief that careful, quantitative study of monkeys with neatly circumscribed cortical lesions and matched experimental experience could throw light on human neurological disorders such as visual agnosia. Following his post-doctoral training with Karl Pribram at the Institute of Living in Hartford, Connecticut, he set up at the Maudsley Hospital in London one of the first European laboratories to perform parallel, mutually informative investigations of monkeys and patients. It was in this tradition that we returned to Ettlinger's approach to studying the nature of visual 'agnosia' in monkeys, but extending the range of tests to avoid the criticism that Ettlinger's tests failed to cover several important sensory attributes (Campion 1987).

The importance of the inferior temporal neocortex in visual discrimination learning and remembering in macaque monkeys was established in the 1950s by several investigators, including George Ettlinger (Mishkin and Pribram 1954; Ettlinger 1959; Ettlinger *et al.* 1968; also reviewed by Dean 1976; Gross 1994). When the region labelled TE in Fig. 3.1 was removed bilaterally, macaque

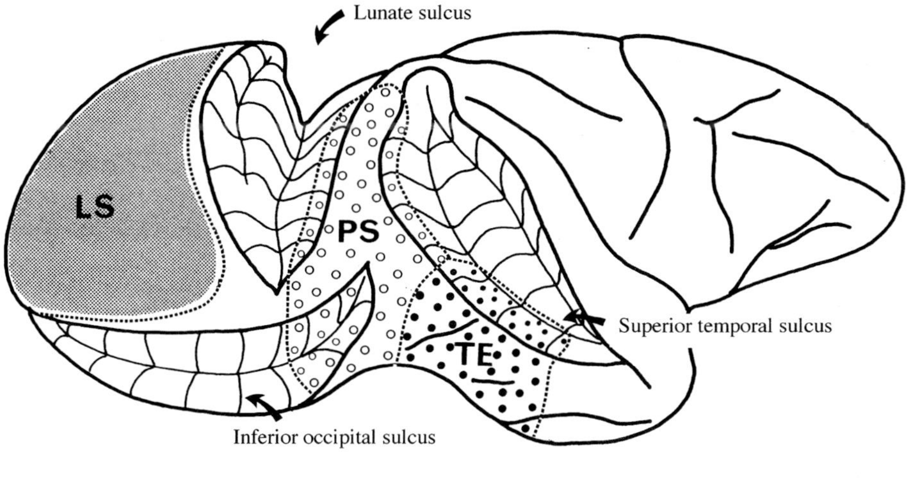

Fig. 3.1 Schematic view of the lateral surface of the right hemisphere of a rhesus macaque, showing the position of the lesions in lateral striate cortex (LS), prestriate cortex (PS), and inferior temporal cortex (TE). Area PS includes both areas V4 and TEO and continues on the ventral surface (not shown here), where it crosses the middle third of the occipito-temporal sulcus. The TE lesion also continues ventrally but ends at the rostral part of the occipito-temporal sulcus, without crossing it. The lunate, inferior occipital, and superior temporal sulci have been opened to reveal their depths. (Adapted from Cowey 1994, with permission.)

monkeys were slow to learn and relearn almost any kind of visual shape discrimination, although they were not impaired at either purely luminance discrimination or on tasks performed in other modalities, indicating that their general learning ability was intact. It is salutary to note that the importance of the ventral temporal lobe in vision was established by Ettlinger and his contemporaries long before we knew about extra-striate visual areas as demonstrated electrophysiologically. Twenty years later it was demonstrated that ablation of prestriate cortex covering the region labelled PS in Fig. 3.1 had similar consequences but perhaps for different reasons, namely that the caudal, prestriate, region was involved in computing the visual image whereas the rostral region was involved in visual memory (Cowey and Gross 1970; Mishkin 1972; Weiskrantz and Saunders 1984). The possible parallel with apperceptive and associative visual agnosia in neurological patients did not escape attention (despite the fact that human associative agnosia is more closely linked to damage of ventral limbic areas than to adjacent temporal neocortex), and macaques with temporal lobe lesions were used to investigate visual object agnosia (e.g. Levine 1982). This has continued to the present day, where the temporal lobes and ventral prestriate cortex are often referred to as the 'ventral processing stream' with its dominant input from the parvocellular (P) geniculate projection and its emphasis on the cortical processing of shape and colour, in contrast to the 'dorsal processing stream', receiving a predominantly magnocellular (M) geniculate input and coding position, motion and, perhaps, depth (reviewed by Ungerleider and Mishkin 1982; Cowey 1994). But the idea that monkeys with damage to parts of the ventral stream might have associative agnosia can still be questioned (e.g. Campion 1987) on the grounds first raised by Bay, namely that the visual disorder reflects subtle changes in visual sensory thresholds of a kind not revealed by conventional measures such as acuity or flicker fusion thresholds or clinical estimates of restriction or insensitivity of the visual fields, all of which are normal in monkeys made 'agnosic' by inferotemporal lesions (Symmes 1965; Cowey and Weiskrantz 1967). We therefore tested normal monkeys and monkeys with inferotemporal, or ventral prestriate, or lateral striate ablation (the latter certain to produce a sensory loss in macular vision) on a variety of visual tasks in order to determine their visual thresholds psychophysically. Although the monkeys with inferotemporal or latero-ventral prestriate ablation were visually 'agnosic' their sensory status was resolutely normal, with the exception of chromatic discrimination, which is irrelevant to achromatic shape perception. Our results vindicate Ettlinger's conclusions about human associative visual agnosia and we regret that he died without knowing about either them or our reasons for performing the experiments.

3.2 General methods

3.2.1 Animals and cortical ablations

Twelve male macaque monkeys, all juvenile at the start of testing, were tested psychophysically and almost daily for several years. They were divided into four groups, each of three animals. The control group received no surgery. The bilateral cortical ablations in the other three groups are shown schematically in Fig. 3.1. In group LS the lateral striate cortex, corresponding to the central 4–5 degrees of the retina (Daniel and Whitteridge 1961) was removed bilaterally, which produces a macular field defect and reduced visual acuity (Cowey and Weiskrantz 1963; Weiskrantz and Cowey 1963). In group TE the cortical removal involved the entire region TE of von Bonin and Bailey (1947). The lesion corresponds closely to that studied in many investigations of visual learning and retention in macaque monkeys (reviewed by Gross 1994). In group PS the lesion embraces all of cortical visual areas V4 and TEO (the latter identical to area PIT, i.e. posterior inferotemporal cortex) and perhaps small parts of area V2 concerned with the central few degrees of vision. This area, designated PS, is identical to the posterior lesions studied by Cowey and Gross (1970), who showed it to be just as effective as lesions of area TE in producing visual agnosia, but possibly of a perceptual rather than mnemonic nature (Cowey 1982). It has recently been proposed, on both anatomical and electrophysiological grounds, that areas V4 and TEO are part of a single complex (Zeki 1996). All lesions were verified histologically and were essentially as shown in Fig. 3.1.

3.2.2 *Testing methods*

The luminance, simple shape, and colour discriminations were carried out in a Wisconsin General Test Apparatus (WGTA), as described by Heywood *et al.* (1988). Each trial was presented manually by the experimenter, who could observe the monkey without being seen. All other tests were carried out in an automatic, remotely controlled apparatus, as follows. The monkey was tested in a transport cage, secured in front of a visual display in a darkened room. In the centre of the cage, facing the display, was a mask with the contours of a monkey's face. When the monkey pressed its face into the mask and kept it there the display was activated and the monkey could obtain a food reward by responding to the positive stimulus in a pair of simultaneously presented stimuli. Head position was monitored by photocells, so that if it withdrew its head, the display disappeared. Attached to the front of the mask was a device for holding spectacle lenses. Each monkey was photorefracted (Atkinson *et al.* 1984) and viewed the display through the appropriate lenses. Several monkeys were hyperopic or myopic and, additionally, astigmatic.

With one exception (Efron shapes) the display consisted of two different 'patterns', each presented on adjacent oscilloscopes (Tektronix, P31 phosphor). These were used in preference to VDUs because of their higher spatial resolution. In front of the monkey were two levers, at arm's length and just below its line of vision to the two cathode ray tubes (CRTs). The monkey learned to reach out and press the lever below the CRT that showed the positive stimulus. Initially the CRTs were also at arm's length but were moved progressively further away until the monkeys performed even at a viewing distance of 114 cm, where 1 cm = 0.5°. Screen luminance was varied by changing the voltage to the Z-axis of the CRTs and was calibrated by a digital photometer, itself calibrated against a beta light whose luminance, and change of luminance with age, were known (Saunders Roe Developments Ltd).

3.2.3 *Measuring thresholds*

This was done by using a modified method of limits. Individual variations are given under each test but, in general, the same stimulus value was used in each block of 20 trials. If the monkey achieved 17/20 or better in a block, the task was made more difficult for the next block; if it scored 16/20, no change was made; if it scored 15/20 or fewer, the task was made easier on the next block. Points of reversal between blocks, or scoring 16/20, were defined as *individual thresholds*. Overall threshold was reached when the mean of 20 (or 30) consecutive individual thresholds was no longer lower than that of the immediately previous 20 (or 30) and when the standard error was not more than 5 per cent of the overall mean. This ensured minimal variance in performance.

Each daily testing session typically involved 100 trials (five 20-trial blocks), and reversals or scores of 16/20 typically occurred no more than twice or thrice per session once the animal's performance had stabilized. It therefore required several weeks of stable performance to reach overall threshold. In practice, 2–3 months of testing were needed on each task, given the initial improvement that invariably precedes steady-state performance.

3.3 Specific tests

3.3.1 Contrast sensitivity

This was the only visual threshold to be tested both before and after operation. The other tests were all post-operative only. The ability to detect the luminance contrast in one-dimensional stationary sinusoidal gratings is often considered to be the best single measure of spatial vision. It is portrayed by the contrast sensitivity function (CSF), which shows sensitivity (i.e. reciprocal of threshold contrast) in relation to spatial frequency (i.e. number of cycles of light and dark bars per degree of visual angle). One oscilloscope displayed a uniform field of 10 candela (cd) m^{-2}. The other showed a vertical sine-wave grating of the same mean luminance but variable contrast. The grating was the positive stimulus and its left or right position on each trial was random. Thirteen different spatial frequencies, from 0.25 to 32.0 cpd were tested, using the following modification of the general procedure described above. For three consecutive days a given spatial frequency was used (= 300 trials in 15 blocks). This was called a run. Every other spatial frequency was then tested before returning to the first one for its second run, and so on. Criterion for each spatial frequency was reached when the third run differed from the second by less than 10 per cent, or the fourth from the third, and so on, and was calculated as the mean of the last two consecutive runs. As the minimum total number of sessions was 39 (3 × 13), but in practice was about 50–70, about 3 to 4 months of testing were needed to achieve stable performance and a complete CSF. The procedure was repeated after operation or after a similar period of time with the control group.

The results are given in Fig. 3.2, where for each group the envelopes of pre- and post-operative performance (or first and second testing for the controls) are shown. Variance for every monkey was necessarily small because of the criterion for establishing a stable threshold and, for clarity, is therefore omitted. There are several noteworthy features. First, every group improved at lower spatial frequencies, presumably reflecting the gradual improvement that is common with protracted psychophysical testing. Secondly, peak sensitivity was in the range 5–10 cpd, which is slightly higher than expected and possibly reflects the effect of having fewer total cycles at low spatial frequencies in small displays. Thirdly, and as predicted, group LS was clearly and significantly impaired at the highest spatial frequencies, with visual acuity, as estimated from the extrapolated curve, reduced from about 40 to 25 cpd. Group PS showed a similar but much smaller high-frequency impairment. However, the last and most important result is that none of the above changes indicates a visuosensory loss that could account for visual agnosia. The largest changes occurred in the group with lateral striate lesions, but the latter do not produce visual discrimination learning and retention impairments (see below). Just as informative, the slightly impaired performance of some monkeys was still better than that of some normal monkeys, which are presumably not agnosic!

3.3.2 Contrast matching

There is more to vision than *detecting* contrast, which describes sensitivity at threshold. For example, we need to be able to discriminate between different contrasts at supra-threshold levels, and this is one of the things that could conceivably be disturbed in agnosia. We accordingly tested the three operated groups—but not the unoperated controls—on a simultaneous visual discrimination between a sinusoidal grating of contrast 0.6 (the positive stimulus) and a grating of the same spatial frequency but lower contrast (the negative stimulus). The contrast of the latter was then systematically varied using the staircase procedure already described and the same criterion for assessing the threshold for 80 per cent correct performance. This was carried out for three different spatial frequencies of the positive stimulus: 1, 4, and 12 cpd. Mean screen luminance was 10 cd m^{-2}.

The result is shown in Fig. 3.3. For every monkey the threshold contrast difference depended on spatial frequency. But the three groups were otherwise similar. The only exception is the larger threshold at 4 cpd for the three monkeys with prestriate lesions, but such a small difference could hardly render them agnosic.

3.3.3 Spatial frequency discrimination

Perhaps 'agnosic' monkeys have difficulty in discriminating between different spatial frequencies even though they can detect and discriminate contrast normally, or nearly so. We therefore tested all 12 monkeys on a simultaneous visual discrimination between two different spatial frequencies of identical physical contrast. Subjective contrast would not be the same at widely different spatial frequencies, if monkeys are like human observers, but this difference should decline and disappear as the two gratings approached one another in spatial frequency. In each session the positive grating was 10, 5, or 1 cpd. The negative grating was 2, 1, or 0.2 cpd, respectively, at the beginning of training and was made progressively more like the positive, using the customary titration procedure with blocks of 20 trials and starting each testing session

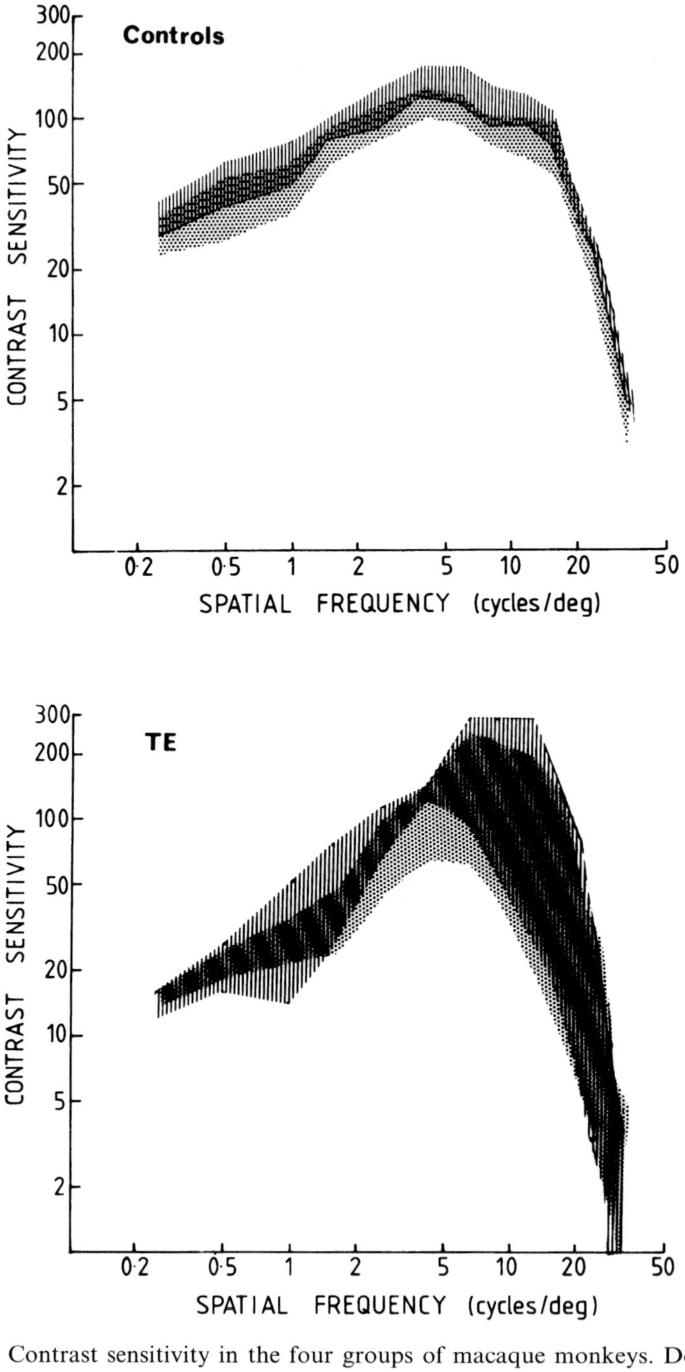

Fig 3.2 Contrast sensitivity in the four groups of macaque monkeys. Dots show the envelope for three animals pre-operatively; vertical lines show the envelope post-operatively or for the second set of measurements for the control group. The overlap in

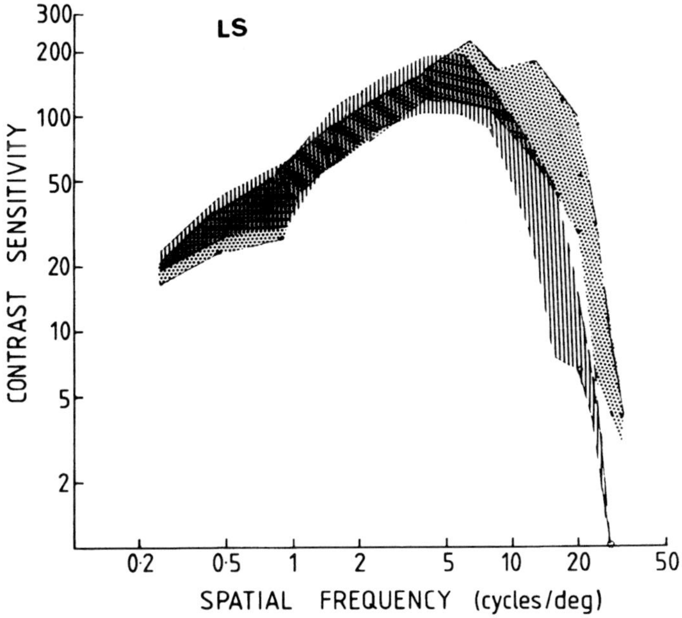

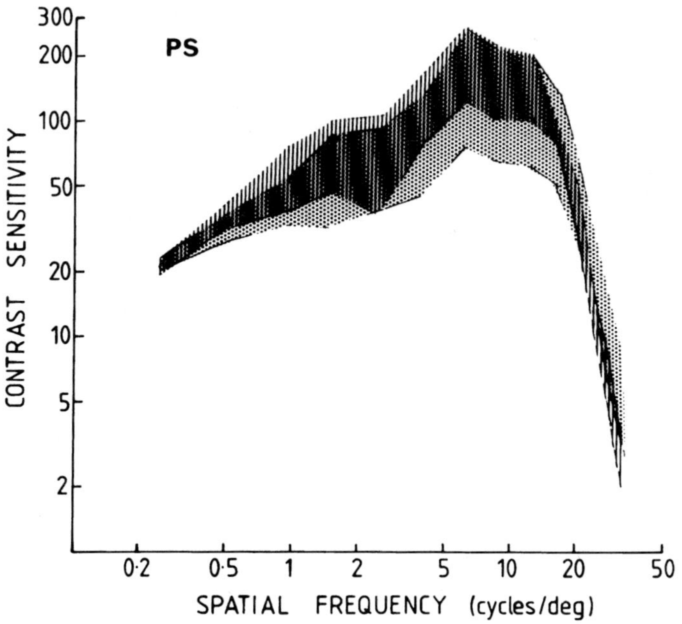

the envelopes is shown by dots plus lines. Only group LS was substantially impaired post-operatively and only at higher spatial frequencies.

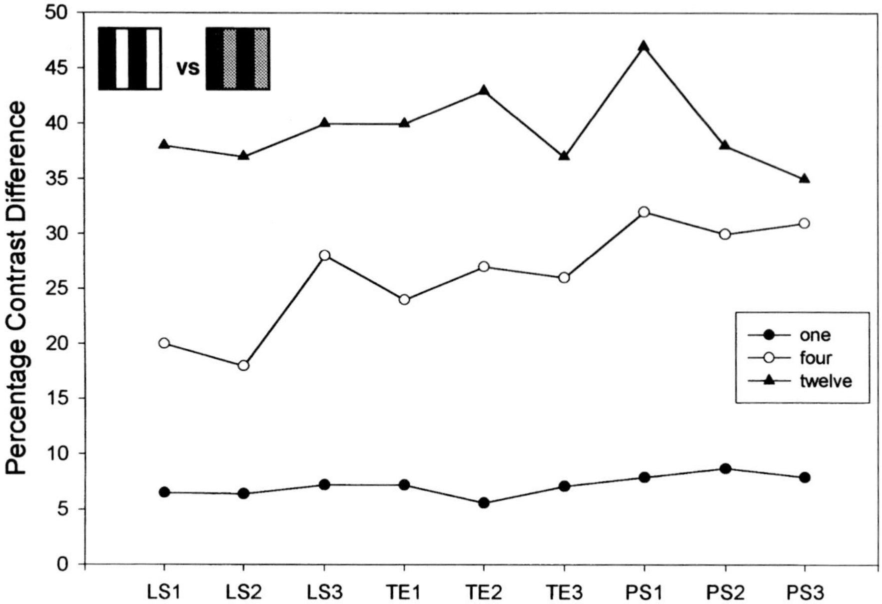

Fig. 3.3 The graph shows the percentage difference in contrast for 80% correct discrimination between two gratings (see inset top left) of identical spatial frequency (1, 4, or 12 cpd). The three control monkeys were not tested on this task.

with the variable spatial frequency determined by performance on the last test block in this condition. The negative stimulus was changed by halving or doubling the *difference* between positive and negative, e.g. with a positive of 5 cpd and an initial negative of 1 cpd, the other possible values of the latter were 3, 4, 4.5, 4.75, 4.87, and 4.93 cpd. For each of the three spatial frequencies of the positive stimulus, testing was continued until 40 reversals or scores of 16/20 were obtained and the overall mean of the last 20 showed no improvement on the preceding 20, and the standard error of the overall mean was less than 5 per cent of the mean. Different spatial frequencies were tested in interleaved sessions, and after criterion was reached on the first spatial frequency, testing continued with the remaining two, and finally with the last one. Although the theoretical minimum number of 20-trial blocks on which a reversal or a score of 16/20 occurred was 40, the actual number—counting from the first reversal point—varied from 40 to 127.

The results of several months of testing are shown in Fig. 3.4, where the threshold difference in spatial frequency of the two gratings is given as a percentage of the frequency of the positive stimulus. Although there are hints of small differences between groups, for example groups TE and PS compared to group LS at 1 and 10 cpd, they were not statistically significant

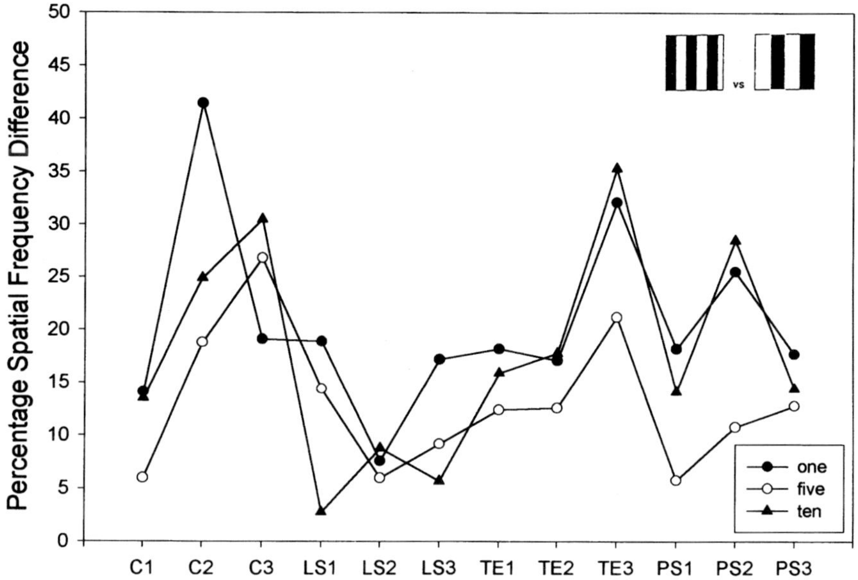

Fig. 3.4 The graph shows for all 12 monkeys the minimum percentage difference in spatial frequency for 80% correct discrimination between two gratings of the same physical contrast. The grating of higher spatial frequency was 1, 5, or 10 cpd.

and the monkey with the highest, i.e. poorest, overall threshold was actually an unoperated control (C2). This result provided no evidence of a sensory impairment that might explain poor form discrimination.

3.3.4 *Vernier acuity*

Object vision could be impoverished if the subject can detect contours normally but cannot align them in the mind's eye, for example judging co-linearity of contours in complex cluttered scenes in order to disentangle one object from another (discussed by Barlow 1986). We tested this by measuring the smallest offset the monkeys could discriminate—a version of vernier acuity. One of the CRTs had an uninterrupted horizontal line across its centre. This was the negative stimulus. In the positive stimulus the same line was 'broken' every 2 cm, by a step change in the Y-axis signal, such that alternate segments of the line were offset and the stimulus resembled a square wave in which the vertical excursion could be made invisible or barely visible by adjusting the sweep speed and brightness. The lines were made as thin as possible (<1 mm) by optimally focusing the CRT beam. Once the monkeys had learned to respond to the interrupted line, the offset was systematically varied according to the schedule described under spatial frequency discrimination, except that performance had to be stable for 60 consecutive individual thresholds rather than 40. The reason for interrupting the line at 2 cm intervals rather than just once was to ensure that monkeys in group LS, which had macular field defects, would be able to see at least some of the offsets, no matter where they fixated the display or how they visually explored it.

Figure 3.5 shows that the LS group was still impaired relative to the other three groups, which did not differ from each other. The impairment in group LS presumably reflects their inability to use the fovea, which is needed for fine discriminations. One puzzling feature of the results is that no monkey had a vernier threshold in the 'hyperacuity' range (i.e. spatial offsets about a log unit better than normal visual acuity), except TE2. We therefore tested three human subjects, including one of the authors (A.C.). All three performed in the hyperacuity range despite having much less practice than the monkeys. Why the monkeys had relatively high vernier thresholds is unclear, but they were certainly not high enough to account for poor pattern vision because the highest thresholds were present after lateral striate lesions, which do not impair the perception or recognition of large patterns and objects.

3.3.5 Efron shapes

Some neurological patients with severe apperceptive agnosia cannot tell the difference between a square and a grossly dissimilar rectangle of the same total area. This was first demonstrated by Efron (1968), after whom the test is

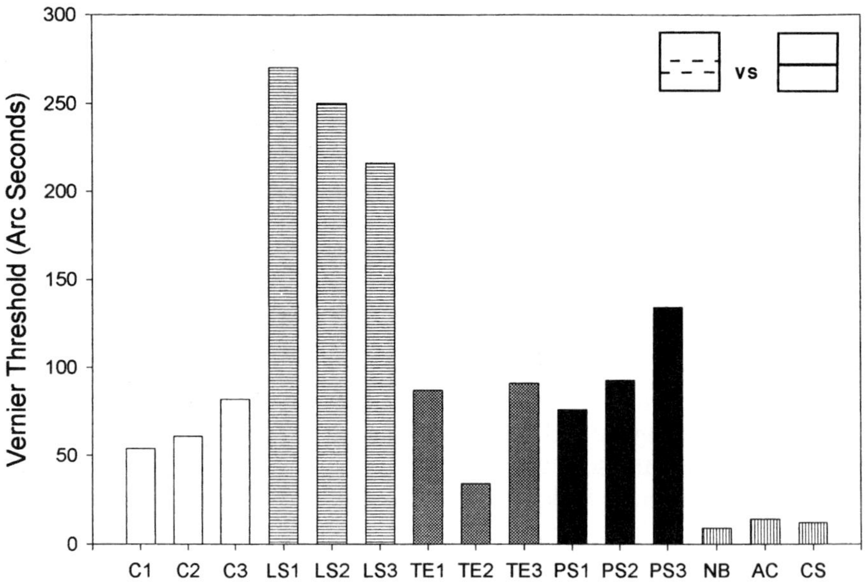

Fig. 3.5 Vernier thresholds, measured with the display shown in the inset at top right. The last three bars refer to three human subjects tested on the same task.

named, and again in several patients by Warrington and her colleagues (reviewed by Warrington 1985), who also refer to this apparent low-level visual deficit as pseudo-agnosia to distinguish it from less severe and perhaps higher-order changes in apperceptive agnosia (for example, not recognizing common objects from unusual views, or not knowing whether two very different views of an object are of the same object). We are less concerned here with possible varieties of non-associative agnosia than in determining whether any of our operated monkeys showed evidence of the Efron deficit.

Instead of the CRTs we used a VDU controlled by a microcomputer. On each trial a white square (50 mm × 50 mm) was presented in the left or right half of the screen. This was the positive stimulus. The negative stimulus, in the other half, was an upright rectangle of almost the same total area, in which the ratio of the long and short sides could vary in 14 steps up to 1.6 (64 mm × 40 mm). The ratio was titrated using the customary procedure until a stable threshold was reached over 60 consecutive reversals or scores of 16/20. Apart from the usual left/right randomization of the positive and negative stimuli, their relative vertical positions were also varied from trial to trial, so that whichever shape had the highest or lowest top or bottom edge, or was closer to the border of the VDI, was not a useful cue.

Figure 3.6 shows that there were no substantial differences in threshold among the four groups. Although groups TE and PS each contained one

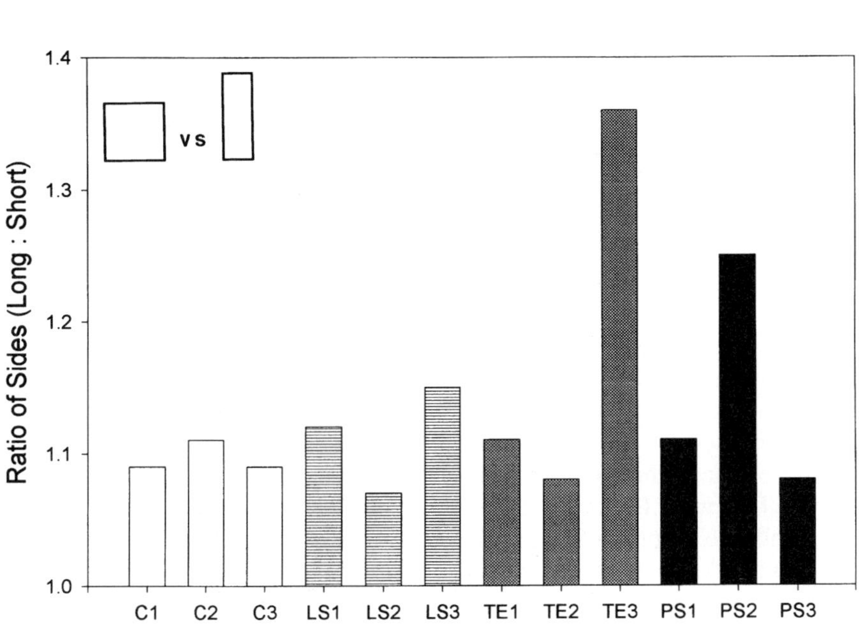

Fig. 3.6 The minimum ratio of the long and short sides of a rectangle needed by the 12 monkeys in order to discriminate it from a square of the same area (inset top left). The positive stimulus, the square, was always 5 cm × 5 cm.

monkey that was markedly poorer than the other 10 monkeys, even these two could discriminate at 80 per cent correct between a square and a rectangle of long/short ratio 1.3, which would be impossible for the kind of agnosic patient described by Efron (1968) and by Warrington (1985). The animals with inferotemporal or prestriate lesions are therefore not agnosic as a result of some gross, low-level, inability to register differences in the shape of simple outlines. However, there was clear evidence of a learning defect. Before the titration began the monkeys had to achieve 90 per cent correct in 200 consecutive trials on the easiest version of the discrimination. The number of errors made by each of the monkeys in this initial stage of the task was: C1 = 66; C2 = 257; C3 = 223; LS1 = 176; LS2 = 225; LS3 = 170; TE1 = 323; TE2 = 339; TE3 = 1015; PS1 = 972; PS2 = 1442; PS3 = 367. Even after the initial discrimination had been mastered the inferotemporal and prestriate groups required more individual thresholds before reaching the beginning of the 60 thresholds over which performance was stable. The numbers were: C1 = 0; C2 = 2; C3 = 37; LS1 = 34; LS2 = 47; LS3 = 5; TE1 = 65; TE2 = 56; TE3 = 84; PS1 = 131; PS2 = 150; PS3 = 74. Translating these numbers into behaviour, the two groups with extra-striate lesions learned the initial discrimination and dealt with its progressive increase in difficulty much more slowly (U-test, $N1 = 6$, $N2 = 6$, $U = 0$, $p = 0.001$, 1-tailed). Unfortunately, this result is compatible either with a shape discrimination learning disorder or with a perceptual disorder whose effects are slowly overcome by learning to monitor the different eye movements elicited when examining the shapes and using that to select the correct shape.

3.3.6 Luminance and shape discriminations

After spending about 2 years demonstrating that monkeys with lesions that are known to impair visual pattern discrimination have essentially normal visual sensory thresholds, we became concerned that perhaps they had recovered from, or had never had, a disorder of shape discrimination. We therefore tested them in a WGTA (see Heywood *et al.* 1988, for details) on a luminance discrimination (white versus black) that should not be impaired by ventral occipito-temporal lesions, and a simple pattern discrimination (+ versus □). For the luminance discrimination the monkey was presented on each trial with two grey plaques side by side on a sloping black board (56 cm wide and 30 cm high), which faced the animal. The plaques rested on a narrow ledge and each covered a foodwell. Between trials an opaque screen was lowered between the animal and the display. The experimenter was concealed behind a one-way vision screen. After the screen was raised the monkey responded through the bars of a transport cage by displacing a plaque laterally and, when its choice was correct, obtained a peanut from the foodwell. There was a white square in the middle of one plaque and a black square in the middle of the other (see Fig. 3.7). For the shape discrimination, both plaques were white but one had an outlined black cross in the centre and the other an outlined square, each

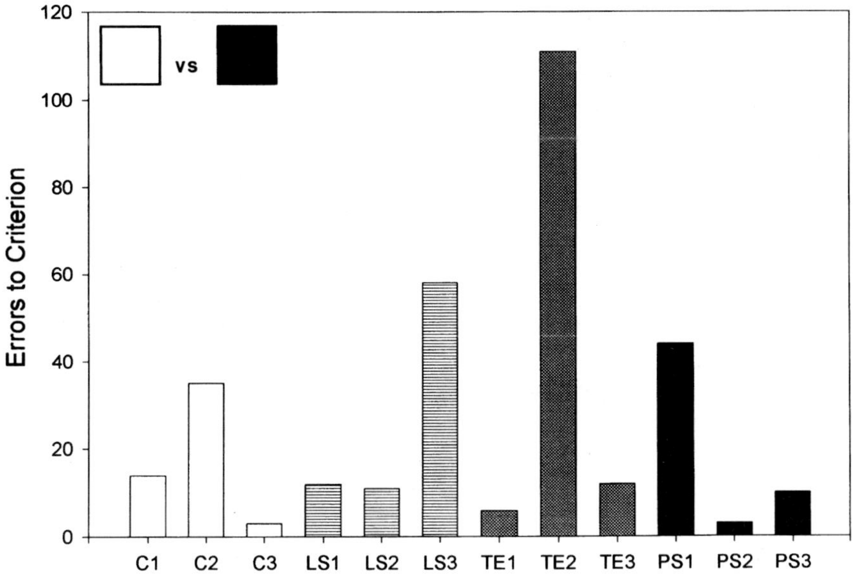

Fig. 3.7 The number of errors made by each monkey to achieve a criterion of 90 correct responses in 100 consecutive trials when discriminating between the white and black plaques.

made from black tape and of identical height, width and total length of contour (see Figure 3.8). The monkeys were tested first on the white versus black discrimination then on cross versus square for 50 trials each day until they reached a criterion of 90 per cent correct responses in 100 consecutive trials.

Figure 3.7 shows that there were no group differences with respect to the number of errors made in reaching criterion on the white/black discrimination, even though monkeys LS3 and TE2 were conspicuously worse than others in their groups. But Fig. 3.8 shows that when then tested on the shape discrimination all six monkeys with either inferotemporal or prestriate lesions made more errors than unoperated monkeys or monkeys with lateral striate lesions, as predicted (*U*-test, $N1 = 6$, $N2 = 6$, $U = 0$, $p = 0.001$, 1-tailed). These tests were carried out nearly 3 years after operation.

3.3.7 Hue discrimination

Lest we give the impression that neither prestriate nor inferotemporal lesions impair anything but shape discrimination learning, it should be mentioned that all 12 monkeys were also tested on hue discrimination or grey discriminations after completing the previous set of tasks (Heywood *et al.* 1988). The stimuli were Munsell colour or grey swatches (7.5 cm × 5 cm) mounted under thin and minimally reflective glass, which was frequently cleaned. In the case of

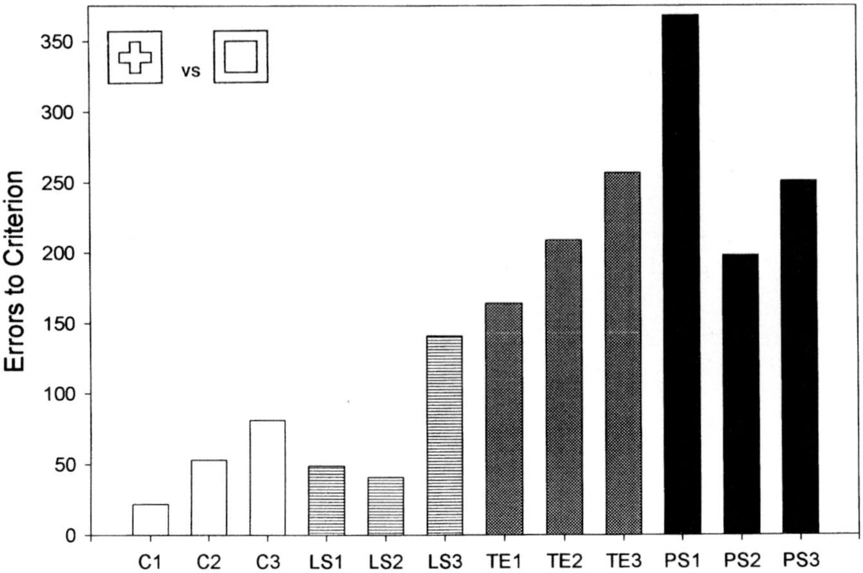

Fig. 3.8 The number of errors made by each monkey to achieve a criterion of 90 correct responses in 100 consecutive trials when discriminating between an outlined black cross and an outlined square on a white background. Monkeys of groups TE and PS were impaired.

coloured stimuli, their brightnesses (= 'value' on Munsell notation) were matched, i.e. they should be equally bright and therefore indiscriminable on the basis of brightness to the average young human observer. They were also matched for 'chroma' (= saturation). The technical specifications of each series of stimuli, using the conventional notation, were as follows. For the initial stages of training a positive red (2.5R/6/12) stimulus was paired with a negative green (10GY/6/12). Following that, the same positive red stimulus was paired with a negative pinkish red (5YR). There were 11 stimuli in each of the yellow, blue, and grey series. The yellow stimuli ranged in hue from 10YR to 2.5GY, in hue steps of 1.25. The blue series ranged in hue from 10G to 5PG in steps of 2.5. The series of achromatic 'greys' varied in brightness by 4.6 to 50.7 per cent and they were selected in order to be as difficult to discriminate from each other as the hues are for human observers.

After learning to discriminate between red versus green and red versus pink and the two extreme hues of each series of yellow, blue, and the extreme brightnesses of the grey series, the monkeys were then successively tested with progressively more similar examples of each series. For example, after learning blue 1 versus blue 11 they were presented with 2 versus 10, 3 versus 9, 4 versus 8, 5 versus 7, and 5 versus 6, the lower (bluer) number being positive in every case. Identical procedures were then followed in the grey and, finally, the yellow ranges. If criterion was not reached within 500 trials on a particular stage, then testing on that series ceased, on the grounds that failing a discrimination was unlikely to be followed by solving an even more difficult one. The results are given in Fig. 3.9 and show that the three monkeys with TE lesions performed poorly on even simple colour discriminations, and in several instances failed to progress to more difficult discriminations. However, as Ettlinger would probably have pointed out, any sensory loss with respect to colour can hardly explain poor learning and retention of visual patterns and objects. When compared with all animals of the other three groups, they were also slightly but significantly impaired with the grey discriminations (*U*-test, $p = 0.02$, 2-tailed), as previously reported in an achromatopsic patient (Heywood *et al.* 1991) and in achromatopsic monkeys (Heywood *et al.* 1995). However, the difference between their performance and that of the monkeys with lateral striate lesions was negligible, yet the latter are not agnosic.

3.4 Discussion

On a series of tests designed to measure detection or discrimination thresholds in four groups of monkeys we found three noteworthy impairments. First, the monkeys with lateral striate lesions had reduced sensitivity to luminance contrast at spatial frequencies above about 10 cpd. Although never previously reported, it presumably reflects the well-known macular field defect caused by removing the macular representation in striate cortex, usually examined by testing visual acuity, i.e. the maximal spatial frequency that can be detected at maximal contrast, and corresponding to the point at which the extrapolated curves of Fig. 3.2 intersect the horizontal axis. It is of considerable interest that there was no reduction in contrast sensitivity at lower spatial frequencies in group LS, but this is not relevant to the major point of our chapter. Secondly, the same group had elevated 'vernier' thresholds, again reflecting their macular field defect. Thirdly, the monkeys with inferotemporal lesions (group TE) were substantially impaired at discriminating between roughly isoluminant colours, even categorically different colours such as red and green. Their defect could be a learning deficit specific for colours, but independent experiments on similar monkeys suggest that they have a specific sensory defect better likened to human cerebral achromatopsia (Heywood *et al.* 1995). Just as important, group PS, in which area V4 was entirely removed, was not achromatopsic, indicating that the region in the human brain now commonly referred to as 'human V4' is either nothing of the sort, or that achromatopsia related to destruction of human V4 actually arises from additional damage to adjacent cortex or white matter.

The most important conclusion to be drawn from the above results, when taken together with the lack of effects of either PS or TE lesions on the other visuosensory tasks, is that they can not explain why such monkeys are visually 'agnosic' in the purely operational sense of performing poorly on a wide range

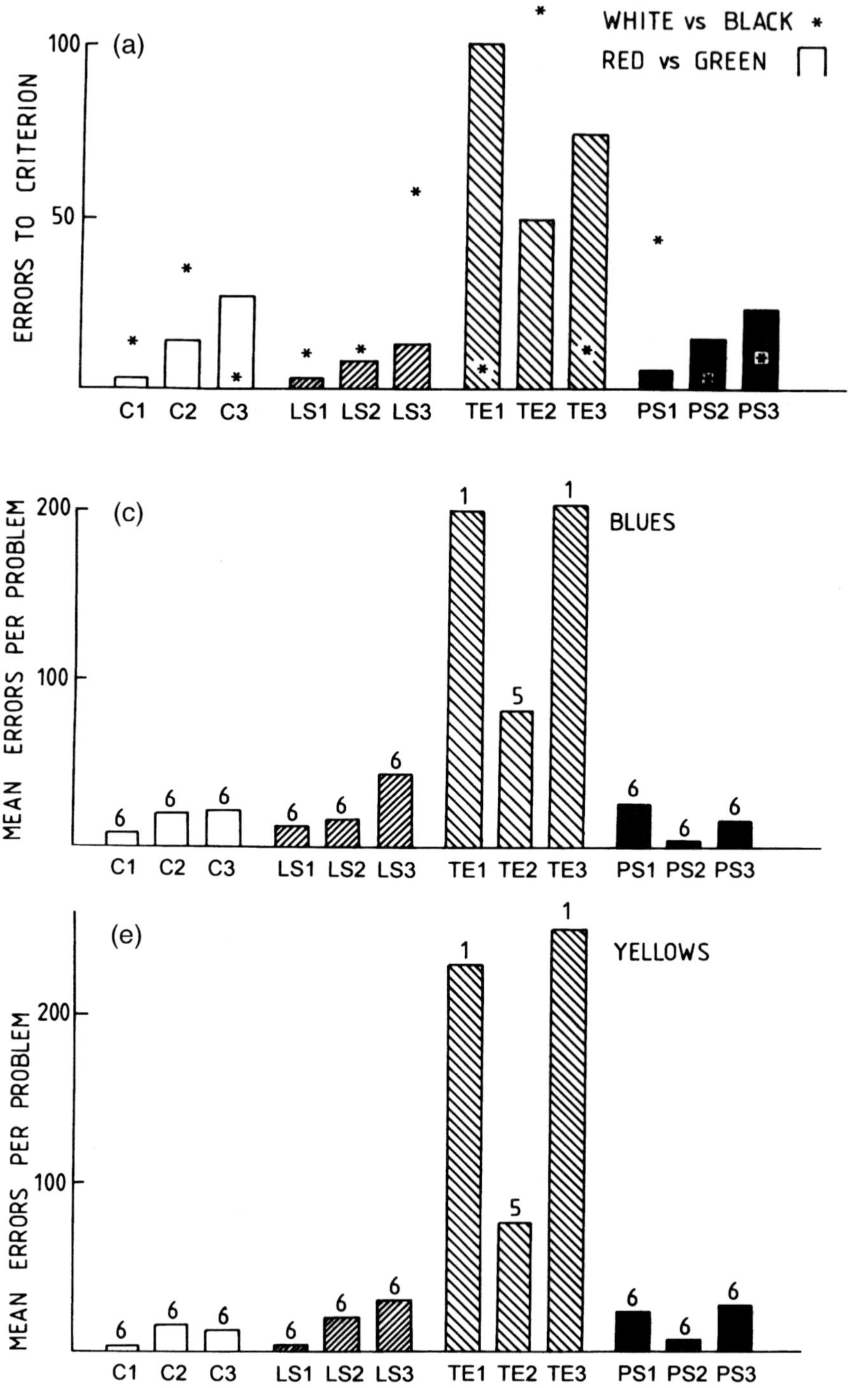
WHITE vs BLACK *
RED vs GREEN
100
50
ERRORS TO CRITERION
(a)
C1 C2 C3 LS1 LS2 LS3 TE1 TE2 TE3 PS1 PS2 PS3
200
100
MEAN ERRORS PER PROBLEM
(c)
BLUES
1 1 5 6 6 6 6 6 6 6 6 6
C1 C2 C3 LS1 LS2 LS3 TE1 TE2 TE3 PS1 PS2 PS3
(e)
YELLOWS
200
100
MEAN ERRORS PER PROBLEM
1 1 5 6 6 6 6 6 6 6 6 6
C1 C2 C3 LS1 LS2 LS3 TE1 TE2 TE3 PS1 PS2 PS3

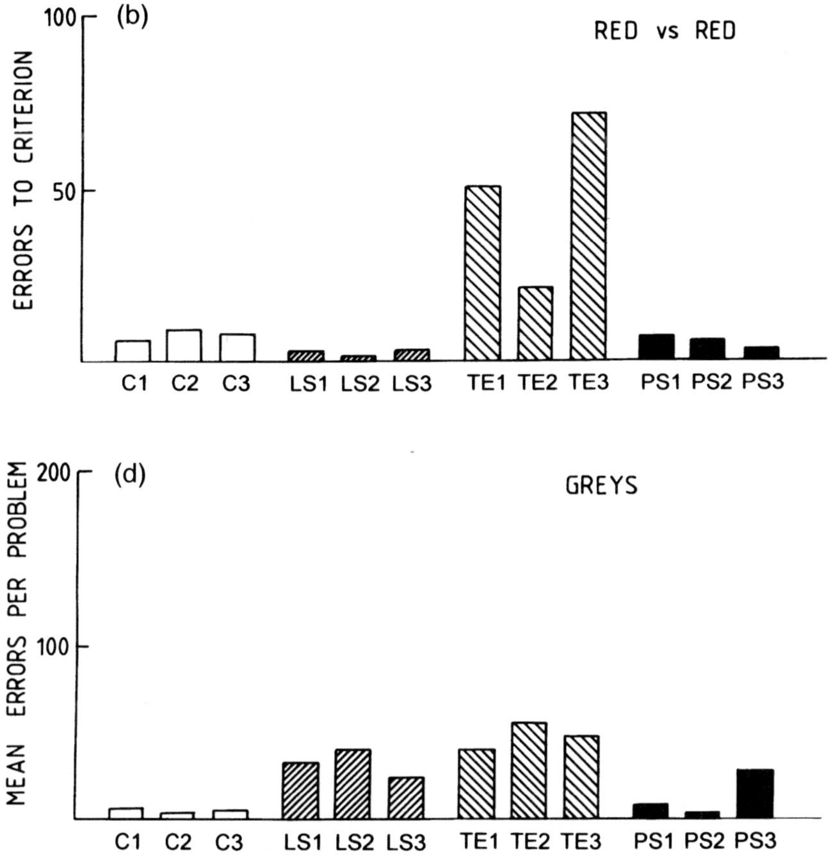

Fig. 3.9 Chromatic and achromatic discriminations. Each of the five sets of histograms shows the number of errors made in learning one or more simultaneous discriminations to a criterion of 90 per cent correct in 100 consecutive trials, with 50 trials per session. (a) Results for red positive versus green negative. For easy comparison, the asterisks repeat the results for white versus black shown in Fig. 3.7. (b) Results of testing with the same positive red stimulus and a pinkish negative stimulus. (c) The results of testing with two different blue stimuli and then making both positive and negative blues progressively more similar to each other in five equivalent Munsell hue steps (see Heywood *et al.* 1988 for details). The bars indicate the mean number of errors made across all problems that were presented (maximum = 6). If a monkey failed to reach criterion within 500 trials on any problem it was not advanced to a more difficult stage in the series. The number above each bar indicates how many levels of difficulty were reached by that animal. (d) The results of the same procedure with achromatic, grey, stimuli. (e) The results with yellow stimuli. Note that the three monkeys with inferotemporal lesions (TE) were substantially impaired with chromatic stimuli, especially at small hue differences (a, b, c, e), whereas they were little different from monkeys with lateral striate lesions with grey stimuli. Note also that group PS (whose lesions involved the whole of visual areas V4 and TEO) was not impaired on fine hue discriminations, unlike patients with cerebral achromatopsia. (Adapted from Cowey 1994, with permission.)

of tests of visual shape discrimination learning and retention. Good colour discrimination is not needed for discriminating achromatic or monochromatic shapes, just as colour television is little better than black and white television in enabling viewers to understand the picture. The lack of an impairment when shape was systematically varied along a single axis (the Efron task) is particularly important in ruling out any gross disturbance of low-level pattern discrimination mechanisms of the kind reported in 'pseudo-agnosia' or apperceptive agnosia. The visual disorder in monkeys must lie elsewhere, as it does in patients with visual associative agnosia as studied by Ettlinger and by De Haan *et al.* (1995), and whose disorder lies in visual memory, and in patients with apperceptive agnosia, whose visual shape constancy is impaired.

What might Ettlinger have said about our results? He would probably have liked the demonstration that a hypothesis was disconfirmed, for he advocated this way of conducting empirical science. And if he had also considered, in his characteristic and occasionally provocative manner, that our results confirmed his own view of the nature of visual agnosia, we would not be displeased.

Acknowledgements

This research was supported by a grant form the Medical Research Council. We thank Nigel Brown for his help over several years with the testing of the monkeys, the design of the apparatus, and the programming of the experiments; Carolyne Le Mare for her help in preparing the figures; and Drs Oliver Braddick and Janette Atkinson for making the photorefractive measurements that allowed us to use appropriate spectacle correction for each monkey.

References

Atkinson, J., Braddick, O. J., and Durden, K. (1984). Screening for refractive errors in 6–9 month-old infants by photorefraction. *British Journal of Ophthalmology*, **68**, 105–12.

Barlow, H. B. (1986). Why have multiple cortical areas? *Vision Research*, **26**, 81–90.

Bay, E. (1953). Disturbances of visual perception and their examination. *Brain*, **76**, 515–51.

Bonin, G. von and Bailey, P. (1947). *The neocortex of* Macaca mulatta. University of Illinois, Urbana.

Campion, J. (1987). Apperceptive agnosia: the specification and description of constructs. In *Visual object processing: a cognitive neuropsychological approach*, (ed. G. W. Humphreys and M. J. Riddoch), pp.197–232. Erlbaum, London.

Cowey, A. (1982). Sensory and non-sensory visual disorders in man and monkey. *Philosophical Transactions of the Royal Society of London, Series B*, **298**, 3–13.

Cowey, A. (1994). Cortical visual areas and the neurobiology of higher visual processes. In *Object representation and recognition*, (ed. M. Farah and G. Ratcliff), pp.1–31. Erlbaum, Hillsdale, New Jersey.

Cowey, A. and Gross, C. G. (1970). Effects of foveal prestriate and inferotemporal lesions on visual discrimination by rhesus monkeys. *Experimental Brain Research*, **11**, 128–44.

Cowey, A. and Weiskrantz, L. (1963). A perimetric study of visual field defects in monkeys. *Quarterly Journal of Experimental Psychology*, **15**, 91–115.

Cowey, A. and Weiskrantz, L. (1967). A comparison of the effects of inferotemporal and striate cortex lesions on the visual behaviour of rhesus monkeys. *Quarterly Journal of Experimental Psychology*, **19**, 246–53.

Daniel. P. M. and Whitteridge, D. (1961). The representation of the visual field on the cerebral cortex in monkeys. *Journal of Physiology*, **159**, 203–21.

Dean, P. (1976). Effects of inferotemporal lesions on the behavior of monkeys. *Psychological Bulletin*, **83**, 41–71.

De Haan, E. H. F., Heywood, C. A., Young, A. W., Edelstyn, N., and Newcombe, F. (1995). Ettlinger revisited: the relation between agnosia and sensory impairment. *Journal of Neurology, Neurosurgery and Psychiatry*, **58**, 350–6.

Efron, R. (1968). *What is perception?* Boston Studies in the Philosophy of Science, Vol. 4, pp. 137–73. Humanities Press, New York.

Ettlinger, G. (1956). Sensory deficits in visual agnosia. *Journal of Neurology, Neurosurgery and Psychiatry*, **19**, 297–308.

Ettlinger, G. (1959). Visual discrimination with a single manipulandum following temporal ablations in the monkey. *Quarterly Journal of Experimental Psychology*, **11**, 164–74.

Ettlinger, G., Iwai, E., Mishkin, M., and Rosvold, H. E. (1968). Visual discrimination in the monkey following serial ablation of inferotemporal and preoccipital cortex. *Journal of Comparative and Physiological Psychology*, **65**, 110–17.

Gross, C. G. (1994). How inferior temporal cortex became a visual area. *Cerebral Cortex*, **5**, 455–69.

Heywood, C. A., Shields, C., and Cowey, A. (1988). The involvement of the temporal lobes in colour discrimination. *Experimental Brain Research*, **71**, 437–41.

Heywood, C. A., Cowey, A., and Newcombe, F. (1991). Chromatic discrimination in a cortically blind observer. *European Journal of Neuroscience*, **3**, 802–12.

Heywood, C. A., Gaffan, D., and Cowey, A. (1995). Cerebral achromatopsia in monkeys. *European Journal of Neuroscience*, **7**, 1064–73.

Levine, D. N. (1982). Visual agnosia in monkey and in man. In *Analysis of visual behavior*, (ed. D. J. Ingle, M. A. Goodale, and R. J. W. Mansfield), pp. 629–70. MIT Press, Cambridge, Mass.

Lissauer, L. (1889). Ein Fall von Seelenblindheit nebst einem Beitrag zur Theorie derselben. *Archiv für Psychiatrie und Nervenkrankheiten*, **21**, 222–70.

Mishkin, M. (1972). Cortical visual areas and their interactions. In *The brain and human behavior*, (ed. A. G. Karczmar and J. C. Eccles), pp. 187–208. Springer, Berlin.

Mishkin, M. and Pribram, K. H. (1954). Visual discrimination performance folowing partial ablations of the temporal lobe. 1. Ventral vs. lateral. *Journal of Comparative and Physiological Psychology*, **47**, 14–20.

Symmes, D. (1965). Flicker discrimination by brain damaged monkeys. *Journal of Comparative and Physiological Psychology*, **60**, 470–3.

Ungerleider, L. G. and Mishkin, M. (1982). Two cortical visual systems. In *Analysis of visual behavior*, (ed. D. J. Ingle, M. A. Goodale, and R. J. W. Mansfield), pp. 549–86. MIT Press, Cambridge, Mass.

Warrington, E. K. (1985). Agnosia: the impairment of object recognition. In *Handbook of Clinical Neurology*, Vol. 1, *Clinical Neuropsychology*, (ed. P. J. Vinken, G. W. Bruyn, and H. L. Klawans), pp. 333–49. Elsevier Science Publishers, New York.

Weiskrantz, L. and Cowey, A. (1963). Striate cortex lesions and visual acuity of the rhesus monkey. *Journal of Comparative Physiology and Psychology*, **56**, 225–31.
Weiskrantz, L. and Saunders, R. C. (1984). Impairments of visual object transforms in monkeys. *Brain*, **107**, 1033–72.
Zeki, S. (1996). Are areas TEO and PIT of monkey visual cortex wholly distinct from the fourth visual complex (V4 complex)? *Proceedings of the Royal Society of London, Series B*, **263**, 1539–44.

4

Cross-modal associations, intramodal associations, and object identification in macaque monkeys

ELISABETH A. MURRAY, LUDISE MALKOVA, and SONIA GOULET

4.1 Introduction

The ability to associate two or more stimuli that are perceived through different modalities of sensory input (vision, somatic sensation, audition, gustation, olfaction, and vestibular signals) undoubtedly affords an adaptive advantage to organisms. Stimulus–stimulus associations may be used to guide behaviour in many ways. For example, a juvenile monkey that associates the sight of its mother's face with the sound of her vocalization would be in a position quickly to approach and seek refuge with the mother, on the basis of auditory sensory information alone, in conditions in which the mother is visually obscured (e.g. temporarily situated in tall grass, behind a tree, or in a group of several individuals). And a monkey that finds a small, round red fruit to be consistently tasty but a small, round green fruit unpalatable would be able to forage more efficiently if it associated the visual properties of the fruit with its gustatory and olfactory properties. In short, stimulus–stimulus associations have considerable predictive power. There are at least three main ways in which this advantage may become manifest. First, knowledge of stimulus–stimulus associations may guide the decision of an organism to approach or avoid a particular stimulus object. That is, a given behavioural response may be facultative or conditional. Secondly, on many occasions the co-occurrence of two sensory events predicts a different outcome from the occurrence of either a different combination of stimuli or of one stimulus alone. In other words, the appropriateness of a certain behaviour may be contingent upon a specific combination or configuration of sensory events, rather than a single sensory event. Thirdly, a single sensory input, if associated in memory with other sensory inputs that often occurred closely together in time, may evoke a memory of a particular object, place, or event. In these three types of situations, which do not necessarily represent mutually exclusive categories, knowledge of stimulus–stimulus associations would confer an adaptive advantage by virtue of promoting the suitability of responses. There are undoubtedly many other ways in which the reader may envisage that the ability to associate stimuli with one another, either within a modality (intramodal) or across sensory modalities (cross-modal), would be advantageous (e.g. in directing of attention, or in the preparation for limb movements).

In this chapter we will first review some of the attempts to investigate the phenomenon of cross-modal sensory–sensory associations in macaque monkeys. We will not attempt an exhaustive examination of the multifarious types of 'cross-modal' associations that are available to monkeys, but, rather, will provide a selective review of studies that have examined objects, including two- and three-dimensional stimuli. Then we will discuss the available evidence concerning the neural basis for cross-modal associations, and its possible relationship with intramodal associations. Finally, we will explore the ways in which both cross-modal and intramodal associations may contribute to object identification.

4.2 Overview of cross-modal associations in monkeys

The term 'cross-modal' performance, used in the context of our discussion of neuropsychological studies examining this phenomenon in monkeys, refers to the ability to use experience gained via one sensory modality to guide performance dependent on stimuli presented through another sensory modality.

Early experiments on monkeys encountered great difficulty in obtaining clear evidence of cross-modal performance (e.g. Ettlinger 1960, 1967). At least two distinct training procedures were used in the 1960s and early 1970s: cross-modal *transfer* and cross-modal *matching*. In transfer, subjects are trained to discriminate two objects in one sensory modality (e.g. somatic sensation, or touch) and then are presented with the same stimuli for discrimination in the other sensory modality (e.g. vision). If the subjects learn faster in the second modality than a control group whose experience in the first modality was with a different pair of stimuli, then cross-modal transfer would be demonstrated (Ettlinger 1960). In cross-modal matching, one of two objects (A or B) is presented to the animal as a sample in a given modality (e.g. touch) and the animal is later rewarded for selecting the same object (A′ or B′) when the two are presented together for choice in the alternative modality (e.g. vision). As originally implemented, only two objects were used repeatedly across trials. As a control, 'true' matching (as just described) was contrasted with 'false' matching (Ettlinger and Blakemore 1967), which involved an identical trial sequence but required the association of arbitrarily paired stimulus objects rather than the association of different sensory qualities derived from one and the same object (e.g. if A is the sample, then choose X′ on the choice test; if B, then Y′). This latter procedure is often referred to as 'symbolic' matching. Neither of these training procedures yielded evidence for cross-modal performance in monkeys.

Davenport, Rogers, and their colleagues (Davenport and Rogers 1970; Davenport *et al.* 1973), who used a large set of objects, later demonstrated that apes are not only able to perform cross-modal matching, but that they could perform it in both directions, i.e. vision-to-touch and touch-to-vision. At that time, it became widely accepted that apes are capable of cross-modal performance but monkeys are not. That monkeys are indeed able to perform cross-modal associations was first demonstrated by Cowey and Weiskrantz (Cowey and Weiskrantz 1975; Weiskrantz and Cowey 1975), who used a training procedure that brought together components of the cross-modal transfer and matching procedures. They used 'cookies' made of edible material which were rendered either palatable or non-palatable by addition of sugar or quinine, respectively. There were two stages of training. In the first stage, monkeys were given repeated experiences, across days, with a large (and equal) number of palatable and non-palatable cookies in the dark. The palatable cookies took one form (say, spherical) and the non-palatable ones another (say, star-shaped). Later, the two shapes that had been experienced only in the dark were presented together in the light, for a choice based on visual cues only. This procedure was repeated using several additional shapes, a different pair for each test. Because tactual, gustatory, and olfactory experience was followed by a single visual choice trial, the task was assumed to measure cross-modal *recognition*. On average, the monkeys chose the palatable shapes significantly more often than the non-palatable shapes; they chose the matching object on roughly 80 per cent of the cross-modal trials. Similar results obtained with the same technique were subsequently reported by Elliot (1977).

Although this procedure appeared to demonstrate true cross-modal performance in monkeys, there were two serious drawbacks. First, the sensory discrimination abilities could not easily be assessed independently of the cross-modal abilities. In the context of studies examining the neural substrates of cross-modal association this kind of assessment is critical, because failure on a cross-modal problem might reflect either disruption of the associative mechanism (the process of interest), or impairment in basic sensory capacities. The second drawback was that a single cross-modal trial required several days of testing.

Later, Jarvis and Ettlinger (1977) elaborated the cross-modal recognition procedure in such a way as to overcome the aforementioned drawbacks. In their task, within-modal discrimination abilities were assessed concurrently with cross-modal abilities, and several problems were administered within a single test session. Monkeys were trained on a series of two-choice discrimination problems, each employing a different pair of objects. Attainment of criterion in one modality was followed immediately by a single choice trial in the alternate modality (i.e. vision-to-touch or touch-to-vision) with the same pair of objects. That is, visual discrimination problems, followed by a single cross-modal trial in touch, were alternated with tactual discrimination problems, followed by a single cross-modal trial in vision. On the visual discrimination trials preceding a (visual-to-tactual) cross-modal recognition trial, a clear plastic barrier immediately in front of the object precluded the monkey from obtaining tactual information during the 'visual' exposure. The monkey displaced the object by pushing directly against the plastic barrier.

Two of the four monkeys trained in this way exhibited significant cross-modal recognition; they scored about 70 per cent correct, which was slightly lower than that obtained by the monkeys trained with the Cowey and Weiskrantz method. In addition to confirming Cowey and Weiskrantz's (1975) finding of successful tactual-to-visual cross-modal recognition in monkeys, Jarvis and Ettlinger also demonstrated, for the first time, successful visual-to-tactual cross-modal recognition.

Finally, Murray and Mishkin (1985), and later Goulet and Murray (1996) and Malkova and Murray (1996), successfully demonstrated cross-modal performance using a tactual-to-visual delayed non-matching-to-sample (DNMS) procedure with a set of 40 highly familiar objects. This procedure differed in three main ways from the procedures used by Cowey and Weiskrantz (1975) and by Jarvis and Ettlinger (1977):

(1) it employed the non-matching rule instead of the matching rule;

(2) the sample was presented only once per trial, so that each choice test evaluated cross-modal performance;

(3) the objects were already highly familiar to the monkeys before cross-modal testing was initiated.

Like the method of Jarvis and Ettlinger, this procedure allows assessment of intramodal recognition abilities. Unlike their procedure, however, it taxes cross-modal *association* rather than cross-modal *recognition*. This is so because the monkeys were given extensive experience with the tactual and visual properties of the individual objects before being required to make a cross-modal choice. The cross-modal matching task of Bolster (1978) and of DiMattia *et al.* (1990) falls in this same (associative) category, according to our classification scheme, because their monkeys received both tactual and visual experience with individual objects, which over the course of training must have become familiar. We hasten to add, however, that the descriptive terms *transfer*, *matching*, *recognition*, and *association*, as used here, apply only to the different cross-modal testing paradigms we have outlined. Whether the cross-modal abilities assessed by these different methods are subserved by one and the same neural mechanism remains to be determined. Further, these terms are not applied consistently throughout the neuropsychological literature. Indeed 'recognition', as used in 'cross-modal recognition', should not be assumed to be the same process as that engaged in 'intramodal recognition', which is discussed later in this chapter. The former arguably relies on an associative process whereas the latter may be mediated by a familiarity judgement based on perceptual matching.

It would be of interest to understand why macaque monkeys fail to exhibit cross-modal abilities using some procedures but not others. In transfer, one might speculate that the monkeys simply could not, or did not, connect one discrimination problem with the next, unless they had extensive experience (learning set). As for matching, we now know that normal monkeys have extreme difficulty in learning the delayed matching- or non-matching-to-sample task with a single pair of repeatedly used objects (Mishkin and Delacour 1975; Murray *et al.* 1996). Thus it is not so surprising that monkeys failed to learn a cross-modal version of delayed matching-to-sample (DMS) with a single pair, as in the original implementation (Ettlinger and Blakemore 1967), yet performed well on DNMS with a larger stimulus set (Murray and Mishkin 1985; Goulet and Murray 1996; Malkova and Murray 1996). Nevertheless, monkeys can learn cross-modal matching with a single pair when they are given the benefit of simultaneously experiencing both the tactual and visual qualities of the individual objects (Bolster 1978; DiMattia *et al.* 1990). As for cross-modal recognition, if several discrimination trials administered in one modality precede the single discrimination trial given in the second modality, the monkeys may grasp only slowly the to-be-applied rule on the infrequently occurring recognition trial. The procedures that have been most successful in demonstrating cross-modal abilities have in common:

(1) the use of a high percentage of trials requiring cross-modal abilities; and

(2) familiar objects with set sizes in the moderate range.

Perhaps these two factors promote learning of the rule and object identification, respectively.

Because we will consider the cross-modal DNMS task further in later sections, we will describe the methods used by Murray and her colleagues (Murray and Mishkin 1985; Goulet and Murray 1996; Malkova and Murray 1996) in detail. The monkeys in the three studies received several stages of training, including visual DNMS, a light-dimming phase of DNMS, tactual DNMS, and then, finally, cross-modal DNMS. The same set of 40 objects, which varied widely in colour, size, shape, texture, and compressibility, was used throughout all phases of training. In addition, the objects were mounted on corks that fitted snugly into the wells of the test tray. This forced the monkeys to grasp and lift, and, thereby, palpate the objects as they displaced them. During the sample presentation portion of the trial, the central well of a three-well test tray was covered with a sample object, which the monkey had to displace in order to obtain a food reward hidden underneath. In the choice part of the trial, presented 10 seconds later, the sample object plus a 'new' object from the set were presented over the lateral wells of the test tray. The monkey had to displace the new object in order to gain another food reward. Choosing the sample led to non-reinforcement and termination of the trial. At the end of a 30-second intertrial interval, the procedure was repeated with a new pair of objects, and so on, until the 20 trials comprising a test session were completed. The 40 objects were paired anew each day in random fashion. After they had attained criterion on both the intramodal DNMS tasks, the monkeys were trained on the cross-modal version, which combined a tactual sample presentation with a visual choice test. To ensure that the monkey's choices on the cross-modal trials would be based on vision alone, the first object touched was scored as the response. Presumably, before being confronted with the cross-modal task, the animals had built up the tactual and visual associations during the course of training on the intramodal versions of DNMS. Then, on cross-modal choice tests, they could use the tactual-to-visual associations to identify the sample and avoid it in favour of the new object. With this procedure, normal cynomolgus and rhesus monkeys both performed at about 80 per cent correct (Goulet and Murray 1996; Malkova and Murray 1996). (It should be noted that the visual DNMS task, as administered in these studies, allowed the monkeys to obtain both tactual and visual information when displacing the objects. That is, no attempt was made to restrict the sensory input to the visual sensory domain during either the sample presentation or choice test portions of the trial. However, as explained earlier, a visual choice was enforced on the tactual-to-visual cross-modal choice tests and was, in fact, routinely made on visual DNMS choice tests.)

4.3 Neural basis for cross-modal associations

Investigation of the neural substrate conferring cross-modal abilities is based mainly on ablation studies, and, to date, the evidence remains inconclusive. Some earlier-identified candidate structures for the mediation of cross-modal associations, defined by sites of convergence of sensory information arising from different sensory modalities, included the cortex of the superior temporal sulcus (STS), the premotor cortex, the inferior parietal cortex, and the anterior cingulate cortex, among others (Jones and Powell 1970; Seltzer and Pandya 1978).

4.3.1 Cross-modal recognition

When cross-modal abilities were assessed using the cross-modal recognition method, no impairment was found in monkeys following lesions of anterior inferotemporal cortex (Sahgal *et al.* 1975), the cortex of the principal sulcus, or anterodorsal part of the head of the caudate nucleus (Petrides and Iversen 1976), the premotor cortex, or inferior parietal cortex (Aitken 1980), the cortex of the superior temporal sulcus, or the dorsolateral prefrontal cortex (Ettlinger and Garcha 1980). By contrast, lesions of foveal prestriate or posterior inferotemporal cortex (Sahgal *et al.* 1975), of arcuate cortex (Petrides and Iversen 1976), or of anterior cingulate cortex (Aitken 1980), or combined lesions of the frontal and parieto-occipital polysensory areas or the cortex within the superior temporal sulcus (Streicher and Ettlinger 1987) have been reported to yield significant impairments in cross-modal recognition in monkeys. However, none of these studies provided evidence that both forms of intramodal matching were intact: thus, they failed to demonstrate a selective cross-modal impairment, i.e. one independent of a deficit in sensory or perceptual abilities.

4.3.2 *Cross-modal associations with familiar objects*

Shindy *et al.* (1994) evaluated the effects of cooling of the dorsolateral prefrontal cortex in monkeys trained on a cross-modal matching task. Monkeys were impaired in the performance of cross-modal (tactual-to-visual and visual-to-tactual) as well as intramodal (tactual-to-tactual) versions of the matching task while their prefrontal cortex was cooled, relative to the non-cooled condition. Because cooling affected performance on the intramodal and cross-modal tasks equally, it seems likely that the impairment reflects the disruption of a general function of the frontal cortex (e.g. response selection or working memory) rather than disruption of cross-modal abilities specifically. Consequently, we will not consider this result further.

In 1985, Murray and Mishkin reported that monkeys with aspiration lesions of the amygdala plus subjacent cortex were severely impaired on a cross-modal (tactual-to-visual) version of delayed non-matching-to-sample. Whereas operated control monkeys scored about 90 per cent correct from the first block of trials, the amygdalectomized monkeys averaged only 55 per cent correct and showed no improvement across 500 trials. This finding was especially striking for two reasons:

(1) the impairment was severe; and

(2) the same monkeys demonstrated good performance on the intramodal versions of the task using the same objects, the same test apparatus, and the same intratrial delays (10 seconds).

On the basis of these results, Murray and Mishkin concluded that the amygdala was responsible for mediating cross-modal stimulus–stimulus associations. Subsequently, Murray and collaborators (Murray 1992; Murray *et al.* 1996; Malkova and Murray 1996) acknowledged that aspiration lesions of the amygdala encroach either directly or indirectly on the entorhinal and perirhinal cortex (rhinal cortex, for short) located ventral to the amygdala. It now appears that there are at least three possibilities regarding the neural substrate(s) responsible for the impairments observed after aspiration lesions of the amygdala:

(1) the amygdala, either as a whole or some of its nuclear constituents;

(2) the anterior portion of the rhinal cortex; and

(3) the amygdala together with the anterior portion of the rhinal cortex.

To test the first possibility, Malkova and Murray (1996) examined the effects of subtotal lesions of the amygdala on cross-modal DNMS. Because the basolateral subdivision of the amygdala receives dense projections from neurones residing in the modality specific neocortical regions subserving vision and touch (Herzog and Van Hoesen 1976; Aggleton *et al.* 1980; Turner *et al.* 1980; Friedman *et al.* 1986; Iwai and Yukie 1987), these authors hypothesized that, within the amygdala, the basolateral subdivision constitutes the most probable location of convergence of tactual and visual information about individual objects. The structure could act either as a site of the formation and/or storage of stimulus–stimulus associations, or as a relay linking representations stored in the modality specific neocortical regions, such as area TE and the posterior insula.

In Malkova and Murray's Experiment 1, macaques were trained to perform visual, tactual, and cross-modal versions of DNMS before they received bilateral injections of ibotenic acid centred in the basolateral subdivision of the amygdala. As a control, a separate group of monkeys received injections aimed at the centromedial amygdala. After surgery, both groups of monkeys showed perfect retention for the preoperatively acquired cross-modal associations. This lack of effect of the subtotal lesions is consistent with the findings of Streicher and Ettlinger (1987), who reported no effect on a cross-modal task with familiar objects after 'small' amygdala lesions made by aspiration.

Because subtotal lesions of the amygdala failed to yield a cross-modal deficit (Streicher and Ettlinger 1987; Malkova and Murray 1996) whereas aspiration lesions of the amygdala plus subjacent cortex (Murray and Mishkin 1985; Malkova and Murray 1996) produced a severe impairment, Goulet and Murray (1996) examined the second possibility outlined above and re-examined the first. They tested the effects of selective removal of the two main components of aspiration lesions of the amygdala, namely, the amygdala and the anterior portion of the rhinal cortex. Once again, monkeys were trained on the two intramodal as well as on the cross-modal versions of DNMS prior to surgery. One group of monkeys received bilateral aspiration lesions of the anterior rhinal cortex, whereas the other group received bilateral injections of the excitotoxin ibotenic acid into the amygdala, designed to spare the underlying rhinal cortex. This time, the plan was to produce cell loss throughout the entire amygdala. A third group of monkeys served as unoperated controls. After recovery from surgery or an equivalent period of rest, monkeys were retested on each version of the task, beginning with cross-modal DNMS.

Although the monkeys with ablations of the anterior rhinal cortex showed the largest drop in cross-modal scores relative to their pre-operative baseline, there was no significant difference between groups on this measure (arithmetical difference between the scores obtained over the last week pre-operatively and the first 3 weeks post-operatively). The scores of monkeys with ablations of the anterior rhinal cortex dropped 15 per cent, on average, whereas those of the amygdalectomized monkeys and controls dropped about 10 per cent and 4 per cent, respectively. However, when monkeys were retested on cross-modal DNMS after having received additional post-operative training with the two intramodal versions of the task, the pattern of results changed dramatically. Whereas both the unoperated monkeys and those with selective amygdala lesions reattained their pre-operative levels of cross-modal non-matching within 100 trials, one monkey with a lesion of the anterior rhinal cortex reattained criterion only after 240 trials, and the other two failed to reach criterion within the training limit of 500 trials. Thus, whereas both the control and amygdalectomized monkeys benefited from additional training with each sensory modality, monkeys with lesions of the anterior rhinal cortex did not. These preliminary results indicate that selective lesions of the amygdala are not sufficient to disrupt cross-modal associations either consistently or permanently. They also strongly suggest that within the medial temporal lobe, the anterior rhinal cortex plays a pivotal role in maintaining cross-modal associations in long-term memory. Histological findings from Goulet and Murray (1996), yet to come, will shed more light on the merits of these interpretations. Nevertheless, we can reasonably hypothesize that the cross-modal deficits observed by Murray and Mishkin (1985) and by Malkova and Murray (1996) after aspiration lesions of the amygdala plus subjacent cortex are largely due to the inadvertent damage to the rhinal cortex, either directly or indirectly, rather than to the amygdala removal *per se*.

It is noteworthy that the structure most commonly thought to be critical for associative memory is, at least in the context of cross-modal stimulus–stimulus associations, unequivocally not necessary. The operated control monkeys studied by Murray and Mishkin (1985), who had received bilateral aspiration lesions of the hippocampus plus subjacent cortex, performed (as already indicated) roughly 90 per cent correct responses on our tactual-to-visual version of DNMS, a score even higher than that later found to be typical of intact monkeys (Goulet and Murray 1996; Malkova and Murray 1996). This lack of effect of hippocampectomy on cross-modal associative memory is consistent with the finding that the hippocampus is likewise not necessary for either retention or new learning of intramodal (visual–visual) stimulus–stimulus associations in monkeys (Murray *et al.* 1993). It appears that the hippocampus, while necessary for certain types of associative memory (e.g. spatial memory and event memory), is not necessary for stimulus–stimulus associative memory.

4.4 Other studies examining cross-modal associative abilities

So far we have focused on the conditional designs employed in assessing cross-modal associative abilities. For example, the tactual-to-visual cross-modal DNMS task can be described formally by the conditional rule *if A is the sample, then choose B′ but not A′; whereas if B is the sample, choose A′ but not B′*. And for the visual stimulus–stimulus task alluded to in the previous paragraph, the conditional rule can be described as *if A is the sample, then choose X but not Y; whereas if B is the sample choose Y but not X*. Although this design has proven useful in assessing associative abilities (see D'Amato *et al.* 1985), there are other experimental paradigms, not yet discussed, that may also shed light on these abilities. For example, Gaffan and his colleagues have investigated visual discrimination learning for auditory secondary reinforcement. In one study (Gaffan and Harrison 1987), the monkeys were confronted with a visual discrimination problem that could only be solved on the basis of the auditory feedback that was provided. Two visual stimuli were simultaneously available for choice on each trial. Selection of the correct visual discriminanda (S+) produced the auditory secondary reinforcer, whereas selection of the incorrect visual stimulus (S−) produced the auditory non-reinforcer. Only when the S+ had been chosen four times in a row was the food reward delivered and the problem successfully completed. Although it is not necessarily so, it may be the case that accurate performance on this task, like that in the conditional designs discussed earlier, requires the association of the two sensory stimuli with each other. In addition, several investigators have examined configural learning. Configural tasks, while having in common with the conditional tasks the requirement to associate two different stimuli, have the additional requirement that these associations be held distinct from, or be represented separately from, any representation of the constituent elements. This is so because the test design calls for one response when confronted with certain combinations of stimuli (based on the 'configural' representation), but another response when confronted with other, overlapping combinations of stimuli or the stimuli presented individually. For example, in the configural task used by Gallagher and Holland (1992) a light (L) signals the availability of reinforcement when it is presented simultaneously with one auditory stimulus (T1), but the non-availability of reward when it is paired with another auditory stimulus (T2). The task involved four main trial types: reinforced trials with LT1 and T2 alone, but non-reinforced trials with LT2 and T1 alone. Thus the discrimination could not be solved on the basis of associations made between reinforcement and each individual stimulus. Rather, the task could be solved only by forming configural or compound representations of the stimuli (LT1, LT2) that are separable from the individual stimuli (L, T1, T2). Such configured representations are needed to solve a wide assortment of discrimination problems for which there is no linear solution. Again, the associative mechanism(s) underlying performance on configural and conditional tasks are not necessarily one and the same. However, this possibility is at least consistent with physiological studies of the anterior inferior temporal cortex of monkeys (discussed in section 4.6), which have revealed neuronal mechanisms that would allow for the maintenance of both individual and associated representations.

Interestingly, what little is known about the neural basis of these types of associative learning is at least consistent with the idea that the rhinal cortex is involved. Although Gaffan and Harrison (1987) had reported earlier that monkeys with aspiration lesions of the amygdala were severely impaired on visual discrimination learning for auditory secondary reinforcement, a more recent study by Malkova *et al.* (1997) found that monkeys with selective, excitotoxic lesions of the amygdala were unimpaired on this task. Thus, some structure(s) in the medial temporal lobe outside the amygdala is required for efficient learning of visual discrimination problems based on auditory sensory feedback. Based on the same logic outlined earlier, the list of potential critical substrates includes the rhinal cortex, among other regions.

Studies on configural learning, too, have faced a recent turn of events surrounding the neural basis for the learning. Although much early work suggested that configural learning was critically dependent on the integrity of the hippocampus (reviewed by Sutherland and Rudy 1989), there are now reports indicating that selective lesions of the hippocampus fail to disrupt the learning of configural associations (e.g. Gallagher and Holland 1992; Alvarado and Rudy 1995). Because some of the earlier studies used cocktails of kainic acid and colchicine to produce cell loss in the hippocampus, a procedure that causes damage to distant interconnected structures including the rhinal cortex (Alvarado and Rudy 1995), the possibility remains that the rhinal cortex mediates configural associations. Future experiments will need to address this possibility directly.

4.5 Relationship of cross-modal association to intramodal recognition and association

It has been assumed that a given brain structure might be critical for cross-modal associations selectively. If so, one would predict that removal of this structure would yield an impairment on cross-modal abilities without disrupting sensory discrimination abilities and without necessarily affecting either intramodal recognition or association abilities. Just this result was obtained by Murray and Mishkin (1985): their monkeys with aspiration lesions of the amygdala plus subjacent cortex were severely impaired on the cross-modal (tactual-to-visual) version of DNMS, yet were able to perform over 90 per cent correct on the both the intramodal recognition tests (visual DNMS, tactual DNMS) using the same test apparatus, the same set of objects, and the same intratrial delay between sample and choice test. If one accepts that the impairment in this group is due to rhinal cortex damage associated with the amygdala removal, as we have argued, this raises another consideration. Whereas monkeys with ablations of the rhinal cortex can perform visual delayed matching and non-matching tasks proficiently when short intratrial delays are used, it is also the case that an impairment in visual recognition memory is revealed when longer delays are interposed between sample and choice (Meunier *et al.* 1993; Eacott *et al.* 1994; Murray *et al.* 1996). Nevertheless, the data of Murray and Mishkin (1985) show clearly that at the time when stimulus recognition is demonstrably intact, stimulus-stimulus association is virtually absent.

The dissociation of intramodal recognition and cross-modal association abilities after aspiration lesions of the amygdala plus subjacent cortex (Murray and Mishkin 1985) is striking, and should be kept in mind. At the same time, however, it should be recognized that the separation of intramodal and cross-modal abilities is not always so clear. First, as just noted, although monkeys with aspiration lesions of the amygdala plus subjacent cortex were indeed able to perform well on tactual DNMS, they took significantly more trials to relearn than monkeys from the comparison group (Murray and Mishkin 1984). Secondly, a similar, though even stronger tactual deficit was observed by Malkova and Murray (1996) in monkeys with similar removals. In their study, only one of three monkeys reattained criterion within the training limit of 1000 trials: the two remaining subjects only reattained criterion after receiving double-sample presentation as a remedial procedure. Thirdly, Goulet and Murray (1996) found that monkeys with ablations of the anterior rhinal cortex required more trials to relearn tactual DNMS than monkeys in the amygdala and control groups, which did not differ from one another. Whereas all the amygdalectomized monkeys and controls relearned tactual DNMS relatively quickly, only one of three monkeys with a lesion of the anterior rhinal cortex made criterion within the training limit of 1000 trials. This is the same group of monkeys that was found to perform poorly when retested on the cross-modal version of DNMS.

Visual recognition abilities are not so clearly linked to cross-modal associative abilities. In the studies cited above, relearning of visual DNMS was only slightly retarded, at least compared to pre-operative scores. Although this relearning was carried out only after post-operative training on cross-modal and/or tactual DNMS, and it is therefore possible that any impairment on visual DNMS would be underestimated, it seems unlikely that the picture would be altered had the measure been made immediately after surgery. Other studies in which the effects on visual DNMS of anterior rhinal cortex lesions have been assessed directly after surgery have yielded no impairment in relearning (Murray *et al.* 1996). The relatively good performance on visual DNMS in the face of poor performance on cross-modal or tactual DNMS can perhaps be ascribed to the greater number of descriptive features available through the visual sensory modality (e.g. shape, size, pattern, hue, saturation, luminance, etc.) relative to touch, and to the innate tendency of primates to rely on the visual sensory system.

As we have seen, intramodal recognition abilities can be spared in the face of deficits in cross-modal associative abilities. However, it appears that the same cannot be said for intramodal *associations*. Two studies shed light on the relationship of cross-modal and intramodal associative abilities. First, Murray *et al.* (1993) found that monkeys with ablations of the rhinal cortex were severely impaired in learning new visual stimulus–stimulus associations. Whereas controls learned a set of 10 new visual stimulus–stimulus pairs in an average of 26 sessions, two monkeys with rhinal cortex ablation were unable to attain criterion within 100 sessions. Secondly, Murray and Gaffan (1994) found that monkeys with aspiration lesions of the amygdala plus subjacent cortex were equivalently impaired on retention of intramodal and cross-modal associations. In their experiment, monkeys were trained pre-operatively on auditory–visual stimulus–stimulus associations, and retention of these associations was assessed after surgery. Monkeys with removals of the amygdala plus subjacent cortex showed poor retention of the auditory–visual associations, and appeared to be just as impaired as the monkeys with similar removals, trained on visual–visual associations, studied by Murray *et al.* (1993). Further, the monkeys relearned the different types of stimulus–stimulus associations at the same, slow rate. This finding would appear to conflict with that of Murray and Mishkin (1985) who reported good performance (after relearning) on intramodal versions of DNMS in monkeys with similar lesions. However, Murray and Mishkin assessed intramodal *recognition* whereas Murray and Gaffan assessed intramodal *association*. If the critical neural substrate for cross-modal associations is the rhinal cortex, as we have suggested, then it would appear that stimulus recognition requires less intact rhinal cortex than stimulus–stimulus association. Further, the results are consistent with the idea that the rhinal cortex subserves intramodal as well as cross-modal long-term associative memory for objects.

4.6 Object identification

One way in which the findings regarding cross-modal and intramodal associations can be brought together involves the concept of object identification. Could it be that when intact monkeys perform both the cross-modal and intramodal associative tasks discussed earlier they are, in fact, engaging an object identification system? Certainly the relatively intact stimulus recognition (at short delays), but impaired stimulus–stimulus association, after rhinal cortex damage in monkeys, suggest at least two separable stages of stimulus processing. Indeed, the dissociation of recognition and association has long been respected in the clinical setting. For example, some visual agnosics have intact perception of objects, but an inability to associate those objects with their purpose or meaning (Farah 1990). In a similar vein, some prosopagnosics have intact perception of faces but a breakdown in the association of faces with biographical memories (Gross and Sergent 1992). Moreover, Warrington and her colleagues (Warrington and Taylor 1973, 1978; Warrington 1982) have reported a small number of subjects with damage to the posterior right hemisphere who are poor at identifying objects presented in unusual views, and in determining whether pictures of objects (e.g. faces or buildings), when presented in two different views, are the same or different. These deficits in object identification (or 'perceptual classification' according to Warrington and her colleagues) cannot be accounted for by deficits in sensory thresholds or figure–ground separation. Taken at face value, these results provide strong support for the notion that there exists a stage of stimulus processing, one supporting object identification, that is beyond that engaged in object recognition or perceptual matching. This higher-order stage has been variously described as one of 'association' (Kosslyn *et al.* 1994, 1995) or 'convergence' (Damasio 1990). Although this proposal might seem to be at odds with the apparent correlation of tactual but not visual recognition abilities with cross-modal performance in monkeys with rhinal cortex damage, it may well be the case that intact monkeys rely heavily on an object identification system when performing tactual DNMS. This might be expected if monkeys had extensive visual experience with the objects, but not if they had been denied such experience. One could evaluate this possibility by directly comparing the tactual recognition abilities of monkeys given either bimodal experience with objects during preliminary training or tactual experience only.

Is there any reason to believe that the rhinal cortex constitutes part of an object identification system? Accumulating evidence from neuroanatomical, ablation, and unit recording studies in monkeys suggests an answer in the affirmative. First, neuroanatomical tract-tracing studies have shown that the perirhinal cortex is the first cortical region within the ventromedial temporal lobe into which a wide assortment of sensory inputs converge (Van Hoesen and Pandya 1975; Turner *et al.* 1980; Friedman *et al.* 1986; Suzuki and Amaral 1994). Further, the predominant inputs to the perirhinal cortex are from the modality-specific, as opposed to polymodal, neocortical fields serving vision, audition, and touch (Suzuki and Amaral 1994). The perirhinal cortex would therefore be in a position to associate together the individual qualities of objects. Secondly, as already discussed, damage to the rhinal cortex disrupts the retention of both cross-modal associations (Goulet and Murray 1996) and intramodal associations (Murray *et al.* 1993), as well as the learning of new intramodal stimulus–stimulus associations (Murray *et al.* 1993). Thirdly, unit-recording studies in monkeys have found cells located in the anterior inferior temporal cortex, including the rhinal cortex, that reflect associative memories. For example, in monkeys that have learned several visual stimulus–stimulus associations, some neurones show responses of similar magnitude to separate presentations of two different items that have been repeatedly paired with one another, but not to other stimuli or to other stimulus pairs. In addition, during the delay period between sample and choice, the neuronal activity of some cells reflects not the stimulus just seen, but the upcoming stimulus that should be chosen on the choice test. These kinds of cells have been termed 'pair-coding' and 'pair-recall' neurones, respectively (Sakai and Miyashita 1991; Sakai *et al.* 1994). As has been suggested elsewhere (Stryker 1991; Sakai *et al.* 1994), such associative mechanisms may underlie the phenomenon of object invariance, the ability to identify an object regardless of viewing angle, size, location of the image on the retina, etc.

Another recent finding implicates the rhinal cortex in associative mechanisms even more directly. Higuchi and Miyashita (1996) studied the effect of rhinal cortex ablation on pair-coding in the following way. Monkeys with transection of the anterior commissure were trained on several pairs of visual stimulus–stimulus associations. After the monkeys had learned a set of stimulus–stimulus associations, the activity of cells in the inferior temporal cortex (the portion lateral to the rhinal cortex) was recorded, and, as expected based on the original study by Sakai and Miyashita (1991), pair-coding neurones were found. The monkeys then received a unilateral ablation of the rhinal cortex, and were retrained on the original stimulus–stimulus associations and on a new set of associations. Finally, single units were recorded in the same region as for the prelesion control. Although neurones responded selectively to the visual stimuli in both the pre-operatively and post-operatively learned sets, there was no evidence of pair-coding for either set. Thus, consistent with the evidence from ablation studies, it appears that the rhinal cortex is critical for the emergence and maintenance of the mechanisms that underlie the learning and retention of visual stimulus–stimulus associations. Higuchi and Miyashita suggested that the neurones projecting from the rhinal cortex 'back' to visual area TE were the critical element of the associative mechanism that had been disrupted. Although these associative coding mechanisms have not yet been invoked to explain the cross-modal associative abilities of monkeys that are the topic of this chapter, the same principles may well apply. For example, neurones in perirhinal cortex may both receive inputs from the granular and dysgranular insular cortex, a region which is devoted to the processing of somatic sensory inputs (Friedman *et al.* 1986; Schneider *et al.* 1993), and also project back to area TE, thereby providing the circuitry to mediate the tactual-to-visual cross-modal non-matching behaviour we have described. Likewise, auditory sensory inputs may project to neurones in perirhinal cortex, which could in turn project back to the insular cortex or area TE. Although it is clear that the projections to perirhinal cortex from somatic sensory, visual, and auditory cortical regions overlap to a large extent (Turner *et al.* 1980; Suzuki and Amaral 1994), and therefore convergence of this sort is possible, it is not yet known whether such specific 'cross-modal' backward projections exist, nor whether such connections actually mediate the formation and retrieval of cross-modal associations.

Other evidence implicating the rhinal cortex in object identification is found in a comparison of visual processing areas in monkeys and humans. The ventral occipito-temporal region of humans (especially the region of the fusiform gyrus) has been implicated in the processing of colour, motion, faces, and objects. Further, this same region seems to be activated when humans are required, as in the studies by Warrington and her colleagues, to identify objects from unusual views (Kosslyn *et al.* 1994). It has been suggested that many visual areas in humans, although located in the caudal portion of the human temporal lobe, are homologous to regions located in the rostral portion of the temporal lobe of non-human primates (Ungerleider and Haxby 1994). In this context, it would not be unreasonable to speculate that the function of the ventromedial occipito-temporal region activated in humans by shapes and unusual views is analogous to that of the rhinal cortex of macaques. At present the precise architectonic fields thought to be activated in object identification in humans (Kosslyn *et al.* 1994) are on the posterior fusiform gyrus (Brodmann's area 37), whereas in monkeys they would appear to reside in Brodmann's areas 35 and 36, so this speculation regarding homology is tentative at best. However, this issue could be addressed experimentally by examining whether the rhinal cortex is necessary for the phenomenon of object invariance in monkeys (see Holmes and Gross 1984; Weiskrantz and Saunders 1984).

4.7 Conclusion and comment

We have reviewed several experimental paradigms that have been used to evaluate cross-modal stimulus–stimulus associative abilities in macaque monkeys, and have explored the potential relationship of both cross-modal and intramodal associative memory with stimulus recognition. It appears that intramodal and cross-modal stimulus–stimulus associative abilities may share a common neural mechanism: the weight of evidence points toward a critical role for the rhinal cortex in the storage of both intramodal and cross-modal associative memories. Whether the rhinal cortex serves as a permanent site of storage of the associative information is, at present, uncertain, but it seems likely given the available evidence. Nevertheless, there are some caveats. First, cross-modal associations in monkeys have been examined with only a small number of tasks, and consequently it is difficult to state with confidence the extent to which the results concerning neural substrates may be generalized—to other tasks or other species. Secondly, lesion studies have emphasized the retention of cross-modal associative memories. As a consequence, there is little known about either new learning or, for that matter, very remote memories. Thirdly, intact object identification may, in many instances, be a prerequisite for any higher-order associative processing based on those objects, e.g. stimulus–affect associations, stimulus–place associations, stimulus associations with motor acts. Thus, to the extent that storage of stimulus information and object identification are disrupted as a consequence of injury to the brain, these types of associations and others may be disrupted as well. We have suggested that the mnemonic contribution of the rhinal cortex may best be characterized as one of object identification, a process through which the visual, tactual, gustatory, olfactory, and auditory properties of objects, as appropriate, are linked together, and through which environmental stimuli are invested with meaning. This idea is consistent with the accumulating evidence that the rhinal cortex serves as the kernel of a system for storing knowledge about objects, analogous to a semantic memory system in humans (Eacott *et al.* 1994; Murray 1996).

Acknowledgements

We thank G. Pixley for help in typing the manuscript and R. Hampton for constructive criticism on an earlier version of the manuscript. This chapter was prepared as a tribute to the memory of George Ettlinger.

References

Aggleton, J. P., Burton, M. J., and Passingham, R. E. (1980). Cortical and subcortical afferents to the amygdala of the rhesus monkey (*Macaca mulatta*). *Brain Research*, **190**, 347–68.

Aitken, P. G. (1980). Lesion effects on tactual to visual cross-modal matching in the monkey. *Neuropsychologia*, **18**, 575–8.

Alvarado, M. C. and Rudy, J. W. (1995). A comparison of kainic acid plus colchicine and ibotenic acid-induced hippocampal formation damage on four configural tasks in rats. *Behavioral Neuroscience*, **109**, 1052–62.

Bolster, R. B. (1978). Cross-modal matching in the monkey (*Macaca fascicularis*). *Neuropsychologia*, **16**, 407–16.

Cowey, A. and Weiskrantz, L. (1975). Demonstration of cross-modal matching in rhesus monkeys, *Macaca mulatta*. *Neuropsychologia*, **13**, 117–20.

Damasio, A. R. (1990). Category-related recognition defects as a clue to the neural substrates of knowledge. *Trends in Neuroscience*, **13**, 95–8.

D'Amato, M. R., Salmon, D. P., Loukas, E., and Tomie, A. (1985). Symmetry and transitivity of conditional relations in monkeys (*Cebus apella*) and pigeons (*Columba livia*). *Journal of the Experimental Analysis of Behavior*, **44**, 35–47.

Davenport, R. K. and Rogers, C. M. (1970). Intermodal equivalence of stimuli in apes. *Science*, **168**, 279–80.

Davenport, R. K., Rogers, C. M., and Steele Russell, I. (1973). Cross-modal perception in apes. *Neuropsychologia*, **11**, 21–8.

DiMattia, B. V., Posley, K. A., and Fuster, J. M. (1990). Cross-modal short-term memory of haptic and visual information. *Neuropsychologia*, **28**, 17–33.

Eacott, M. J., Gaffan, D., and Murray, E. A. (1994). Preserved recognition memory for small sets, and impaired stimulus identification for large sets, following rhinal cortex ablations in monkeys. *European Journal of Neuroscience*, **6**, 1466–78.

Elliot, R. C. (1977). Cross-modal recognition in three primates. *Neuropsychologia*, **15**, 183–6.

Ettlinger, G. (1960). Cross-modal transfer of training in monkeys. *Behaviour*, **16**, 56–65.

Ettlinger, G. (1967). Analysis of cross-modal effects and their relationship to language. In *Brain mechanisms underlying speech and language*, (ed. F. L. Darley and C. H. Millikan), pp. 53–60. Grune and Straton, New York.

Ettlinger, G. and Blakemore, C. B. (1967). Cross-modal matching in the monkey. *Neuropsychologia*, **5**, 147–54.

Ettlinger, G. and Garcha, H. S. (1980). Cross-modal recognition by the monkey: The effects of cortical ablations. *Neuropsychologia*, **18**, 685–92.

Farah, M. J. (1990). *Visual agnosia: Disorders of object recognition and what they tell us about normal vision*. MIT Press, Cambridge, MA.

Friedman, D. P., Murray, E. A., O'Neill, J. B., and Mishkin, M. (1986). Cortical connections of the somatosensory fields of the lateral sulcus of macaques: Evidence for a corticolimbic pathway for touch. *Journal of Comparative Neurology*, **252**, 323–47.

Gaffan, D. and Harrison, S. (1987). Amygdalectomy and disconnection in visual learning for auditory secondary reinforcement by monkeys. *Journal of Neuroscience*, **7**, 2285–92.

Gallagher, M. and Holland, P. C. (1992). Preserved configural learning and spatial learning impairment in rats with hippocampal damage. *Hippocampus*, **2**, 81–8.

Goulet, S. and Murray, E. A. (1996). Neural substrate of intramodal and cross-modal memory in rhesus monkeys. *International Journal of Psychology*, **31**, 307.

Gross, C. G. and Sergent, J. (1992). Face recognition. *Current Opinion in Neurobiology*, **2**, 156–61.

Herzog, A. G. and Van Hoesen, G. W. (1976). Temporal neocortical afferent connections to the amygdala in the rhesus monkey. *Brain Research*, **115**, 57–69.

Higuchi, S. and Miyashita, Y. (1996). Formation of mnemonic neuronal responses to visual paired associates in inferotemporal cortex is impaired by perirhinal and entorhinal lesions. *Proceedings of the National Academy of Sciences*, **93**, 739–43.
Holmes, E. J. and Gross, C. G. (1984). Stimulus equivalence after inferior temporal lesions in monkeys. *Behavioral Neuroscience*, **98**, 898–901.
Iwai, E. and Yukie, M. (1987). Amygdalofugal and amygdalopetal connections with modality-specific visual cortical areas in macaques (*Macaca fuscata*, *M. mulatta*, and *M. fascicularis*). *Journal of Comparative Neurology*, **261**, 362–8.
Jarvis, M. J. and Ettlinger, G. (1977). Cross-modal recognition in chimpanzees and monkeys. *Neuropsychologia*, **15**, 499–506.
Jones, E. G. and Powell, T. P. S. (1970). An anatomical study of converging sensory pathways within the cerebral cortex of the monkey. *Brain*, **93**, 793–820.
Kosslyn, S. M., Alpert, N. M., Thompson, W. L., Chabris, C. F., Rauch, S. L., and Anderson, A. K. (1994). Identifying objects seen from different viewpoints: A PET investigation. *Brain*, **117**, 1055–71.
Kosslyn, S. M., Alpert, N. M., and Thompson, W. L. (1995). Identifying objects at different levels of hierarchy: A positron emission tomography study. *Human Brain Mapping*, **3**, 107–32.
Malkova, L. and Murray, E. A. (1996). Effects of partial versus complete lesions of the amygdala on cross-modal associations in rhesus monkeys. *Psychobiology*, **24**, 255–64.
Malkova, L., Gaffan, D., and Murray, E. A. (1997). Excitotoxic lesions of the amygdala fail to produce impairment in visual learning for auditory secondary reinforcement but interfere with reinforcer devaluation effects in rhesus monkeys. *Journal of Neuroscience*, **17**, 6011–20.
Meunier, M., Bachevalier, J., Mishkin, M., and Murray, E. A. (1993). Effects of visual recognition on combined and separate ablations of the entorhinal and perirhinal cortex in rhesus monkeys. *Journal of Neuroscience*, **13**, 5418–32.
Mishkin, M. and Delacour, J. (1975). An analysis of short-term visual memory in the monkey. *Journal of Experimental Psychology: Animal Behavior Processes*, **1**, 326–34.
Murray, E. A. (1992). Medial temporal lobe structures contributing to recognition memory: The amygdaloid complex versus the rhinal cortex. In *The amygdala: Neurobiological aspects of emotion, memory, and mental dysfunction* (ed. J. A. Aggleton), pp. 453–701. Wiley Liss, New York.
Murray, E. A. (1996). What have the ablation studies told us about the neural substrate of stimulus memory? *Seminars in the Neurosciences*, **8**, 13–22.
Murray, E. A. and Gaffan, D. (1994). Removal of the amygdala plus subjacent cortex disrupts the retention of both intramodal and cross-modal associative memories in monkeys. *Behavioral Neuroscience*, **108**, 494–500.
Murray, E. A. and Mishkin, M. (1984). Severe tactual as well as visual memory deficits follow combined removal of the amygdala and hippocampus in monkeys. *Journal of Neuroscience*, **4**, 2565–80.
Murray, E. A. and Mishkin, M. (1985). Amygdalectomy impairs cross-modal associations in monkeys. *Science*, **228**, 604–6.
Murray, E. A., Gaffan, D., and Mishkin, M. (1993). Neural substrates of visual stimulus–stimulus association in rhesus monkeys. *Journal of Neuroscience*, **13**, 4549–61.
Murray, E. A., Gaffan, E. A., and Flint, R. W. Jr (1996). Anterior rhinal cortex and amygdala: dissociation of their contributions to memory and food preference in rhesus monkeys. *Behavioral Neuroscience*, **110**, 30–42.
Petrides, M. and Iversen, S. D. (1976). Cross-modal matching and the primate frontal cortex. *Science*, **192**, 1023–4.

Sahgal, A., Petrides, M., and Iversen, S. D. (1975). Cross-modal matching in the monkey after discrete temporal lobe lesions. *Nature*, **257**, 672–4.

Sakai, K. and Miyashita, Y. (1991). Neural organization for the long-term memory of paired associates. *Nature*, **354**, 152–5.

Sakai, K., Naya, Y., and Miyashita, Y. (1994). Neuronal tuning and associative mechanisms in form representation. *Learning and Memory*, **1**, 83–105.

Schneider, R. J., Friedman, D. P., and Mishkin, M. (1993). A modality-specific somatosensory area within the insula of the rhesus monkey. *Brain Research*, **621**, 116–20.

Seltzer, B. and Pandya, D. N. (1978). Afferent cortical connections and architectonics of the superior temporal sulcus and surrounding cortex in the rhesus monkey. *Brain Research*, **149**, 1–24.

Shindy, W. W., Posley, K. A., and Fuster, J. M. (1994). Reversible deficit in haptic delay tasks from cooling prefrontal cortex. *Cerebral Cortex*, **4**, 443–50.

Streicher, M. and Ettlinger, G. (1987). Cross-modal recognition of familiar and unfamiliar objects by the monkey: The effects of ablation of polysensory neocortex of the amygdaloid complex. *Behavioural Brain Research*, **23**, 95–107.

Stryker, M. P. (1991). Temporal associations. *Nature*, **354**, 108–9.

Sutherland, R. J. and Rudy, J. W. (1989). Configural association theory: the role of the hippocampal formation in learning, memory, and amnesia. *Psychobiology*, **17**, 129–44.

Suzuki, W. A. and Amaral, D. G. (1994). Perirhinal and parahippocampal cortices of the macaque monkey: Cortical afferents. *Journal of Comparative Neurology*, **350**, 497–533.

Turner, B. H., Mishkin, M., and Knapp, M. (1980). Organization of amygdalopetal projections from modality-specific cortical association areas in the monkey. *Journal of Comparative Neurology*, **191**, 515–43.

Ungerleider, L. G. and Haxby, J. V. (1994). 'What' and 'where' in the human brain. *Current Opinion in Neurobiology*, **4**, 157–65.

Van Hoesen, G. W. and Pandya, D. N. (1975). Some connections of the entorhinal (area 28) and perirhinal (area 35) cortices of the rhesus monkey. I. Temporal lobe afferents. *Brain Research*, **95**, 1–24.

Warrington, E. K. (1982). Neuropsychological studies of object recognition. *Philosophical Transactions of the Royal Society of London*, **298**, 15–33.

Warrington, E. K. and Taylor, A. M. (1973). The contribution of the right parietal lobe to object recognition. *Cortex*, **9**, 152–64.

Warrington, E. K. and Taylor, A. M. (1978). Two categorical stages of object recognition. *Perception*, **7**, 695–705.

Weiskrantz, L. and Cowey, A. (1975). Cross-modal matching in the rhesus monkey using a single pair of stimuli. *Neuropsychologia*, **13**, 257–61.

Weiskrantz, L. and Saunders, R. C. (1984). Impairments of visual object transforms in monkeys. *Brain*, **107**, 1033–72.

5

Visual processing in the primate parietal lobe

A. DAVID MILNER and H. CHRIS DIJKERMAN

> the parietal system of the monkey . . . is involved in 'spatial sensory-motor coordinations and attention' . . . but not in 'spatial vision' nor in 'spatial perception' (Ettlinger 1990, p. 329)

5.1 Historical introduction

George Ettlinger was one of the first scientists to examine in detail the behavioural consequences of posterior parietal lesions in the monkey, in work done mainly during the 1950s and 1960s. As shown in Fig. 5.1, the region studied included what we now know to be a large number of distinct cortical areas, but at that time it was considered to include only three: namely areas 5, 7, and (part of) 19 of Brodmann (1909) (or areas PE, PF, and PG, plus part of OA, of Bonin and Bailey 1947). In accordance with the general assumptions of the time, the posterior parietal cortex (PPC) was regarded as being principally an association area for the somaesthetic sense modality, in much the same way that the inferior temporal cortex (ITC) had been established as an association area for vision (Mishkin and Pribram 1954). For example, Wilson (1957) had shown that monkeys were impaired at tactual but not visual discrimination learning after PPC lesions, while the converse was true after ITC lesions.

However, Ettlinger and others then began publishing evidence that visual functions, as well as tactual ones, were affected by PPC lesions. In the first of these papers, Ettlinger and Wegener (1958) tested monkeys on a forerunner of the 'landmark' task (see section 5.3.2 below). The monkeys were required to learn a discrimination based on the presence or absence of pegs on the two sides of a pegboard located between two covered foodwells. They had to learn that on trials when pegs were missing from the right side, the right foodwell was baited, and vice versa, and they were tested either visually or through touch (i.e. in the dark). Monkeys showed a clear impairment on this task when retested on it after bilateral PPC lesions. Bates and Ettlinger (1960) went on to show that the presence of a small separation between the position of a solid shape and the site of the choice response (i.e. the foodwell) was sufficient to elicit a severe impairment in the relearning of a discrimination between two shapes. Again this was shown to hold good under both visual and tactual testing conditions. One influential interpretation of findings of this kind was that PPC lesions might disrupt a 'supramodal' spatial processing system, causing a deficit not only on tactual discrimination tasks (which might be

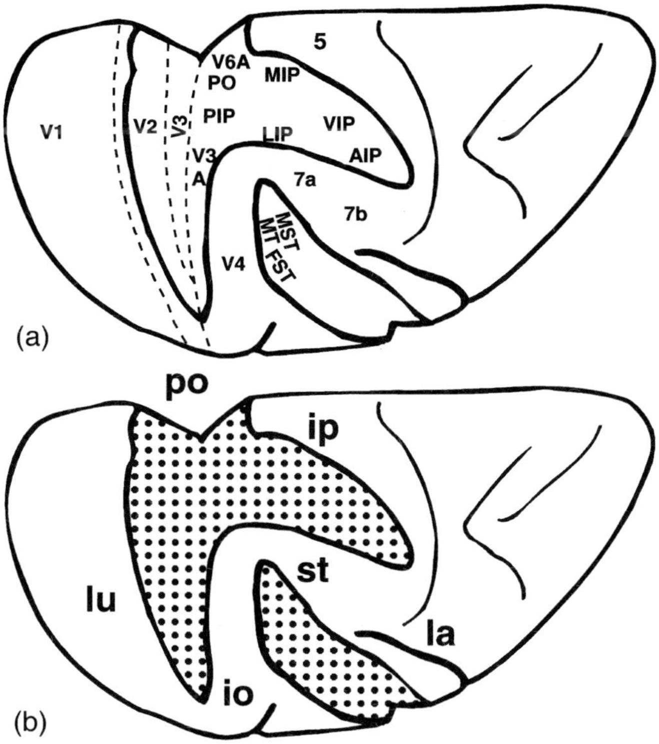

Fig. 5.1 (a) A dorsolateral view of the parietal lobe of the monkey. All of the areas marked, other than areas V1, V2, V3, and most of V4, would generally have been included in the classical 'posterior parietal region' of the cortex (PPC), though some authors would have used a more constricted definition. Likewise, all of these same areas would now be regarded as parts of the 'dorsal stream'. The lunate, parieto-occipital, superior temporal, and intraparietal sulci are shown in exploded form. (b) The same view, identifying the sulci: io, inferior occipital sulcus; ip, intraparietal sulcus; la, lateral sulcus; lu, lunate sulcus; po, parieto-occipital sulcus; st, superior temporal sulcus. Adapted from Sakata *et al.* (1997).

assumed to be inherently 'spatial' in nature, given the need for haptic exploration) but also on visual tasks (Semmes 1965).

George Ettlinger was unusual in taking seriously the behaviour of his lesioned monkeys *outside* the formal testing apparatus, and he regularly recorded their difficulties in reaching accurately to grasp food objects in their home cages, as well as the spatial errors they made when jumping between transport cage and home cage. The misreaching after bilateral parietal lesions was attributed by Bates and Ettlinger (1960) to a disturbance of 'visual orientation', the phraseology adopted by Holmes (1918) in his descriptions of soldiers who had suffered from parietal gunshot wounds in the First World War. In other words, Ettlinger followed Holmes in suggesting that parietal misreaching might be due to perceptual mislocalization, though he argued on internal correlational evidence that the impairments on tasks that involved stimulus–response separation could not be attributed to the same basic disorder. But later observations changed Ettlinger's mind about the cause of the misreaching in his monkeys. With Kalsbeck (Ettlinger and Kalsbeck 1962), he made unilateral PPC lesions, and observed misreaching only with the contralateral hand, irrespective of the visual hemifield in which the target was presented. As Ettlinger and Kalsbeck convincingly argued, this finding precluded an interpretation in terms of a Holmesian perceptual mislocalization.

Despite these early findings of visual impairments after PPC lesions, it was not until the 1970s that speculation began about possible input pathways that might supply visual information to this region in the monkey. In 1972, Mishkin pointed out that there was a divergence among the cortico-cortical projections from primary visual cortex (V1), such that those passing to the dorsal regions of prestriate cortex represented peripheral parts of the visual field, while those passing more ventrally represented central parts. He suggested that this separation would be consistent with a specialization of dorsal prestriate and/or posterior parietal regions for visuospatial processing, versus a specialization of ventral (occipito-temporal) regions for pattern processing. He argued that lesion studies supported this model, citing the results of his student Pohl (1973). Pohl used a 'landmark' task, in which a single cylindrical object was placed at a variable location between two foodwells, and its relative location provided the cue as to which of the two wells contained food on a given trial. Pohl contrasted his results on this task with those on standard visual discrimination tasks (with no stimulus–response separation), and argued that the two tasks dissociated in opposite directions between monkeys given either PPC (specifically area 7) or ITC lesions. Over the following 20 years, the landmark task came to be regarded as a diagnostic assay of visuospatial perceptual deficit in monkeys, and it is therefore discussed in some detail below (section 5.3.2). One of the few researchers to have questioned this diagnostic status of the task was George Ettlinger, in one of the last papers he wrote (Ettlinger 1990).

5.2 The dorsal stream

5.2.1 Anatomical considerations

The clearest and most persuasive statement of the notion of two cortical visual streams emanating from area V1 came with the publication in 1982 of Ungerleider and Mishkin's seminal paper entitled 'Two cortical visual systems'. The authors described anatomical studies that confirmed and extended previous demonstrations by Zeki (1969, 1971, 1980) that V1 sends discrete neuronal projections directly to a number of cortical targets. These targets include the area now generally called MT (Zeki's V5), located in the fundus and posterior bank of the caudal third of the superior temporal sulcus, and area V3A. We now know that V1 also projects directly to the posterior intraparietal area (PIP) and the parieto-occipital area (PO) (Colby *et al.* 1988) and to the lateral portion of the medial superior temporal area (area MST) (Boussaoud *et al.* 1990).

A great deal of further cortico-cortical anatomy has been carried out over the intervening years, but it may be summarized as showing that the areas which together subsume the old Brodmann areas 5 and 7 (including parts or all of areas MST, MIP, LIP, VIP, AIP, 7a, and MDP) all receive major cortical visual inputs via the V1 projections described in the previous paragraph. In fact, as can be seen in Fig. 5.1, the region of parieto-preoccipital cortex included in the early lesion studies of Ettlinger and others more or less corresponds to the entire 'dorsal stream' as we now know it. In addition, as we shall see in the next section, several dorsal-stream areas (unlike areas in the 'ventral stream') have discrete areas in the frontal cortex that are reciprocally linked with them, particularly within the agranular premotor region.

The integrity of the dorsal stream as a discrete processing system is further reinforced by its subcortical connections. Most areas of posterior parietal cortex (including areas FST and MST) are reciprocally linked with the medial pulvinar nucleus of the thalamus (e.g. Boussaoud *et al.* 1992), which in turn receives inputs from the intermediate and deep laminae of the superior colliculus (e.g. Benevento and Standage 1983). These laminae are closely implicated in oculomotor control (Sparks and Hartwich-Young 1989). The majority of dorsal-stream areas also send direct projections *back* to those same intermediate and deep layers (e.g. Lynch *et al.* 1985). In addition, many dorsal-stream areas send heavy projections to nuclei in the dorsolateral region of the pons (Galletti *et al.* 1982; Glickstein *et al.* 1980, 1985; May and Andersen 1986; Boussaoud *et al.* 1992). These pontine nuclei, through their close links with the cerebellum, seem likely to play a critical role in the subcortical organization of visuomotor skills (Glickstein *et al.* 1985).

In contrast, the inferior temporal cortex sends few if any projections to either the intermediate or deep layers of the superior colliculus, or to pontine nuclei (Glickstein *et al.* 1985; Baizer *et al.* 1993; Schmahmann and Pandya 1993). Instead, it has strong reciprocal connections with the amygdala (Baizer *et al.* 1993), a structure lying deep within the temporal lobe that is known to be intimately concerned in the process of learning to associate visual stimuli with reward (e.g. Gaffan *et al.* 1988). The posterior parietal cortex has very few such interconnections with the amygdala.

Thus the consensus 15 years on from Ungerleider and Mishkin's explicit proposal of the idea of two separate cortical visual streams is that they do indeed exist. The dorsal stream is a cluster of interconnecting areas quasi-separate from the ventral stream (Morel and Bullier 1990; Baizer *et al.* 1991; Baleydier and Morel 1992), although cross-connections ensure that it is by no means fully insulated from that other stream (Felleman and Van Essen 1991; Webster *et al.* 1994).

5.2.2 Neurophysiological evidence

Ungerleider and Mishkin's functional interpretation of the divergence of the dorsal and ventral visual streams leant heavily on two lines of evidence. One was the behavioural evidence using the landmark task, but the other was the newly reported series of findings from single-neurone recordings from within area 7. Beginning with the work of Hyvärinen and Poranen (1974), this new source of evidence of PPC function in vision had only become available with the advent of techniques for monitoring neuronal activity in active un-anaesthetized monkeys. Using standard procedures where the animal was maintained under anaesthesia, parietal neurones had been found to be largely 'silent' to visual stimulation, unlike those in occipital areas (V1, V2, V3) or areas within the ventral stream (e.g. inferior temporal cortex). As these initial studies during the 1970s soon revealed, the reasons for this neuronal silence were twofold. First, many of the neurones were not significantly activated by visual stimuli except when the monkey performed particular motor responses towards the stimuli (Hyvärinen and Poranen 1974; Mountcastle *et al.* 1975); and secondly, many PPC neurones were found to respond most strongly when the monkey was selectively attending to the stimulus (Bushnell *et al.* 1981). Such neuronal properties could not have been discovered in sleeping monkeys.

Six major classes of visually responsive neurones were identified in these early studies. Different subsets of cells respond selectively when the monkey:

(1) makes a *saccade* towards a stimulus in a particular location;
(2) when it *pursues* a stimulus moving in a particular direction;
(3) when it *fixates* a stationary visual stimulus in one part of space;
(4) when it *reaches* for a stimulus in a particular location; and
(5) when it *grasps* a stimulus object of a specific kind.

In addition, there are *'light-sensitive'* neurones which do not appear to have any association with particular motor acts.

Although there was scepticism in certain quarters for some years as to whether these various PPC neurones should properly be regarded as 'visuomotor' in nature (e.g. Bushnell *et al.* 1981), it is now generally accepted that they play a pivotal role in the transformation of information from visually based to motor-based coordinates (e.g. Andersen 1995; Kalaska 1996).

More recent research has shed a great deal of further light on these six groups of visually responsive neurones. 'Saccade' neurones, for example, are now known to be concentrated heavily in a discrete area within the lateral intraparietal sulcus (LIP), though other saccade cells, with slightly different properties, are located in area 7a (Andersen *et al.* 1992) and area PO (Galletti *et al.* 1991). Area LIP has strong reciprocal connections with the frontal eye field, long known to be involved in the control of eye movements, and also another site where visual saccade neurones can be recorded (Bruce and Goldberg 1985). 'Pursuit' neurones have been found not only in areas 7a (Lynch *et al.* 1977) and VIP (Colby *et al.* 1993), but also in large numbers in the lateral portion of area MST, a major source of input into 7a, and itself a major recipient of outputs from area MT. Almost all neurones in area MT are selectively responsive to the direction of stimulus movement—often in three dimensions. Although pursuit neurones have not yet been reported in the frontal lobe, other evidence indicates that a region neighbouring the frontal eye field is very likely to form part of the neuronal circuit for visual pursuit (Gottlieb *et al.* 1993).

In a similar vein, reaching-related neurones have been found in the frontal premotor cortex (in the inferior sector F4, Gentilucci *et al.* 1988; and also in the more dorsal sector F2, Johnson *et al.* 1996) as well as in PPC (area MIP, Johnson *et al.* 1996). Non-visual reaching neurones are found in area V6A (Galletti *et al.* 1997). These two parietal regions are both connected with F2 (Johnson *et al.* 1993; Matelli *et al.* 1995).

Clearly many of these eye- and hand-movement-related neurones must depend critically on a reliable coding of egocentric spatial location, if for example they are to ensure that a saccade is accurately directed. This coding process has been investigated extensively in recent years. One mechanism for spatial coding in posterior parietal areas has emerged from work by Duhamel *et al.* (1992). This group has shown that some LIP cells shift their receptive field transiently just before the animal makes a saccadic eye movement. As a result, stimuli that *will* fall on that receptive field after the eye movement is completed, actually influence the cell's activity *before* the eye movement occurs. In addition, many cells will respond when an eye movement brings the site of a *previously* flashed stimulus into the cell's receptive field. Taken together, these results suggest that a network of cells in the posterior parietal cortex anticipates the retinal consequences of saccadic eye movements and updates the cortical representation of visual space to provide a continuously accurate coding of the location of objects in the world.

In another important series of studies, Andersen and his colleagues discovered that many cells in areas 7a and LIP have 'gaze-dependent' responses. In other words, where the animal is looking (i.e. the position of the eye in the orbit) determines the amplitude of the neurone's response to a visual stimulus in its receptive field (e.g. Andersen *et al.* 1990). Similar observations were made by Galletti and Battaglini (1989) in area V3A. Such modulation or 'gating' by gaze direction could permit the computation of the head-related coordinates of the target stimulus independent of eye position. In other words, it could be used to transform the retinal coordinates of the stimulus into head-based coordinates. This might be done by networks of cells acting collectively (Andersen *et al.* 1990; Andersen 1995). Furthermore, a study by Brotchie *et al.* (1995) has shown that the monkey's *head* position influences the visual and saccade-related responses of some neurones in a manner similar to the way that the eye position in the orbit affects them. Both neck proprioceptive and vestibular signals have been suggested to play a role here (Brotchie *et al.* 1995). The modulation of neuronal responses by head position would therefore allow the representation of space in body-centred coordinate systems, again through the concerted action of assemblies of neurones (Andersen 1995).

The work of other research groups, however, suggests that while the visual control of saccadic eye movements may use such ensemble-based coding, other visuomotor systems may use head-based spatial information explicitly coded in individual neurones. In particular, a region provisionally known as V6A, which lies in the dorsal part of the anterior bank of the parieto-occipital sulcus, adjacent to the parieto-occipital area (area PO or V6), appears to contain neurones that code for location in craniocentric as well as in retinocentric coordinates with gaze modulation (Galletti *et al.* 1995). Since this area also contains neurones that are associated with reaching movements (Galletti *et al.* 1997), it may be assumed to play a role in the transformation of visual position into arm movements. If so, then it is possible that an explicit coding of head-centred location characterizes the visual control of reaching, while neuronal assemblies are used to provide the necessary visual control of saccadic eye movements. Area V6A may be the major source of the parietal projections to the superior parts of premotor cortex (area F2, Matelli *et al.* 1995), where recent research suggests that neurones take into account eye position in the control of hand movements (Boussaoud 1995). There is also good evidence that most visual cells related to arm movements found in the more ventral premotor sector (F4) are coded in head-based coordinates (Fogassi *et al.* 1996), and that area VIP, which is connected with F4 (Matelli *et al.* 1994), also contains visual cells whose receptive fields are coded in head-based coordinates (Duhamel *et al.* 1997).

Thus, evidence for the coding of visual location in multiple ways within the dorsal stream, for different motor purposes, is becoming increasingly clear (cf. Colby and Duhamel 1997). But all of these forms of spatial coding, of course, would only be of value over rather short time spans, since every time the animal moved its *body*, the usefulness of the coding would be lost. In other words, *any* form of egocentric spatial coding would be useful for guiding action in the present, but not for storing spatial information for use very far in the future. It would provide useful information about object location for calibrating the amplitude and direction of an immediate movement of the eye, head, or limb, but not for the long-term storage of information about the relative location of that object *vis-à-vis* other objects in the world.

These different coding strategies would provide saccade and reach neurones with all the visual information they need to direct the monkey's eye or arm towards the target of interest. Indeed, many neurones in LIP appear to encode the intended saccade itself (Gnadt and Andersen 1988; Andersen 1995; Mazzoni *et al.* 1996), and many in area 5 encode the intended direction of visually guided arm movements and the spatial configuration of the arm

(Kalaska 1996). Thus the parietal lobe not only plays a role in the analysis of sensory information but also in the preparation of movements. Recent compelling evidence of separate visuomotor channels within PPC has been provided by Snyder *et al.* (1997). They trained monkeys to respond (after a brief delay) to targets in different locations either by *reaching* (if the target came on green), or by *moving the eyes* (if the target came on red). They found that during the delay most PPC neurones were selectively activated according to the type of movement about to be made by the animal: some before an eye but not a hand movement, others before a hand but not an eye movement. This proves without room for serious doubt that most PPC neurones that code visual location are not doing so as 'general-purpose' visuospatial units, but rather are dedicated to transforming information about locations into particular responses to those locations.

Behavioural studies show that directing the arm or eye towards a target is a two-stage process in both response domains, with an initial movement towards the 'ballpark' region of egocentric space, followed by corrective adjustments to capture the precise location of the target (e.g. Goodale *et al.* 1986). This two-stage process is a highly adaptive one, as it provides an efficient means for the animal or human to capture a target which may move (within a certain range) after the initial programming of the movement. The visual information used to compute the corrective movements can be processed without the intervention of awareness (Goodale *et al.* 1986). It is reasonable to assume that the visual guidance of the entire act of reaching, or of directing a saccade, is mediated by the dorsal stream.

But as well as the many neurones in posterior parietal cortex that require egocentric spatial coding for their visuomotor properties, there are others that code little or no information about spatial location: these are the so-called 'manipulation' cells. They have been studied in detail only in the past few years (Taira *et al.* 1990; Sakata *et al.* 1997). Many manipulation neurones are not only visually selective for the size, orientation, and shape of an object, but also for the appropriate motor act performed in grasping or otherwise manipulating it; others respond equally well even when the monkey is merely passively fixating the object. Manipulation neurones are largely concentrated in an area located rostrally within the intraparietal sulcus (area AIP). Rather similar visuomotor 'grasp' cells have been found in premotor cortex (Rizzolatti *et al.* 1988), in the rostral sector of inferior area 6 (area F5), a part of the frontal lobe known to be reciprocally connected with AIP (Matelli *et al.* 1986, 1994). Sakata *et al.* (1992) have proposed that these premotor neurones provide a feedback message to enable a 'matching' process between sensory input and motor output to take place in posterior parietal cortex. An alternative idea is that they provide a 'vocabulary' of motor elements for constructing possible motor grasps, which operates by matching the 'affordances' of the object as analysed by AIP neurones (Gallese *et al.* 1997).

The existence of all of these separate classes of visuomotor neurones strongly supports the idea that the PPC contains quasi-independent modules that each play a distinct visuomotor role in prehension. Such a modular architecture fits well with proposals for separate visual control subsystems serving the proximal ('transport' or reaching) component of prehensive acts and the distal ('grasp') component (Arbib 1981; Jeannerod 1986). Indeed, as suggested by Arbib (1981), the modularity may go still further, and extend to subunits *within* the distal component, with quasi-separate visual channels for the control of the wrist and of the digits during grasping behaviour. Thus Sakata and his colleagues have found some visual neurones in the posterior part of the lateral bank of the intraparietal sulcus that are selective for stimulus orientation, often in three dimensions, but others that are selective only for size or three-dimensional shape (Shikata *et al.* 1996; Sakata *et al.* 1997). If these are genuinely separate subpopulations, they might form part of distinct visuomotor channels for controlling (1) wrist rotations (in preparation for grasping differently oriented objects) and (2) grip size and grip type (in preparation for grasping objects of different sizes and shapes).

The ground-breaking investigations by Sakata and his co-workers into the properties of manipulation neurones have forced a revision of Ungerleider and Mishkin's (1982) model of the two cortical visual systems. All of the other categories of visually driven neurones in the PPC could be regarded as coding static or dynamic spatial information about the visual scene, and therefore their properties were consistent with a dedicated role of the dorsal stream in spatial perception. But the coding of *intrinsic* stimulus features in PPC neurones (unknown at the time of Ungerleider and Mishkin's 1982 paper) now shows quite clearly that (1) not all object processing takes place in the ventral stream, and that (2) not all dorsal-stream processing is spatial.

A revised model has therefore been proposed which accepts the reality of the two streams, but characterizes the dorsal stream as dealing with the visual processing that is needed to guide action, and the ventral stream as subserving the visual processing needed to serve recognition and memory (Goodale and Milner 1992; Jeannerod and Rossetti 1993; Milner and Goodale 1993). This new perspective on the two cortical visual streams provides a framework within which to understand a wide array of behavioural consequences that follow not only lesions of the dorsal stream, but also lesions within the ventral stream (Milner and Goodale 1995).

5.3 Neurobehavioural studies

5.3.1 Visuomotor deficits

Impairments of visuomotor control following parietal lesions in monkeys have been known for over 100 years, as a result of the series of studies carried out by Ferrier (1890). For example, he described a monkey with bilateral ablation of the 'angular gyrus' (the prelunate gyrus plus area 7) as follows: 'Vision gradually improved, but continued to be very imperfect, especially for minute objects, which it rarely, if ever, seized quite precisely; groping at them with the whole hand, and reaching short, or over, or to the side' (Ferrier 1890, p. 57).

Ettlinger's research showed that this parietal misreaching in monkeys is a genuinely *visuomotor* deficit rather than a deficit in either motor execution or spatial perception. A simple *motor* disorder was ruled out by the fact the same animals were able, once they had grasped a food object, to bring it to the mouth efficiently and accurately (Ettlinger and Wegener 1958); and, as mentioned in section 5.1, a purely *perceptual* disorder was ruled out by the fact that after unilateral removals of PPC, the inaccurate reaching was invariably restricted to the contralesional arm (but see section 5.4 below). In other words, the animal was able to process visual information about the target location well enough to guide accurate reaching with the *ipsilesional* arm (Ettlinger and Kalsbeck 1962). That the role of the PPC in mediating accurate visual reaching depends on inputs from primary visual cortex is indicated by the observation that similar misreaching with the contralesional arm is found after removal of the ipsilateral occipital lobe and transection of the posterior corpus callosum (Jason 1983).

Although the 'PPC syndrome' in monkeys includes misreaching with the arm and misdirected jumping with the whole body, along with faulty visually controlled eye movements, there are also visuomotor impairments that go beyond the spatial domain. In particular, as Ferrier's early descriptions indicated, monkeys with posterior parietal lesions fail to shape and orient their hands and fingers appropriately when reaching to pick up a food object. It took almost a century after its discovery by Ferrier for this deficit in the visual control of precision grasp to be assessed quantitatively. This was achieved by Haaxma and Kuypers (1975), who made smaller lesions in inferior parietal cortex designed to disconnect occipital from frontal areas. They used a board in which food morsels had to be dislodged from small grooves set at different angles, thus requiring the hand to be oriented correctly in order for the finger and thumb to grasp the food. Haaxma and Kuypers reported that their monkeys encountered severe difficulties in this task when using their contralesional hand. Yet discrimination training procedures showed that the same animals were well able to distinguish the different orientations of the grooves; and indeed there was no visuomotor impairment when the monkey used the hand ipsilateral to a unilateral lesion. Buchbinder *et al.* (1980) reported a similar contralesional deficit (described as 'irreversible') on this same task, following two-stage dorsal-stream lesions which variably included the dorsal prestriate cortex, area PO, and posterior parts of area 7a. Yet they found no deficit in a control monkey given a large bilateral inferotemporal lesion, despite a severe impairment in visual discrimination.

Other reports (e.g. Faugier-Grimaud *et al.* 1978) confirmed the observation that this disorder in the shaping of the fingers in preparation for grasping was strictly linked to the contralesional hand after a unilateral posterior parietal lesion. Just as in misreaching, this clearly rules out a perceptual deficit, since evidently the orientation and shape of the object are well enough perceived when the ipsilesional hand is responding. Faugier-Grimaud *et al.* also showed that the distal difficulty was not purely motor, since objects were grasped normally in response to tactile stimulation. But although it is striking how similarly the visuomotor impairments in the grasp and transport components of prehension are restricted to the contralesional hand in these monkeys, it does not follow that damage to a single system is causing both deficits. In fact, recent elegant studies by Gallese *et al.* (1997) show clearly that the grasp component can be interfered with selectively. These investigators used microinjections of muscimol to create transient inactivation of area AIP, the part of PPC where most visually guided manipulation neurones have been found (Sakata *et al.* 1997: see section 5.2.2). Gallese *et al.* found a lack of preshaping of the contralateral hand and fingers to fit the shape, size, and orientation of the target object, yet no interference with reaching accuracy. Similar results have also now been reported by Wiesendanger *et al.* (1997).

In short, the visuomotor properties of neurones in the posterior parietal cortex fit well with the changes in reaching and grasping under visual control in monkeys following lesions to this part of the brain. In contrast, neurones within the ventral stream of cortical processing are not associated with particular behavioural acts directed at the optimal stimulus of the neurone; and lesions to these areas (V4, inferior temporal cortex, etc.) do not disrupt visuomotor control. We will consider in the next section whether the changes in visuomotor behaviour that follow PPC lesions can explain the results of formal tests designed to measure visuospatial perception.

5.3.2 *Visuospatial deficits*

The landmark task

The most commonly used test of visuospatial perception in monkeys has been the so-called 'landmark task'. This task requires the monkey to learn to choose between two foodwells on the basis of the location of a 'landmark' object placed at some point between the two. The task has two versions, but both have an identical first stage of training in which the landmark is placed directly adjacent to one of the two foodwells (randomly). The first task for the monkey is to learn to choose this adjacent foodwell. In one version the monkey is then required to learn the reversal (i.e. to choose consistently the foodwell that is *not* adjacent to the landmark) and then having learned this, to revert to the original task, and so on, through several such reversals. In the other version of the landmark task, the monkey is always rewarded for choosing the foodwell nearer to the landmark, but the landmark is shifted inwards from the rewarded foodwell, i.e. closer to the midpoint between the two. In this second version, most of the training is performed preoperatively, and postoperatively the monkeys may only be retested on the final stage of the task, i.e. where a so-called S–R separation has been introduced.

Pohl (1973) used both versions of the landmark task. Using the reversal version, he found that monkeys with bilateral ablations of PPC performed poorly compared with unoperated controls, particularly on later reversals. Animals with lesions of the inferior temporal cortex, however, were also significantly impaired, tending to do worst on the earlier reversals (Fig. 5.2, left). In a later study, Ungerleider and Brody (1977) also used this landmark reversal task, and they too found that both parietal and temporal lesions caused significant impairment on the task. In this case the pattern was reversed, with the later reversals tending to be more impaired after ITC lesions and the earlier ones more impaired after PPC lesions (Fig. 5.2, right). The evidence from the landmark reversal task thus demonstrates that the ventral and dorsal streams of visual processing both make contributions—of comparable importance—to the behavioural performance of the animals.

In his second experiment, Pohl (1973) used the S–R separation version of the task, and in this case posterior parietal damage was clearly more severe in its effects than inferior temporal damage. Nevertheless the ITC lesion did cause a modest decline in performance relative to the preoperative level. Subsequent investigators have generally replicated Pohl's finding of a parietal deficit on this S–R separation version of the task (e.g. Milner *et al.* 1977; Latto 1986). In addition, Mishkin and Ungerleider (1982) reported a deficit following a

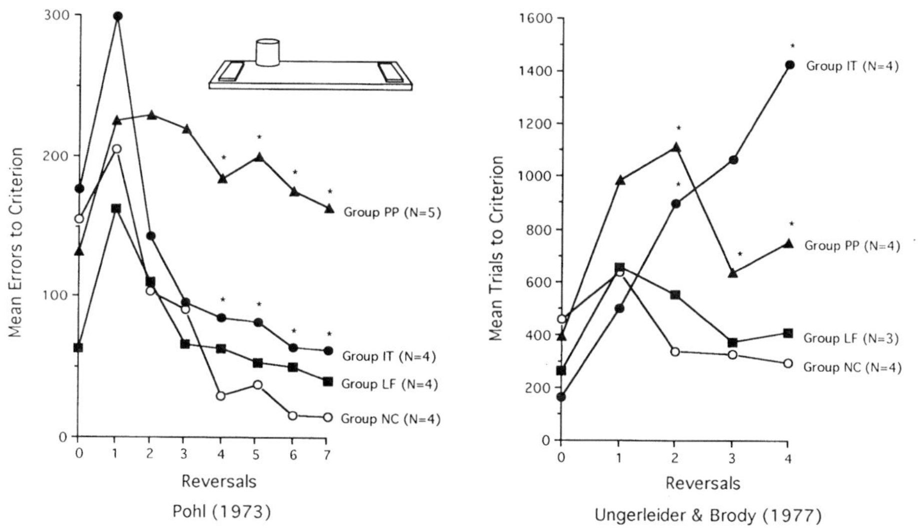

Fig. 5.2 The performance of monkeys with different bilateral cortical lesions on the landmark reversal task in the experiments of Pohl (1973) and Ungerleider and Brody (1977). The asterisks mark where the performance of the monkeys with lesions was significantly different from that of the normal monkeys ($p < .05$). Although the monkeys with parietal lesions were impaired in both experiments, so were the monkeys with inferotemporal lesions. Animals with dorsolateral frontal lesions were impaired in neither experiment. (Adapted from Pohl 1973 and Ungerleider and Brody 1977.)

combined unilateral lesion of posterior parietal cortex and the contralateral area V1. This result confirms that occipital inputs to the posterior parietal area, i.e. dorsal-stream projections, are important for the task (just as occipito-temporal projections are crucial for visual discrimination learning: Ettlinger 1959).

Only the three studies reported by Pohl (1973) and by Ungerleider and Brody (1977) have included monkeys with inferior temporal lesions, but it is clear from these that the common belief that such animals are unimpaired on the landmark task is incorrect. Two of the three experiments demonstrated a significant and substantial impairment, and the third showed a clear though mild impairment.

It has generally been assumed that the landmark impairment following PPC lesions is due to failures of visuospatial perception, while that after ITC lesions must be due to something else altogether. It is certainly true, as we saw in the previous section, that visual location is processed in the PPC for the purposes of guiding saccadic and manual movements towards target objects. And equally it is certain that the landmark task cannot be performed without some ability to process the relative spatial location of the landmark with respect to the foodwells. It is less obvious, however, whether the *relative* spatial information that is needed for this task would be available from the outputs of PPC neurones. There is currently no evidence from our knowledge of the coding of individual stimulus location in PPC cells whether any relational information *between* stimuli could be recovered. One major problem could be that computing the relative locations of two objects—A and B—logically requires that A and B are identified as being different individual objects by the system. The ventral stream, on the other hand, would have no difficulty with that, making it easy to envisage such relational coding being computed there. It is thus perhaps not absurd to speculate that ITC cortex may play the major role in the visuospatial computations needed in the landmark task.

But before any spatial perceptual system can guide a monkey's performance on the landmark task, the monkey first has to *look* at the landmark on a given trial before responding. Unfortunately, even normal monkeys are disinclined to do that, making it hardly surprising that most are slow to learn the task. It is a common and frustrating experience familiar to many behavioural researchers that monkeys tend to concentrate their attention on the likely source of reward—in this case the foodwells—and notice little else. Needless to say, when a monkey ignores the landmark, its choice of foodwells on that trial cannot fail to fall close to chance. One way that has been used to induce monkeys to pay attention to the landmark is to bait it with a desirable morsel such as a raisin. Normal monkeys do much better on the task when this is done (Sayner and Davis 1972; Milner *et al.* 1977). Presumably, the monkey guides its hand visually when taking the bait, and this act of directed gaze enables the monkey to code the position of the landmark in its immediate memory. Unhappily, the improvement caused by such baiting does not last long once the baiting is discontinued. On the other hand, many monkeys spontaneously develop a persistent habit of touching the landmark prior to choosing a foodwell, even in the absence of baiting (Milner *et al.* 1977). This remarkable habit is hard to explain unless it delivers more frequent rewards in the task: in other words, by leading to better performance it is reinforced and therefore learnt. These two different lines of evidence lead one to conclude that the simple act of responding manually to the landmark *ipso facto* improves the choice performance of normal monkeys.

In other words, while a basic level of spatial perception must be needed to permit a monkey to choose correctly in the landmark task, the *primary* need is for the monkey to orient towards the landmark using its head and eyes, facilitated perhaps by a forelimb movement towards it. Yet we know from numerous neurophysiological studies that PPC neurones are associated with visually guided eye and hand movements, and we know further that PPC lesions cause a slowing of saccadic reactions (Lynch and McLaren 1989), as well as slowing and spatial errors in reaching with the hand (Ettlinger 1977). Furthermore, in the landmark task itself, PPC lesions reduce the frequency of any habitual touching of the landmark prior to choice (Milner *et al.* 1977). These considerations suggest that the reason why PPC-lesioned monkeys fail on the landmark task may simply be that they fail *even more than normal monkeys* to look at the landmark before choosing a foodwell.

These ideas lead to two straightforward predictions. First, it would be predicted that using some means of attracting the PPC-lesioned monkey's gaze to the landmark should help it to perform the task. Precisely such an effect was reported by Milner *et al.* (1977): baiting the landmark improved choice accuracy in PPC-lesioned as well as normal monkeys. Similarly, Cowey (personal communication) has found that while a landmark consisting of a steady light on a TV screen revealed the usual parietal deficit, the use of a flashing light permitted the same monkey to perform without impairment. Secondly, it would be predicted that posterior parietal lesions should cause a deficit in *any* task where the informative cue is separated from the choice foodwells, even when the correct choice depends on the nature rather than the location of the separated cue. Several investigators have indeed reported such a deficit (Bates and Ettlinger 1960; Mendoza and Thomas 1975; Lawler and Cowey 1987). It is important to emphasize that in these cases the spatial location of the separated cue had no significance for the task, so that any difficulty in spatial discrimination (Pohl 1973; Ungerleider and Mishkin 1982) could not explain the results.

In conclusion, the most parsimonious explanation of the landmark task deficit following PPC lesions is that it results from a marked reduction in the likelihood that the monkey will orient towards the landmark prior to making its choice response. This would cause impaired performance on the task irrespective of the animal's ability to perceive the relative location of the landmark. In fact, since baiting raises the performance of PPC monkeys to the same level as controls tested under *un*baited conditions (Milner *et al.*

1977), the lesioned animals seem not to have lost the spatial perceptual ability needed for solving the task.

Other visuospatial tasks

Of course, the fact that PPC lesions reduce the ability of monkeys to use visual information to control their actions does not imply that they cause no other visual impairment. For example, unilateral PPC lesions undoubtedly interfere with selective visual attention in these animals, causing them to show 'extinction' (i.e. a tendency to respond only to the ipsilesional one of two simultaneous stimuli: Lynch and McLaren 1989). Not surprisingly, bilateral lesions have much more profound attentional consequences, and monkeys at first appear to be almost oblivious of their visual surroundings (e.g. Bates and Ettlinger 1960). Accordingly, a narrowing of visual selective attention has been suggested as a contributory cause of the landmark impairment after PPC lesions (Mendoza and Thomas 1975; Lawler and Cowey 1987). It might also explain the learning deficit found by Latto (1986) in a task that required the monkey to choose the middle one of three identical plaques, spaced about 7 cm apart. Such problems in redirecting selective attention would fit well with the fact that the responses of many PPC neurones vary in strength as a function of the locus of the monkey's attention (Bushnell *et al.* 1981; Robinson *et al.* 1995; Colby *et al.* 1996).

George Ettlinger and his colleagues observed that PPC-lesioned monkeys had particular difficulties with finding their way around in a familiar visual environment which could not be accounted for by such general attentive problems. For example, they might fail to find their home cage when released into a common housing area (Ettlinger and Wegener 1958; Bates and Ettlinger 1960; Sugishita *et al.* 1978). This raises the possibility that the monkeys have a problem in topographical orientation within the three-dimensional space of the housing area. Ettlinger and his co-workers, however, were satisfied that the failures could be adequately attributed to the confusion created in the monkey when inaccurate jumps towards its cage resulted in its finding itself in unfamiliar places in the room. These jumping errors were observed to be as great as 30 cm. In other words, an equally plausible explanation of the findings can be framed in terms of disordered visuomotor guidance.

Others have attacked this question experimentally. In one direct test of route finding, monkeys were run pre- and post-operatively on a locomotor maze (Traverse and Latto 1986). They reported that in two of their four monkeys with PPC lesions, relearning was poor; and it seems unlikely that inaccurate visuomotor control could explain this finding. Nevertheless, the two monkeys who were impaired on this retention task went on to learn a *new* route faster than controls, suggesting that whatever their problem was, it was not one of route finding *per se*. In a subsequent study, Barrow and Latto (1996) found impaired retention of one of two routes in two out of three monkeys after bilateral inferior parietal lesions. The two PPC monkeys that performed poorly on the maze were also those that showed the most severe misreaching. The authors point out that these monkeys could not have suffered from topographical disorientation, since their errors tended to consist of incorrect moves in the direction of the correct goal. They suggest instead that the monkeys' difficulty was in responding to 'local spatial cues', presumably causing them to fail to follow rules of the kind 'cue A means turn right'.

It is also possible to test monkeys on small-scale route-finding, by training them to negotiate a manual maze in which a baited object has to be extricated along one particular path in order for the monkey to retrieve the bait. And indeed such maze learning has been found to be impaired after posterior parietal lesions (Milner *et al.* 1977). But the authors also tested their monkeys' dexterity in guiding a similar 'stylus' along a route that lacked blind alleys, and found a comparable and correlated impairment. They concluded on grounds of parsimony that the difficulty in negotiating both mazes should be attributed to poor visuomotor co-ordination. Currently there is therefore no clear evidence for a route-learning impairment independent of difficulties in visuomotor guidance following PPC lesions.

In a more recent experiment, bilateral cooling of the posterior parietal cortex in two monkeys impaired performance on a cued spatial delayed response task (Quintana and Fuster 1993). In this task the colour of a central cue determined whether a key 30° to the left or one 30° to the right had to be touched following a delay of 5 or 12 seconds. It seems likely that a monkey's strategy in solving this task would be to bridge the delay by making a conditioned orienting movement of the eyes towards the correct key, using this to guide the subsequent manual response. But previous work has shown that lesions of PPC cause delayed oculomotor responses towards peripheral targets (Lynch and McLaren 1989), which could be expected to disrupt such a strategy. This account would also explain why PPC cooling had no effect in a variant of the task in which an orienting strategy could not be used (because the monkey could not predict whether a spatial or a colour choice would have to be made after the delay).

5.4 Optic ataxia and the human parietal lobe

Ever the comparative neuropsychologist, George Ettlinger was troubled (Drewe *et al.* 1970; Ettlinger 1977) by the results he and his colleagues obtained when they tested monkeys for their reaching ability after unilateral PPC lesions (Ettlinger and Kalsbeck 1962), as they seemed to conflict in their pattern with those following unilateral parietal lesions in humans. It will be recalled that the reaching disability was invariably restricted to the monkey's contralesional hand, and appeared to be present throughout the visual field. Yet ever since Brain (1941), several authors had described the typical pattern of misreaching errors in humans with unilateral parietal damage as being mainly in the contralesional visual field, irrespective of which hand was used (e.g. Ratcliff and Davies-Jones 1972). Misreaching in humans had been described originally both by Bálint (1909) and Holmes (1918), but their interpretations were rather different, as shown by their terminology. The term used by Bálint was 'optic ataxia', stressing his visuomotor account, while Holmes wrote of 'disturbances of visual orientation', which was intended to convey his belief in a basic disorder of spatial perception. The species difference began to look as if monkeys might show only optic ataxia, but humans something more akin to spatial disorientation.

Later, however, a number of variants on the 'usual' human pattern were reported. Accordingly, in a subsequent paper, Ettlinger (1984) retracted his worries, citing several reports (e.g. Perenin and Vighetto 1983) all of which described patients who misreached with the contralesional hand in both visual fields, though additionally with the ipsilesional hand in the contralesional field. It remains rare in humans, however, for misreaching to be entirely confined to one arm, and yet to be present throughout the visual field, as in Bálint's original (1909) description of optic ataxia, and as in experimental monkeys. Generally when only one arm is affected, the misreaching is found to be confined to a single half-field, either ipsilaterally or contralaterally (Rondot 1989). However Pause *et al.* (1989) have recently described two cases who showed optic ataxia with the contralateral hand throughout the visual field (i.e. the 'monkey' pattern).

In addition, recent studies have shown that the classic pattern reported by Ettlinger and others in the monkey is not universal. Stein (1978), for example, reported that *temporary deactivation* of area 7a in monkeys by cooling caused misreaching in contralesional space only. Thus the parallels between human and monkey reaching data are broadly clear, and suggest that the systems for carrying out visual-to-motor transformations of spatial information are inherited in basically unchanged form from our primate ancestors. The data from group studies (Ratcliff and Davies-Jones 1972; Perenin and Vighetto 1988; Rondot 1989) show that the lesions causing optic ataxia in humans almost invariably include posterior parts of the intraparietal sulcus and adjacent superior parietal lobule. This may not be so different from the termination territory of the dorsal stream in the monkey, which now appears to include parts of area 5 on the superior border of the intraparietal sulcus, as well as the more traditionally 'visual' area 7 (see also Passingham, Chapter 15 of this volume). It is important to note, however, that the inferior parietal lobule has expanded and apparently acquired new functions in the human brain (Milner 1997). This inferior region in humans was given designations (areas 39 and 40) by Brodmann that were totally absent from his mapping of the monkey cerebral cortex (Brodmann 1909); and furthermore, lesions there lead to deficits in visual cognition such as unilateral spatial neglect (Vallar and Perani 1986), which are difficult to demonstrate after PPC lesions in monkeys (Milner 1987).

Just like monkeys with PPC lesions, optic-ataxic patients also betray problems in the visual control of their distal musculature, appearing clumsy in their attempts to grasp objects that they see quite clearly. The reasons for this incoordination have been illuminated by careful analyses of the visually guided hand and finger movements of these patients. In the first of an important series of studies carried out in Lyon, Tzavaras and Masure (1976) made video recordings of two patients with optic ataxia as they attempted to extricate a small object lodged in a groove that was presented at different angles from trial to trial (after Haaxma and Kuypers 1975: see section 5.3.1). One of these patients failed to reach accurately towards the object, and also failed to orient his finger–thumb grip correctly; both kinds of errors were made only when he used his right (contralesional) hand to reach for targets located within the right hemifield. In later studies Perenin and colleagues (e.g. Perenin and Vighetto 1983) recorded a similar failure to rotate the hand appropriately in patients with optic ataxia, in this case as they attempted to project the hand into an open slot. Perenin and Vighetto (1988) subsequently reported quantitative data on both the spatial and orientation errors in this task in 10 patients with optic ataxia. They found that the subjects all made errors in hand rotation as they reached towards the oriented slot, and that the incidence of these errors, in relation to the hand and visual hemifield affected, closely followed the deficits seen in reaching accuracy.

Optic-ataxic patients, then, fail on two components of normal grasping: the arm fails to extend correctly in space, and the wrist fails to rotate accurately to match the orientation of the object to be grasped. The third major component of an efficient normal grasp is that the hand has to open in anticipation of the width of the object. In practice the hand begins to open almost as soon as it starts to move towards the object, reaching a maximum 'grip aperture' about two-thirds of the way there, which is closely correlated with the size of the object (Jeannerod 1986; Jakobson and Goodale 1991). Jeannerod (1986) filmed two optic-ataxic patients while they reached out to pick up a small wooden sphere, and found that, unlike normal subjects, there was no clear anticipatory adjustment of the grip size, and indeed it was usually the palmar surface of the hand that first contacted the object. The abnormality was particularly marked when the patients were unable to see their hand as it moved. Similar results have been described more recently in patients with bilateral parietal lesions who had recovered from Bálint's syndrome (Jakobson *et al.* 1991; Jeannerod *et al.* 1994). Each showed only weak evidence for grip scaling.

To complete the picture, humans with Bálint's syndrome following bilateral parietal lesions invariably show anomalies of visually guided eye movements (Guard *et al.* 1984; Pierrot-Deseilligny *et al.* 1986). Careful studies by Pierrot-Deseilligny *et al.* (1991) have demonstrated an association between reliable slowing of visually elicited saccades and unilateral parietal lesions that include the posterior parts of the intraparietal sulcus. This localization has been confirmed by imaging studies (Pierrot-Deseilligny and Müri 1997). Furthermore, as in monkeys, posterior parietal lesions result in deficient smooth pursuit movements (Pierrot-Deseilligny *et al.* 1986; Heide *et al.* 1996). However, Heide *et al.* (1996) reported that abnormalities in foveal smooth pursuit occurred after parietal lesions only when the damage included the area around the temporo-parieto-occipital junction (the intersection between Brodmann areas 39, 37, and 19). This area corresponds to the likely location of the human homologues of areas MT and MST (Watson *et al.* 1993), where lesions in monkeys also result in smooth pursuit deficits (Dürsteler and Wurtz 1988).

In summary, the visuomotor effects of posterior parietal lesions in monkeys and humans are remarkably similar. That is, what has become known as the 'Bálint–Holmes' syndrome occurs in monkeys as well as in humans; and it appears to result from a disruption of the dorsal stream. We may reasonably infer that the area that forms the common denominator of damage that causes the syndrome in humans constitutes an essential part of the dorsal stream in humans. In turn, we have argued that the deficits seen in the monkey after PPC lesions can be understood readily in terms of the electrophysiology and neuroanatomy of dorsal-stream areas in the monkey. Therefore considerations of comparative neuropsychology, the driving force of George Ettlinger's scientific life, lead us to the conclusion that similar neural mechanisms must underlie visuomotor function in the human occipito-parietal region as well.

Acknowledgements

The authors are grateful to Professor C. Galletti for his helpful comments on the first draft of this paper.

References

Andersen, R. A. (1995). Encoding of intention and spatial location in the posterior parietal cortex. *Cerebral Cortex*, **5**, 457–69.

Andersen, R. A., Bracewell, R. M., Barash, S., Gnadt, J. W., and Fogassi, L. (1990). Eye position effects on visual, memory, and saccade-related activity in areas LIP and 7A of macaque. *Journal of Neuroscience*, **10**, 1176–96.

Andersen, R. A., Brotchie, P. R., and Mazzoni, P. (1992). Evidence for the lateral intraparietal area as the parietal eye field. *Current Opinion in Neurobiology*, **2**, 840–6.

Arbib, M. A. (1981). Perceptual structures and distributed motor control. In *Handbook of physiology, Section I: The nervous system*, Vol. 2: *Motor control* (ed. V.B. Brooks), Part 2, pp. 1449–80. Williams and Wilkins, Baltimore, MD.

Baizer, J. S., Ungerleider, L. G., and Desimone, R. (1991). Organization of visual inputs to the inferior temporal and posterior parietal cortex in macaques. *Journal of Neuroscience*, **11**, 168–90.

Baizer, J. S., Desimone, R., and Ungerleider, L. G. (1993). Comparison of subcortical connections of inferior temporal and posterior parietal cortex in monkeys. *Visual Neuroscience*, **10**, 59–72.

Baleydier, C. and Morel, A. (1992). Segregated thalamocortical pathways to inferior parietal and inferotemporal cortex in macaque monkey. *Visual Neuroscience*, **8**, 391–405.

Bálint, R. (1909). Seelenlähmung des 'Schauens', optische Ataxie, räumliche Störung der Aufmerksamkeit. *Monatsschrift für Psychiatrie und Neurologie*, **25**, 51–81.

Barrow, C. J. and Latto, R. (1996). The role of inferior parietal cortex and fornix in route following and topographic orientation in cynomolgus monkeys. *Behavioural Brain Research*, **75**, 99–112.

Bates, J. A. V. and Ettlinger, G. (1960). Posterior parietal ablations in the monkey. *Archives of Neurology*, **3**, 177–92.

Benevento, L. A. and Standage, G. P. (1983). The organization of projections of the retinorecipient and nonretinorecipient nuclei of the pretectal complex and layers of the superior colliculus to the lateral pulvinar and medial pulvinar in the macaque monkey. *Journal of Comparative Neurology*, **217**, 307–36.

Bonin, G. V. and Bailey, P. (1947). *The neocortex of Macaca mulatta*. University of Illinois Press, Urbana, IL.

Boussaoud, D. (1995). Primate premotor cortex: modulation of preparatory neuronal activity by gaze angle. *Journal of Neurophysiology*, **73**, 886–90.

Boussaoud, D., Ungerleider, L. G., and Desimone, R. (1990). Pathways for motion analysis: cortical connections of the medial superior temporal and fundus of the superior temporal visual areas in the macaque. *Journal of Comparative Neurology*, **296**, 462–95.

Boussaoud, D., Desimone, R., and Ungerleider, L. G. (1992). Subcortical connections of visual areas MST and FST in macaques. *Visual Neuroscience*, **9**, 291–302.

Brain, W. R. (1941). Visual disorientation with special reference to lesions of the right cerebral hemisphere. *Brain*, **64**, 244–72.

Brodmann, K. (1909). *Vergleichende Lokalisationslehre der Grosshirnrinde in ihren Prinzipien dargetellt auf Grund des Zellenbaues*. Barth, Leipzig.

Brotchie, P. R., Andersen, R. A., Snyder, L. H., and Goodman, S. J. (1995). Head position signals used by parietal neurons to encode locations of visual stimuli. *Nature*, **375**, 232–5.

Bruce, C. J. and Goldberg, M. E. (1985). Primate frontal eye fields: I. Single neurons discharging before saccades. *Journal of Neurophysiology*, **53**, 603–35.

Buchbinder, S. B., Dixon, Y. W., Wang, H., May, J. G., and Glickstein, M. (1980). The effects of cortical lesions on visual guidance of the hand. *Society for Neuroscience Abstracts*, **6**, 675.

Bushnell, M. C., Goldberg, M. E., and Robinson, D. L. (1981). Behavioral enhancement of visual responses in monkey cerebral cortex. I. Modulation in posterior parietal cortex related to selective visual attention. *Journal of Neurophysiology*, **46**, 755–72.

Colby, C. L. and Duhamel, J. R. (1997). Spatial representations for action in parietal cortex. *Cognitive Brain Research*, **5**, 105–15.

Colby, C. L., Gattas, R., Olson, C. R., and Gross, C. G. (1988). Topographic organization of cortical afferents to extrastriate visual area PO in the macaque: a dual tracer study. *Journal of Comparative Neurology*, **269**, 392–413.

Colby, C. L., Duhamel, J. R., and Goldberg, M. E. (1993). Ventral intraparietal area of the Macaque: anatomic location and visual response properties. *Journal of Neurophysiology*, **69**, 902–14.

Colby, C. L., Duhamel, J.-R., and Goldberg, M. E. (1996). Visual, presaccadic, and cognitive activation of single neurons in monkey lateral intraparietal area. *Journal of Neurophysiology*, **76**, 2841–51.

Drewe, E. A., Ettlinger, G., Milner, A. D., and Passingham, R. E. (1970). A comparative review of the results of neuropsychological research on man and monkey. *Cortex*, **6**, 129–63.

Duhamel, J.-R., Colby, C. L., and Goldberg, M. E. (1992). The updating of the representation of visual space in parietal cortex by intended eye movements. *Science*, **255**, 90–2.

Duhamel, J.-R., Bremmer, F., Ben Hamed, S., and Graf, W. (1997). Spatial invariance of visual receptive fields in parietal cortex neurons. *Nature*, **389**, 845–8.

Dürsteler, M. R. and Wurtz, R. H. (1988). Pursuit and optokinetic deficits following chemical lesions of cortical areas MT and MST. *Journal of Neurophysiology*, **60**, 940–65.

Ettlinger, G. (1959). Visual discrimination following successive temporal ablations in monkeys. *Brain*, **82**, 232–50.

Ettlinger, G. (1977). Parietal cortex in visual orientation. In *Physiological aspects of clinical neurology*, (ed. F. C. Rose), pp. 93–100. Blackwell, Oxford.

Ettlinger, G. (1984). Humans, apes and monkeys: the changing neuropsychological viewpoint. *Neuropsychologia*, **22**, 685–96.

Ettlinger, G. (1990). 'Object vision' and 'spatial vision': the neuropsychological evidence for the distinction. *Cortex*, **26**, 319–41.

Ettlinger, G. and Kalsbeck, J. E. (1962). Changes in tactile discrimination and in visual reaching after successive and simultaneous bilateral posterior parietal ablations in the monkey. *Journal of Neurology, Neurosurgery and Psychiatry*, **25**, 256–68.

Ettlinger, G. and Wegener, J. (1958). Somaesthetic alternation, discrimination and orientation after frontal and parietal lesions in monkeys. *Quarterly Journal of Experimental Psychology*, **10**, 177–86.

Faugier-Grimaud, S., Frenois, C., and Stein, D. G. (1978). Effects of posterior parietal lesions on visually guided behavior in monkeys. *Neuropsychologia*, **16**, 151–68.

Felleman, D. J. and Van Essen, D. C. (1991). Distributed hierarchical processing in the primate cerebral cortex. *Cerebral Cortex*, **1**, 1–47.

Ferrier, D. (1890). *Cerebral localisation (The Croonian Lectures)*. Smith, Elder, London.

Fogassi, L., Gallese, V., Fadiga, L., Luppino, G., Matelli, M., and Rizzolatti, G. (1996). Coding of peripersonal space in inferior premotor cortex (area F4). *Journal of Neurophysiology*, **76**, 141–57.

Gaffan, E. A., Gaffan, D., and Harrison, S. (1988). Disconnection of the amygdala from visual association cortex impairs visual reward-association learning in monkeys. *Journal of Neuroscience*, **8**, 3144–59.

Gallese, V., Fadiga, L., Fogassi, L., Luppino, G., and Murata, A. (1997). A parietal-frontal circuit for hand grasping movements in the monkey: evidence from reversible inactivation experiments. In *Parietal lobe contributions to orientation in 3D space*, (ed. P. Thier and H.-O. Karnath), pp. 255–70. Springer-Verlag, Heidelberg.

Galletti, C. and Battaglini, P. P. (1989). Gaze-dependent visual neurons in area V3A of monkey prestriate cortex. *Journal of Neuroscience*, **9**, 1112–25.

Galletti, C., Maioli, M. G., Squatrito, S., and Battaglini, P. P. (1982). Corticopontine projections from the visual area of the superior temporal sulcus in the macaque monkey. *Archives Italiennes de Biologie*, **120**, 411–17.

Galletti, C., Battaglini, P. P., and Fattori, P. (1991). Functional properties of neurons in the anterior bank of the parieto-occipital sulcus of the macaque monkey. *European Journal of Neuroscience*, **3**, 452–61.

Galletti, C., Battaglini, P. P., and Fattori, P. (1995). Eye position influence on parieto-occipital area PO (V6) of the macaque monkey. *European Journal of Neuroscience*, **7**, 2486–501.

Galletti, C., Fattori, P., Kutz, D. F., and Battaglini, P. P. (1997). Arm movement-related neurons in the visual area V6A of macaque superior parietal lobule. *European Journal of Neuroscience*, **9**, 410–414.

Gentilucci, M., Fogassi, L., Luppino, G., Matelli, M., Camarda, R., and Rizzolatti, G. (1988). Functional organization of inferior area 6 in the macaque monkey. I. Somatotopy and the control of proximal movements. *Experimental Brain Research*, **71**, 475–90.

Glickstein, M., Cohen, J. L., Dixon, B., Gibson, A., Hollins, M., Labossiere, E., and Robinson, F. (1980). Corticopontine visual projections in macaque monkeys. *Journal of Comparative Neurology*, **190**, 209–29.

Glickstein, M., May, J. G., and Mercier, B. E. (1985). Corticopontine projection in the macaque: the distribution of labelled cortical cells after large injections of horseradish peroxidase in the pontine nuclei. *Journal of Comparative Neurology*, **235**, 343–59.

Gnadt, J. W. and Andersen, R. A. (1988). Memory related motor planning activity in posterior parietal cortex of macaque. *Experimental Brain Research*, **70**, 216–20.

Goodale, M. A. and Milner, A. D. (1992). Separate visual pathways for perception and action. *Trends in Neurosciences*, **15**, 20–5.

Goodale, M. A., Pélisson, D., and Prablanc, C. (1986). Large adjustments in visually guided reaching do not depend on vision of the hand or perception of target displacement. *Nature*, **320**, 748–50.

Gottlieb, J. P., Bruce, C. J., and MacAvoy, M. G. (1993). Smooth eye movements elicited by microstimulation in the primate frontal eye field. *Journal of Neurophysiology*, **69**, 786–99.

Guard, O., Perenin, M. T., Vighetto, A., Giroud, M., Tommasi, M., and Dumas, R. (1984). Syndrome pariétal bilatéral proche d'un syndrome de Balint. *Revue Neurologique (Paris)*, **140**, 358–67.

Haaxma, R. and Kuypers, H. G. J. M. (1975). Intrahemispheric cortical connexions and visual guidance of hand and finger movements in the rhesus monkey. *Brain*, **98**, 239–60.

Heide, W., Kurzidim, K., and Kompf, D. (1996). Deficits of smooth pursuit eye movements after frontal and parietal lesions. *Brain*, **119**, 1951–69.

Holmes, G. (1918). Disturbances of visual orientation. *British Journal of Ophthalmology*, **2**, 449–68.

Hyvärinen, J. and Poranen, A. (1974). Function of the parietal associative area 7 as revealed from cellular discharges in alert monkeys. *Brain*, **97**, 673–92.

Jakobson, L. S. and Goodale, M. A. (1991). Factors affecting higher-order movement planning: a kinematic analysis of human prehension. *Experimental Brain Research*, **86**, 199–208.

Jakobson, L. S., Archibald, Y. M., Carey, D. P., and Goodale, M. A. (1991). A kinematic analysis of reaching and grasping movements in a patient recovering from optic ataxia. *Neuropsychologia*, **29**, 803–9.

Jason, G. W. (1983). Misreaching in monkeys after combined unilateral occipital lobectomy and splenial transection. *Experimental Neurology*, **81**, 114–25.

Jeannerod, M. (1986). The formation of finger grip during prehension: a cortically mediated visuomotor pattern. *Behavioural Brain Research*, **19**, 99–116.

Jeannerod, M. and Rossetti, Y. (1993). Visuomotor coordination as a dissociable visual function: experimental and clinical evidence. In *Visual perceptual defects, Baillière's Clinical Neurology*, Vol.2, No.2, (ed. C. Kennard), pp. 439–60. Baillière Tindall, London.

Jeannerod, M., Decety, J., and Michel, F. (1994). Impairment of grasping movements following bilateral posterior parietal lesion. *Neuropsychologia*, **32** 369–80.

Johnson, P. B., Ferraina, S., and Caminiti, R. (1993). Cortical networks for visual reaching. *Experimental Brain Research*, **97**, 361–5.

Johnson, P. B., Ferraina, S., Bianchi, L., and Caminiti, R. (1996). Cortical networks for visual reaching: physiological and anatomical organization of frontal and parietal lobe arm regions. *Cerebral Cortex*, **6**, 102–19.

Kalaska, J. F. (1996). Parietal cortex area 5 and visuomotor behavior. *Canadian Journal of Physiology and Pharmacology*, **74**, 483–98.

Latto, R. (1986). The role of inferior parietal cortex and the frontal eye-fields in visuo-spatial discriminations in the macaque monkey. *Behavioural Brain Research*, **22**, 41–52.

Lawler, K. A. and Cowey, A. (1987). On the role of posterior parietal and prefrontal cortex in visuo-spatial perception and attention. *Experimental Brain Research*, **65**, 695–8.

Lynch, J. C. and McLaren, J. W. (1989). Deficits of visual attention and saccadic eye movements after lesions of parietooccipital cortex in monkeys. *Journal of Neurophysiology*, **61**, 74–90.

Lynch, J. C., Mountcastle, V. B., Talbot, W. H., and Yin, T. C. T. (1977). Parietal lobe mechanisms for directed visual attention. *Journal of Neurophysiology*, **40**, 362–89.

Lynch, J. C., Graybiel, A. M., and Lobeck, L. J. (1985). The differential projection of two cytoarchitectural subregions of the inferior parietal lobule of the macaque upon the deep layers of the superior colliculus. *Journal of Comparative Neurology*, **235**, 241–54.

Matelli, M., Camarda, R., Glickstein, M., and Rizzolatti, G. (1986). Afferent and efferent projections of the inferior area-6 in the macaque monkey. *Journal of Comparative Neurology*, **251**, 281–98.

Matelli, M., Luppino, G., Murata, A., and Sakata, H. (1994). Independent anatomical circuits for reaching and grasping linking the inferior parietal sulcus and inferior area 6 in macaque monkey. *Society for Neuroscience Abstracts*, **20**, 404.4.

Matelli, M., Luppino, G., D'Amelio, M., Fattori, P., and Galletti, C. (1995). Frontal projections of a visual area (V6A) of the superior parietal lobule in macaque monkey. *Society for Neuroscience Abstracts*, **21**, 169.8.

May, J. G. and Andersen, R. A. (1986). Different patterns of corticopontine projections from separate cortical fields within the inferior parietal lobule and dorsal prelunate gyrus of the macaque. *Experimental Brain Research*, **63**, 265–78.

Mazzoni, P., Bracewell, R. M., Barash, S., and Andersen, R. A. (1996). Motor intention activity in the Macaque's lateral intraparietal area. I. Dissociation of motor plan from sensory memory. *Journal of Neurophysiology*, **76**, 1439–56.

Mendoza, J. E. and Thomas, R. K. (1975). Effects of posterior parietal and frontal neocortical lesions in the squirrel monkey. *Journal of Comparative and Physiological Psychology*, **89**, 170–82.

Milner, A. D. (1987). Animal models for the syndrome of spatial neglect. In *Neurophysiological and neuropsychological aspects of spatial neglect*, (ed. M. Jeannerod), pp. 259–88. Elsevier, Amsterdam.

Milner, A. D. (1997). Neglect, extinction, and the cortical streams of visual processing. In *Parietal lobe contributions to orientation in 3D space*, (ed. P. Thier and H.-O. Karnath), pp. 3–22. Springer-Verlag, Heidelberg.

Milner, A. D. and Goodale, M. A. (1993). Visual pathways to perception and action. In *Progress in brain research*, Vol. 95, (ed. T. P. Hicks, S. Molotchnikoff, and T. Ono), pp. 317–37. Elsevier, Amsterdam.

Milner, A. D. and Goodale, M. A. (1995). *The visual brain in action*. Oxford University Press, Oxford.

Milner, A. D., Ockleford, E. M. and Dewar, W. (1977). Visuo-spatial performance following posterior parietal and lateral frontal lesions in stumptail macaques. *Cortex*, **13**, 350–60.

Mishkin, M. (1972). Cortical visual areas and their interaction. In *The brain and human behavior*, (ed. A. G. Karczmar and J. C. Eccles), pp. 187–208. Springer-Verlag, Berlin.

Mishkin, M. and Pribram, K. H. (1954). Visual discrimination performance following partial ablations of the temporal lobe: I. Ventral vs. lateral. *Journal of Comparative and Physiological Psychology*, **47**, 14–20.

Mishkin, M. and Ungerleider, L. G. (1982). Contribution of striate inputs to the visuospatial functions of parieto-preoccipital cortex in monkeys. *Behavioural Brain Research*, **6**, 57–77.

Morel, A. and Bullier, J. (1990). Anatomical segregation of two cortical visual pathways in the macaque monkey. *Visual Neuroscience*, **4**, 555–78.

Mountcastle, V. B., Lynch, J. C., Georgopoulos, A. P., Sakata, H., and Acuña, C. (1975). Posterior parietal association cortex of the monkey: command function of operations within extrapersonal space. *Journal of Neurophysiology*, **38**, 871–908.

Pause, M., Kunesch, E., Binkofski, F., and Freund, H.-J. (1989). Sensorimotor disturbances in patients with lesions of the parietal cortex. *Brain*, **112**, 1599–625.

Perenin, M.-T. and Vighetto, A. (1983). Optic ataxia: a specific disorder in visuomotor coordination. In *Spatially oriented behavior*, (ed. A. Hein and M. Jeannerod), pp. 305–26. Springer-Verlag, New York.

Perenin, M.-T. and Vighetto, A. (1988). Optic ataxia: a specific disruption in visuomotor mechanisms. I. Different aspects of the deficit in reaching for objects. *Brain*, **111**, 643–74.

Pierrot-Deseilligny, C. and Müri, R. (1997). Posterior parietal cortex control of saccades in humans. In *Parietal lobe contributions to orientation in 3D space*, (ed. P. Thier and H.-O. Karnath), pp. 135–48. Springer-Verlag, Heidelberg.

Pierrot-Deseilligny, C., Gray, F., and Brunet, P. (1986). Infarcts of both inferior parietal lobules with impairment of visually guided eye movements, peripheral visual inattention and optic ataxia. *Brain*, **109**, 81–97.

Pierrot-Deseilligny, C., Rivaud, S., Gaymard, B., and Agid, Y. (1991). Cortical control of reflexive visually-guided saccades. *Brain*, **114**, 1473–85.

Pohl, W. (1973). Dissociation of spatial discrimination deficits following frontal and parietal lesions in monkeys. *Journal of Comparative and Physiological Psychology*, **82**, 227–39.

Quintana, J. and Fuster, J. M. (1993). Spatial and temporal factors in the role of prefrontal and parietal cortex in visuomotor integration. *Cerebral Cortex*, **3**, 122–32.

Ratcliff, G. and Davies-Jones, G. A. B. (1972). Defective visual localization in focal brain wounds. *Brain*, **95**, 49–60.

Rizzolatti, G., Camarda, R., Fogassi, L., Gentilucci, M., Luppino, G., and Matelli, M. (1988). Functional organization of inferior area 6 in the macaque monkey. II. Area F5 and the control of distal movements. *Experimental Brain Research*, **71**, 491–507.

Robinson, D. L., Bowman, E. M., and Kertzman, C. (1995). Covert orienting of attention in macaques. II. Contributions of parietal cortex. *Journal of Neurophysiology*, **74**, 698–712.

Rondot, P. (1989). Visuomotor ataxia. In *Neuropsychology of visual perception*, (ed. J. W. Brown), pp. 105–9. Erlbaum, Hillsdale, NJ.

Sakata, H., Taira, M., Mine, S., and Murata, A. (1992). Hand-movement-related neurons of the posterior parietal cortex of the monkey: their role in the visual guidance of hand movements. In *Control of arm movement in space*, (ed. R. Caminiti, P. B. Johnson, and Y. Burnod), pp. 185–98. Springer-Verlag, Berlin.

Sakata, H., Taira, M., Murata, A., Gallese, V., Tanaka, Y., Shikata, E., and Kusunoki, M. (1997). Parietal visual neurons coding 3-D characteristics of objects and their relation to hand action. In *Parietal lobe contributions to orientation in 3D space*, (ed. P. Thier and H.-O. Karnath), pp. 237–54. Springer-Verlag, Heidelberg.

Sayner, R. B. and Davis, R. T. (1972). Significance of sign in an S-R separation problem. *Perceptual and Motor Skills*, **34**, 671–6.

Schmahmann, J. D. and Pandya, D. N. (1993). Prelunate, occipitotemporal, and parahippocampal projections to the basis pontis in rhesus monkey. *Journal of*

Comparative Neurology, **337**, 94–112.
Semmes, J. (1965). A non-tactual factor in astereognosis. *Neuropsychologia*, **3**, 295–315.
Shikata, E., Tanaka, Y., Nakamura, H., Taira, M., and Sakata, H. (1996). Selectivity of the parietal visual neurones in 3D orientation of surface of stereoscopic stimuli. *NeuroReport*, **7**, 2389–94.
Snyder, L. H., Batista, A. P., and Andersen, R. A. (1997). Coding of intention in the posterior parietal cortex. *Nature*, **386**, 167–70.
Sparks, D. L. and Hartwich-Young, R. (1989). The deep layers of the superior colliculus. In *The neurobiology of saccadic eye movements*, (ed. R. H. Wurtz and M. E. Goldberg), pp. 213–55. Elsevier, Amsterdam.
Stein, J. (1978). Effects of parietal lobe cooling on manipulative behaviour in the monkey. In *Active touch*, (ed. G. Gordon), pp. 79–90. Pergamon Press, Oxford.
Sugishita, M., Ettlinger, G., and Ridley, R. M. (1978). Disturbance of cage-finding in the monkey. *Cortex*, **14**, 431–8.
Taira, M., Mine, S., Georgopoulos, A. P., Mutara, A., and Sakata, H. (1990). Parietal cortex neurons of the monkey related to the visual guidance of hand movements. *Experimental Brain Research*, **83**, 29–36.
Traverse, J. and Latto, R. (1986). Impairments in route negotiation through a maze after dorsolateral frontal, inferior parietal or premotor lesions in cynomolgus monkeys. *Behavioural Brain Research*, **20**, 203–15.
Tzavaras, A. and Masure, M. C. (1976). Aspects différents de l'ataxie optique selon la latéralisation hémisphérique de la lésion. *Lyon Médical*, **236**, 673–83.
Ungerleider, L. G. and Brody, B. A. (1977). Extrapersonal spatial orientation: the role of posterior parietal, anterior frontal, and inferotemporal cortex. *Experimental Neurology*, **56**, 265–80.
Ungerleider, L. G. and Mishkin, M. (1982). Two cortical visual systems. In *Analysis of visual behavior*, (ed. D. J. Ingle, M. A. Goodale, and R. J. W. Mansfield), pp. 549–86. MIT Press, Cambridge, MA.
Vallar, G. and Perani, D. (1986). The anatomy of unilateral neglect after right-hemisphere stroke lesions. A clinical / CT-scan correlation study in man. *Neuropsychologia*, **24**, 609–22.
Watson, J. D. G., Myers, R., Frackowiak, R. S. J., Hajnal, J. V., Woods, R. P., Mazziotta, J. C. *et al.* (1993). Area V5 of the human brain: evidence from a combined study using positron emission tomography and magnetic resonance imaging. *Cerebral Cortex*, **3**, 79–94.
Webster, M. J., Bachevalier, J., and Ungerleider, L. G. (1994). Connections of inferior temporal areas TEO and TE with parietal and frontal cortex in macaque monkeys. *Cerebral Cortex*, **4**, 470–83.
Wiesendanger, M., Kazennikov, O., Perrig, S., Rouiller, E., and Kermadi, I. (1997). Reaching, grasping, and bimanual coordination with special reference to the posterior parietal cortex. In *Parietal lobe contributions to orientation in 3D space*, (ed. P. Thier and H.-O. Karnath), pp. 271–88. Springer-Verlag, Heidelberg.
Wilson, M. (1957). Effects of circumscribed cortical lesions upon somesthetic and visual discrimination in the monkey. *Journal of Comparative and Physiological Psychology*, **50**, 630–5.
Zeki, S. M. (1969). Representation of central visual fields in prestriate cortex of monkey. *Brain Research*, **14**, 271–91.
Zeki, S. M. (1971). Convergent input from striate cortex (area 17) to the cortex of the superior temporal sulcus in the rhesus monkey. *Brain Research*, **28**, 338–40.
Zeki, S. M. (1980). A direct projection from area V1 to area V3A of rhesus monkey visual cortex. *Proceedings of the Royal Society of London*, **B207**, 499–506.

6

Memory and the human temporal lobes

JOHN M. OXBURY and SUSAN M. OXBURY

6.1 Introduction

In 1966 George Ettlinger, together with the psychologist Colin Blakemore and the neurosurgeon Murray Falconer, described their investigation of whether any correlation exists between pre-operative intelligence and the severity of mesial temporal sclerosis in temporal lobe specimens excised to treat intractable epilepsy (Blakemore *et al.* 1966). No significant correlation was found and the paper is now little remembered. It was, however, the forerunner of what has become one of the potentially most interesting techniques for exploring the relationship between certain aspects of human memory and temporal lobe structures.

Mesial temporal sclerosis was the term introduced by the Maudsley epilepsy surgery group (Falconer *et al.* 1964) to describe the neuronal loss and gliosis often found in the hippocampus, especially the Sommer sector (CA1), along with the amygdala and the cortex of the hippocampal and fusiform gyri, and sometimes also in the lateral temporal lobe cortex, on histological examination of *en-bloc* temporal lobectomy specimens from people treated surgically for intractable epilepsy. It is the most common pathology associated with severe intractable temporal lobe epilepsy (Margerison and Corsellis 1966). *Hippocampal sclerosis* is part of the condition, consisting of neuronal loss and gliosis in the various zones of the hippocampus which, when severely affecting the Sommer sector along with the end-folium (CA4, CA5) and the dentate gyrus (see Fig. 6.1), is referred to as *Ammon's horn sclerosis*. The aetiology is uncertain (Mathern *et al.* 1995) but it is the cause of the epileptic seizures in many cases of intractable temporal lobe epilepsy, probably because abnormal patterns of electrical discharges arise from distorted synapses and neurotransmitter release; surgical excision of the abnormal hippocampus along with amygdala and hippocampal gyrus, as in amygdalo-hippocampectomy (Yasargil *et al.* 1985), often leads to alleviation of the epilepsy. George Ettlinger and his colleagues were unfortunate not to use a pre-operative memory parameter for correlation with the degree of mesial temporal sclerosis because, had they done so, they might have achieved a positive result. Meyer and Yates (1955) had already noted a pre-operative impairment of verbal learning in people who were subsequently to have a left temporal lobectomy. There had not, however, been reports of memory impairment in groups of patients prior to right temporal lobectomy, although it was recognized that this could follow such operations (Milner 1962). Furthermore, at that time neither the pre-operative verbal memory deficit nor the post-operative non-verbal memory impairment were specifically associated with damage to medial temporal lobe structures. It might, therefore, have seemed to Ettlinger and his

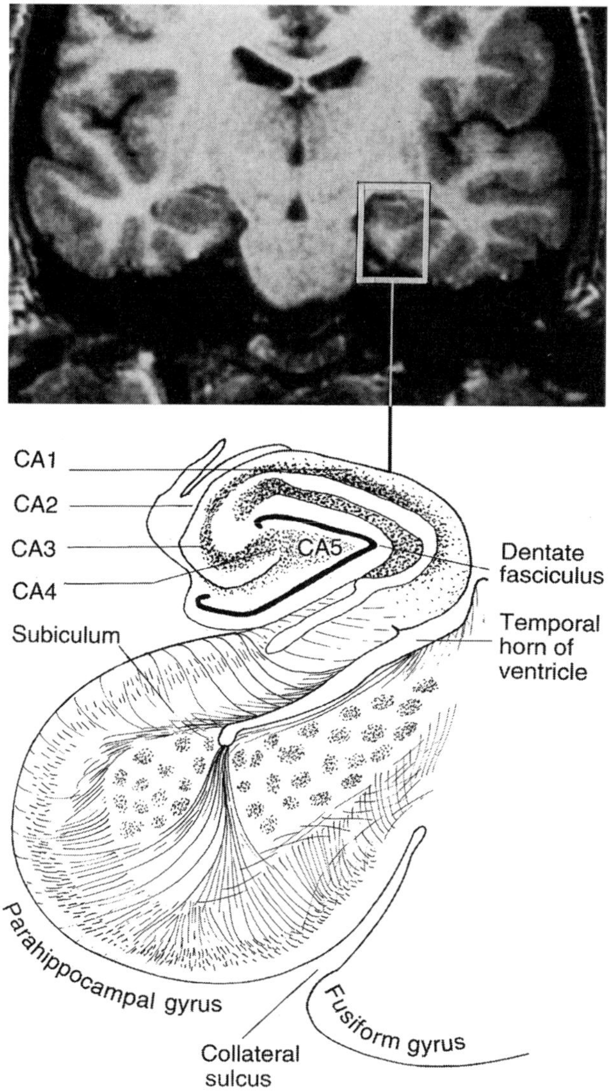

Fig. 6.1 Above is a magnetic resonance coronal T1 image through the temporal lobes. The boxed area shows a hippocampus atrophied by Ammon's horn sclerosis. It can be compared to the normal hippocampus on the other side. The stylized figure below shows the normal relationship of the medial temporal lobe structures including the hippocampal zones.

colleagues that it would be more rewarding to correlate pathology and an overall measure of cognitive function, rather than a restricted memory measure, unless the correlation was to be restricted to left-sided cases.

Ideas concerning the relationship between the human temporal lobes and memory have been nourished by data derived from diverse sources. The outstanding landmark is the report of Scoville (1954), and especially Scoville and Milner (1957), that surgical excision of the medial temporal lobe structures bilaterally could result in a very severe and permanent anterograde amnesic syndrome with some degree of retrograde loss. One of these patients, H.M., has co-operated as a subject in a multitude of experimental investigations of memory during the more than 40 years since he became amnesic (Milner *et al.* 1968; Corkin 1984; Milner 1985; Keane *et al.* 1995). Prior to the original reports of Scoville and Milner, suggestions of temporal lobe involvement in memory function had arisen from descriptions of experiential and mnestic symptoms during temporal lobe epileptic seizures and during intra-operative electrical stimulation of cerebral cortex (Jackson 1888; Penfield and Jasper 1954) but cases of amnesia due to pathology restricted to the medial temporal lobe structures had not been generally recognized (Brierley 1966). Since then, neurophysiological studies have advanced by correlating seizure symptoms with electrical discharges recorded via electrodes situated within the brain substance, usually during clinical assessment prior to surgical treatment for intractable epilepsy (Gloor 1990; Palmini *et al.* 1992; Fish *et al.* 1993; Manford *et al.* 1996). The findings have strengthened the view that the establishing and maintaining of human memories are especially dependent on the hippocampus and/or amygdala, although clearly these structures cannot function except in conjunction with neocortex. Space does not permit a more detailed consideration of the use of neurophysiological techniques to unravel the anatomical basis of memory. Likewise, there will be no discussion of functional imaging, which in essence uses positron emission tomography (PET) or functional magnetic resonance imaging (fMRI) to locate the site(s) of increased brain metabolism coincident with, and therefore presumably the cerebral structures underlying, a defined psychological process. Suffice it to say that activation of medial temporal lobe structures has been detected during verbal memory retrieval (Nyberg *et al.* 1996).

6.2 Effects of surgical excisions

The year after Scoville's 1954 report, Meyer and Yates (1955) reported that left-sided *en-bloc* temporal lobectomy accentuated the verbal learning deficit which they had found to exist pre-operatively, but did not cause any other persistent cognitive decline. Scoville's operation on H.M. had removed, bilaterally, the medial temporal pole, the amygdala, the entorhinal cortex (this corresponds to Brodmann area 28 which occupies most of the parahippocampal gyrus), and the rostral perirhinal cortex (this being the cortical area,

35, on the banks of the collateral sulcus which separates the hippocampal and fusiform gyri), along with the anterior 2–2.5 cm or so of the dentate gyrus, the hippocampus, and the subicular complex. The posterior 2 cm of hippocampus were not removed but shrank, and likewise some of the posterior perirhinal and parahippocampal gyrus cortex was not removed (Keane *et al.* 1995). The left-sided *en-bloc* excisions carried out by Murray Falconer on the patients reported by Meyer and Yates would probably have removed the anterior 5–6 cm of temporal lobe, including the majority of the amygdala and the anterior one-third to one-half of the hippocampus with the overlying hippocampal gyrus; the right-sided removals may have been larger. So, the removal of medial structures in a left-sided *en-bloc* temporal lobectomy is usually somewhat less than was removed on each side in the Scoville operation, although the amount of these structures removed in a selective amygdalo-hippocampectomy approximates the latter.

On rare occasions, severe amnesia follows an unilateral temporal lobe excision (Penfield and Milner 1958; Dimsdale *et al.* 1964; Rausch *et al.* 1985; Loring *et al.* 1994). Such an occurrence is attributed to the presence of pathology, usually hippocampal sclerosis, in the medial structures of the contralateral (unoperated) temporal lobe (Penfield and Mathieson 1974; Warrington and Duchen 1992) which was not detected or was not considered to be significant pre-operatively but which post-operatively resulted in a state akin to a bilateral excision of the medial structures. Also, a severe amnesic state can arise from the new development of severe pathology restricted to the hippocampus contralateral to a successful temporal lobectomy carried out years previously without causing memory impairment (Oxbury, S. *et al.* 1997). Some degree of pathology in the hippocampus contralateral to a medial temporal lobe excision does not, however, inevitably lead to severe amnesia (Henke and Wieser 1996). Indeed, autopsy data presented by Margerison and Corsellis (1966) indicate that approximately one-third of those with intractable temporal lobe epilepsy who have one severely sclerosed hippocampus (and it is these who are most successfully treated by surgical excision) have a lesser degree of sclerosis in their other hippocampus. This is probably so in around one-half of those treated surgically and should be taken into account when interpreting their pre- and post-operative neuropsychological test profiles.

Meyer and Yates' (1955) observation that the verbal learning deficit was accentuated by left temporal lobe excisions was confirmed and extended by Milner (1958, 1962, 1967), and further confirmation came from many others in subsequent years (reviewed by Oxbury, J. and Oxbury, S. 1989; Oxbury, S. 1997). Mostly, verbal memory was tested by requiring recall of narrative material, usually presented only once (e.g. story recall or logical memory, from the Wechsler Memory Scale, WMS), and/or by requiring the learning over several trials of word pairs or word lists which include unrelated material (e.g. the Paired Associate Learning Test, PALT, from the WMS). Milner's data indicated that post-operative verbal memory capacity was inversely related to the extent of both the hippocampal excision and the neocortical excision, although inspection of Table 12 in Milner (1967) suggests that the former could have been the more important. However, which structure seems the more important may depend upon the testing technique used (Jones-Gotman 1991). Furthermore, it is difficult to say to what extent poor performance post-operatively represented a 'post-operative deficit' because pre-operative performance was not reported. Thus post- versus pre-operative change could not be assessed to determine whether 'deficit' had accrued post-operatively or whether poor post-operative performance was simply a continuation of a poor performance that had existed pre-operatively. Other investigators (e.g. Katz *et al.* 1989; Wolf *et al.* 1993) have not found the degree of verbal memory change across surgery to be a function of the extent of the total excision, nor of either the medial or the lateral excisions considered independently. A comparison of our own patient groups (Oxbury, J. M. *et al.* 1995; Renowden *et al.* 1995) has shown that the extent of the change in verbal memory capacity after left-sided surgery is not dependent upon whether the operation was a selective amygdalo-hippocampectomy or an *en-bloc* lobectomy (Table 6.1). Cognitive outcome was, however, better after selective amygdalo-hippocampectomy than after *en-bloc* lobectomy in that only the former group had a significantly increased verbal IQ and improved on a non-verbal memory measure (Rey–Osterrieth figure, delayed reproduction).

Table 6.1 *Pre-operative and 2-year post-operative performance of 24 patients, all with mesial temporal sclerosis as the sole pathology, who underwent either left-sided* en-bloc *temporal lobectomy (*n *= 13, median age = 20 years) or left-sided selective amygdalo-hippocampectomy (*n *= 11, median age = 19 years)*

	L. Temporal lobectomy		L. Selective amygdalo-hippocampectomy	
	Pre-op.	Post-op.	Pre-op.	Post-op.
Verbal IQ	88.7	88.2	86.6	91.6*
Performance IQ	96.3	106.5***	94.8	106.6***
PALT				
initial	12.9	11.1	13.3	13.7
trial 3	8.2	7.4	8.2	8.4
delayed	6.9	6.1	7.6	7.7
Paragraph recall (WMS)				
initial	7.4	6.1*	8.5	7.4*
delayed	4.2	3.6	5.8	7.2
Rey-Osterrieth				
delayed	19.5	18.9	16.3	20.7**

*, Pre-op. versus post-op. change significant at $p < 0.05$.
**, Pre-op. versus post-op. change significant at $p < 0.01$.
***, Pre-op. versus post-op. change significant at $p < 0.001$.
PALT, Paired Associate Learning Test; WMS, Wechsler Memory Scale.

In contrast to the verbal memory deterioration consequent upon left temporal lobe excisions, non-verbal memory impairments have been reported post-operatively in people whose epilepsy was treated by right temporal lobectomy (e.g. Milner 1962; Kimura 1963; Smith and Milner 1981; Feigenbaum *et al.* 1996). However, this non-verbal deficit after right-sided excisions is less consistently seen than the verbal impairment after left excisions.

It is difficult to elucidate the relationship between memory and individual medial temporal lobe structures simply by studying the effects of surgical excisions. One reason is that, in general, it is impossible to excise one structure without damaging others. Another is the problem of how to be sure what precisely has been removed, despite a detailed surgical description, unless each case undergoes post-operative MRI with this particular question in mind. The *en-bloc* anterior temporal lobectomy usually removes around 35–40 g of brain on the left or around 40–45 g on the right, including all or most of the amygdala, about half of the hippocampus and hippocampal gyrus, and variable quantities of the inferior and lateral neocortex. Not only the hippocampus but also the amygdala and the rhinal/perirhinal cortex (that is, mainly, hippocampal gyrus with parts of the fusiform gyrus) have been suggested as important structures subserving memory in the monkey (Mishkin 1982; Meunier *et al.* 1993) although their role in man is more doubtful (Miller *et al.* 1995; Oxbury, S. *et al.* 1997). The operation of selective amygdalo-hippocampectomy as described by Yasargil *et al.* (1985) excises unilaterally the hippocampus, amygdala, and parahippocampal gyrus—no more than 5 g in weight—via an incision in the depth of the Sylvian fissure to gain entry to the temporal horn of the lateral ventricle. Yet even this removes the major part of all of these structures together, thereby making it impossible to differentiate their separate functions. Furthermore, the surgery results in secondary damage in other parts of the temporal lobe and may disconnect temporal neocortex from other brain areas (Renowden *et al.* 1995); the disruption to the temporal lobe appears greater if entry to the temporal horn is through an incision in a gyrus as described by Niemeyer (1958). Consequently, interest has been rekindled in the time-honoured method of studying groups of patients with relatively uniform and well-understood pathology in an attempt to establish the neuroanatomical basis of a cognitive dysfunction—in this case the relationship between a depletion of hippocampal neurones and memory impairment.

6.3 Verbal memory in hippocampal sclerosis and correlations with neuronal density

Techniques for examining the association between pre-operative memory capacity and temporal lobe pathology, especially the state of the hippocampus, which were foreshadowed by George Ettlinger and his colleagues in 1966, have developed considerably during the past decade. Some studies have correlated memory test performance with an overall measure of hippocampal sclerosis as found in the excision specimens (e.g. Oxbury, J. and Oxbury, S. 1989; Saling *et al.* 1993). Others have correlated memory with neuronal densities in specific hippocampal zones (e.g. Rausch and Babb 1987; Sass *et al.* 1990, 1992*a,b*; Matkovic *et al.* 1995*a,b,c*). This latter technique is of interest because different zones are affected to a different degree by whatever the process is that leads to hippocampal sclerosis (Margerison and Corsellis 1966; Sagar and Oxbury 1987; Mathern *et al.* 1995). Yet other studies have taken MRI measures of hippocampal volume, which have been shown by Lencz *et al.* (1992) to correlate significantly with neuronal densities in hippocampal subfields (CA1, CA3, hilar, and dentate, but not CA2), to gauge the extent of the sclerosis and then correlated this with pre-operative memory capacity (reviewed by Baxendale 1995).

In 1984, at the meeting of the International Neuropsychology Symposium in Beaune, we reported that the pre-operative verbal memory of patients whose subsequent *en-bloc* temporal lobectomy specimens contained a sclerotic hippocampus with a severe depletion of neurones (the Ammon's horn sclerosis, AHS, group), irrespective of side, was impaired compared to that of those with only a minor or no depletion (the 'normal' hippocampus group). This significant pathology-dependent difference, which was manifest on both story recall (logical memory) and PALT, exceeded any difference attributable to laterality, which did not itself achieve statistical significance (Oxbury, J. and Oxbury, S. 1986, 1989). Subsequent *en-bloc* temporal lobectomy was followed by a marked deterioration of the verbal memory capacity of those from whom 'normal' left hippocampus was removed and a considerably lesser deterioration when either left hippocampus with severe neuronal depletion or 'normal' right hippocampus was removed. Removal of a right hippocampus severely depleted of neurones was not usually followed by any deterioration. We noted that bitter complaints of memory impairment came from those whose memory was good prior to left-sided surgery and whose excision specimens contained relatively well-preserved hippocampal neurones; in contrast, such complaints were unusual from those whose left hippocampus had been severely depleted of neurones pre-operatively. This finding has been confirmed on a number of occasions since then (e.g. Hermann *et al.* 1992; Sass *et al.* 1994). A post-operative decline in non-verbal memory, measured on maze learning, was detected only after removal of 'normal' hippocampus, the change being greater after right excisions than after left (Oxbury, J. and Oxbury, S. 1986). We concluded that both temporal lobes, not solely the left, have a role in verbal memory, but with a different organization on the two sides and, no doubt, to a different degree. There seemed to be evidence for involvement in verbal memory of both the hippocampus/amygdala system and the neocortex on the left, but of the former only on the right. Likewise, the findings suggested that not only the right hippocampus but also the left was involved in non-verbal (maze) learning.

At much the same time, McMillan *et al.* (1987) reported that left and right groups whose subsequent excision specimens showed hippocampal sclerosis, of any degree, did not differ pre-operatively on immediate or delayed WMS logical memory. More recently, Saling *et al.* (1993) obtained related but slightly different results from their comparison of left and right temporal lobectomy patients selected pre-operatively on the basis of MRI evidence of hippocampal sclerosis, who had severe neuronal depletion confirmed by post-operative histology. Pre-operatively both groups were mildly impaired on the recall of prose passages (WMS) but they did not differ significantly from each other. The left group, however, performed worse than the right group and normal controls on PALT (WMS). Saling and his colleagues concluded that the laterality of verbal memory is conditional upon task specificity, presumably because different tasks impose different cognitive demands. Our initial analysis (Oxbury, J. and Oxbury, S. 1986, 1989), which was based on 30 patients, did not reveal any significant pre-operative differences attributable to laterality of the pathology. A subsequent analysis from our group, however, based on a larger number of patients (54), all with mesial temporal sclerosis of some degree as the sole pathology and all with good post-operative seizure outcome, showed (Table 6.2) that pre-operatively the left group performed significantly worse than the right on PALT (initial, trial 3, and delayed) but not on story recall (Matkovic *et al.* 1997). Also, in this study, the right group was inferior

Table 6.2 *Pre-operative performance of 54 patients, all with mesial temporal sclerosis as the sole pathology, IQ > 70, and good post-operative outcome, prior to left (n = 21) or right (n = 33) temporal lobe epilepsy surgery (mean ages left = 20.1 years, right = 20.3 years)*

	Left	Right
Full-scale IQ	91.4	95.2
PALT		
initial learning	13.8	15.5*
trial 3	8.1	9.0*
delayed recall	7.3	8.8*
Paragraph recall (WMS)		
initial	8.3	9.2
delayed	5.2	8.1
Maze learning		
trials	3.5	4.4*
errors	0.5	1.4*
Benton DE[a]	−0.9	0.8*
Rey–Osterrieth figure		
delayed reproduction	18.9	17.9

*, Difference significant at $p < 0.05$ on *t*-rest.
[a] DE, The expected errors (based on age and IQ) minus the actual errors made.

to the left, pre-operatively, on the Benton visual retention test and maze learning, but not on delayed recall of the Rey–Osterrieth figure or on a face memory task.

Rausch and Babb (1987) were pioneers in examining the relationship between memory and neuronal densities in specific hippocampal zones and other substructures in the temporal lobe. They took left temporal lobectomy patients whose sole pathology was some degree of neuronal loss with sclerosis and correlated pre-operative performance on the two WMS verbal tests, and on the WMS visual reproduction task (immediate and delayed), with neuronal densities in multiple sites in the hippocampus, parahippocampal gyrus, and lateral temporal lobe cortex. The PALT measures correlated significantly with neuronal density in the CA1 hippocampal zone and delayed paragraph recall correlated significantly with hippocampal gyrus neuronal density. (Zola-Morgan *et al.* (1986) had shown that a virtually complete loss of pyramidal neurones in CA1 bilaterally, without other significant cerebral damage, is sufficient to cause severe amnesia.) Visual reproduction performance did not correlate significantly with the density in any of the left temporal lobe sites that were examined by Rausch and Babb. Furthermore, there were no significant correlations with intelligence, a finding which, incidentally, replicates the early finding of George Ettlinger and his colleagues (Blakemore *et al.* 1966). Sass and his colleagues have also correlated pre-operative memory test performance with neuronal densities in specific hippocampal subfields. Using a word-list learning task they found that both left and right groups were impaired, the left more severely than the right. There were significant correlations between test scores and pyramidal neurone densities in CA3 and the hilus on the left, but not with CA1, CA2, or the dentate granule cells; and there was no significant correlation with any subfield on the right (Sass *et al.* 1990). Further studies (Sass *et al.* 1992*a*,*b*) revealed similar correlations between performance on one verbal memory measure (percent retained on delayed paragraph recall) and neuronal densities in each of CA3 and the hilus on the left. There were no significant correlations with any subfield on the right, nor was there any significant correlation between performance on the WMS visual reproduction and neuronal density in any subfield on either side.

Matkovic has measured the neuronal densities in the hippocampal subfields and the dentate gyrus in excision specimens from the Oxford series of temporal lobectomy and selective amygdalo-hippocampectomy patients who had mesial temporal sclerosis as their sole pathology, and these densities have been related to various clinical and neuropsychological parameters (Matkovic *et al.* 1995*a*,*b*,*c*; Oxbury, J. M. *et al.* 1996). The 54 patients (33 right, 21 left) all fulfilled the following criteria: full-scale IQ > 70, English as their first language, and seizure outcome in Engel Class I or II (see Engel *et al.* 1993). In the verbal memory sphere, there were significant correlations between PALT trial 3 and CA4 on the left ($p < 0.05$), but not on the right, and between delayed story recall (WMS logical memory) and CA1 ($p < 0.05$) and CA2-3 ($p < 0.05$) both on the right. With non-verbal memory tests there were significant correlations between the Benton scores and CA4 on the right, and between recall of the Rey–Osterrieth figure and both CA4 on the right and CA1 on the left.

6.4 Conclusions

There is strong evidence that at least some aspects of verbal memory are impaired in association with a depletion of neurones in the left hippocampus. Correlations have been made between performance on verbal learning tasks and neuronal density in various hippocampal subfields, particularly CA1 (Rausch and Babb 1987), CA3 (Sass *et al.* 1990), and CA4 (Matkovic *et al.* 1995b, 1997). In contrast, significant correlations between verbal learning and neuronal densities in subfields of the right hippocampus have not been found. Furthermore, the pre-operative verbal learning of those with left hippocampal sclerosis is significantly worse than that of those with right hippocampal sclerosis (Saling *et al.* 1993; Matkovic *et al.* 1997), even though the verbal learning of those with right hippocampal sclerosis is not normal, being worse than that of people with severe epilepsy but a relatively intact right hippocampus (Oxbury, J. and Oxbury, S. 1989). The impairment of those with right hippocampal sclerosis suggests that the right hippocampus is involved in verbal learning, although it could be attributed to concomitant mild left hippocampal neurone depletion often associated with the severe right-sided loss.

The situation is different with the recall of narrative material, which is also a test of verbal memory but does not consistently correlate with left hippocampal subfield densities. Rausch and Babb (1987) found that performance on story recall did not correlate with the neuronal density in any left hippocampal subfield, but did correlate with hippocampal gyrus neuronal density. Sass *et al.* (1992*a*) obtained a relatively weak correlation between a delayed recall measure and neuronal densities in left CA3 and the hilus (CA4). However, Matkovic *et al.* (1995*b*) found no correlation between any story recall measure and neuronal density in any left hippocampal subfield, although there was a correlation between delayed recall and neuronal densities in CA1 and CA2–3 on the right. Furthermore, compared to verbal learning, it is more difficult to demonstrate pre-operative differences on story recall consistently between left- and right-sided groups with severe hippocampal neurone depletion, even though both groups are impaired compared to those without such depletion (Oxbury, J. and Oxbury, S. 1989; Saling *et al.* 1993). Indeed, Saling *et al.* (1995) have suggested that if language competence is partialled out, the pre-operative difference between the two groups is restricted to the learning of unrelated words, and also that subsequent left temporal lobectomy impairs performance on verbal memory tasks that are open to semantic structuring during the acquisition phase, but is not followed by a decline in the ability to learn unrelated words. One interpretation of this is that the hippocampus plays the major part in word learning but that the acquisition and retention of more 'semantically loaded' material requires participation of the parahippocampal gyrus or more laterally situated cortex.

In conclusion, the development of techniques that are essentially an extension of what was being attempted by George Ettlinger and his colleagues 30 years ago has led to the current position which suggests:

(1) that the left–right dichotomy between verbal and non-verbal memory may not be as sharp as was originally thought;

(2) that within the left hippocampus at least, a different role may be definable for the separate subfields; and

(3) that in the verbal sphere, and perhaps also the non-verbal, both the hippocampus and the cortex may be involved in memory to a different extent depending upon the nature of the material.

We think George would have been interested by these developments and that they would have appealed to his belief in the need for integrating different approaches to dissecting the structural basis of cognition.

References

Baxendale, S. A. (1995). The hippocampus: functional and structural correlations. *Seizure*, **4**, 105–17.

Blakemore, C. B., Ettlinger, G., and Falconer, M. A. (1966). Cognitive abilities in relation to frequency of seizures and neuropathology of the temporal lobes in man. *Journal of Neurology, Neurosurgery, and Psychiatry*, **60**, 268–72.

Brierley, J. B. (1966). The neuropathology of amnesic states. In *Amnesia*, (ed. C. W. M. Whitty and O. L. Zangwill), pp. 150–80. Butterworths, London.

Corkin, S. (1984). Lasting consequences of bilateral medial temporal lobectomy: clinical course and experimental findings in HM. *Seminars in Neurology*, **4**, 249–59.

Dimsdale, H., Logue, V., and Piercy, M. (1964). A case of persistent impairment of recent memory following right temporal lobectomy. *Neuropsychologia*, **1**, 287–98.

Engel, J., Van Ness, P. C., Rasmussen, T. B., and Ojemann, L. M. (1993). Outcome with respect to epileptic seizures. In *Surgical treatment of the epilepsies*, (2nd edn), (ed. J. Engel), pp. 609–35. Raven Press, New York.

Falconer, M. A., Serafetinides, E. A., and Corsellis, J. A. (1964). Etiology and pathogenesis of temporal lobe epilepsy. *Archives of Neurology*, **10**, 233–48.

Feigenbaum, J. D., Polkey, C. E., and Morris, R. G. (1996). Deficits in spatial working memory after unilateral temporal lobectomy in man. *Neuropsychologia*, **34**, 163–76.

Fish, D. R., Gloor, P., Quesney, F. L., and Olivier, A. (1993). Clinical responses to electrical brain stimulation of the temporal and frontal lobes in patients with epilepsy. *Brain*, **116**, 397–414.

Gloor, P. (1990). Experiential phenomena of temporal lobe epilepsy. Facts and hypotheses. *Brain*, **113**, 1673–94.

Henke, K. and Wieser, H. G. (1966). Bilateral medial temporal lobe damage without amnesic syndrome; a case report. *Epilepsy Research*, **24**, 147–61.

Hermann, B. P., Wyler, A. R., Somes, G., Berry, A. D., and Dohan, F. C. (1992). Pathological status of the mesial temporal lobe predicts memory outcome from left anterior temporal lobectomy. *Neurosurgery*, **31**, 652–7.

Jackson, H. J. (1888). On a particular variety of epilepsy ('intellectual aura'), one case with symptoms of organic brain disease. *Brain*, **11**, 179–207.

Jones-Gotman, M. (1991). Presurgical neuropsychological evaluation for localisation and lateralisation of seizure focus. In *Epilepsy surgery*, (ed. H. Luders), pp. 469–75. Raven Press, New York.

Kartsounis, L.D., Rudge, P., Stevens, J. M. (1995). Bilateral lesions of CA1 and CA2 fields of the hippocampus are sufficient to cause a severe amnesic syndrome in humans. *Journal of Neurology, Neurosurgery, and Psychiatry*, **30**, 763–71.

Katz, A., Awad, I. A., Kong, A. K., Chelune, G. J., Naugle, R. I., Wyllie, E. *et al.* (1989). Extent of resection in temporal lobectomy for epilepsy. II. Memory changes and neurologic complications. *Epilepsia*, **30**, 763–71.

Keane, M. M., Gabrieli, J. D. E., Mapstone, H. C., Johnson, K. A., and Corkin, S. (1995). Double dissociation of memory capacities after bilateral occipital-lobe or medial temporal-lobe lesions. *Brain*, **118**, 1129–114.

Kimura, D. (1963). Right temporal lobe damage. *Archives of Neurology*, **8**, 264–71.

Lencz, T., McCarthy, G., and Bronen, R. A. (1992). Quantitative magnetic resonance imaging in temporal lobe epilepsy: relationship to neuropathology and neuropsychological function. *Annals of Neurology*, **31**, 629–37.

Loring, D. W., Herman, B. P., Meador, K. J., Lee, G. P., Gallagher, B. B., King, D. W. *et al.* (1994). Amnesia after unilateral temporal lobectomy: a case report. *Epilepsia*, **35**, 757–63.

McMillan, T. M., Powell, G. E., Janota, I., and Polkey, C. E. (1987). Relationships between neuropathology and cognitive functioning in temporal lobectomy patients. *Journal of Neurology, Neurosurgery, and Psychiatry*, **50**, 167–76.

Manford, M., Fish, D. R., and Shorvon, S. D. (1996). An analysis of clinical seizure patterns and their localising value in frontal and temporal lobe epilepsies. *Brain*, **119**, 17–40.

Margerison, J. H. and Corsellis, J. A. N. (1966). Epilepsy and the temporal lobes. A clinical, electroencephalographic and neuropathological study of the brain in epilepsy with particular reference to the temporal lobes. *Brain*, **89**, 499–530.

Mathern, G. W., Babb, T. L., Vickrey, B. G., Melendez, M., and Pretorius, J. K. (1995). The clinical-pathogenic mechanisms of hippocampal neuron loss and surgical outcomes in temporal lobe epilepsy. *Brain*, **118**, 105–18.

Matkovic, Z., Oxbury, J. M., Morris, J. H., Hiorns, R. W., and Adams, C. B. T. (1995*a*). Neuron loss in hippocampal sclerosis: its relationship to clinical features and outcome after surgical treatment. *Epilepsia*, **36**, (Suppl. 3), p. S55.

Matkovic, Z., Oxbury, S. M., Hiorns, R. W., Morris, J. H., Carpenter, K., Adams, C. B. T. *et al.* (1995*b*). Hippocampal neuronal density correlates with preoperative verbal memory in patients with temporal lobe epilepsy. *Epilepsia*, **36**, (Suppl. 3), S121.

Matkovic, Z., Oxbury, S. M., Hiorns, R. W., Morris, J. H., Carpenter, K., Adams, C. B. T. *et al.* (1995*c*). Hippocampal neuron density correlates with preoperative non-verbal memory in patients with temporal lobe epilepsy. *Epilepsia*, **36**, (Suppl. 3), S93.

Matkovic, Z., Oxbury, S. M., Hiorns, R. W., Oxbury, J. M., Morris, J. H., Carpenter, K. *et al.* (1997). Verbal memory in patients with mesial temporal lobe epilepsy: role of the left and right hippocampi, (in preparation).

Meunier, M., Bachevalier, J., Mishkin, M., and Murray, E. A. (1993). Effects on visual recognition of combined and separate ablation of the rhinal and perirhinal cortex in rhesus monkeys. *Journal of Neuroscience*,**13**, 5418–32.

Meyer, V. and Yates, A. J. (1955). Intellectual changes following temporal lobectomy for psychomotor epilepsy: preliminary communication. *Journal of Neurology, Neurosurgery, and Psychiatry*, **18**, 44–52.

Miller, L. A., Lai, R., and Munoz, D. G. (1995). Mesial temporal pathology and human memory. *Epilepsia*, **36**, (Suppl. 3), S93.

Milner, B. (1958). Psychological defects produced by temporal lobe excision. *Proceedings of the Association for Research in Nervous and Mental Disease*, **35**, 244–57.

Milner, B. (1962). Laterality effects in audition. In *Interhemispheric relations and cerebral dominance*, (ed. V. B. Mountcasle), pp. 177–95. John Hopkins Press, Baltimore.

Milner, B. (1967). Brain mechanisms suggested by studies of temporal lobes. In *Brain mechanisms underlying speech and language*, (ed. F. C. Darley), pp. 122–45. Grune and Stratton, New York.

Milner, B. (1985). Memory and the human brain. In *How we know. Nobel conference XX*, (ed. M. Shafto), pp. 31–59. Harper and Row, New York.

Milner, B., Corkin, S., and Teuber, H.-L. (1968). Further analysis of the hippocampal amnesic syndrome: 14-year follow-up study of HM. *Neuropsychologia*, **6**, 215–34.

Mishkin, M. (1982). A memory system in the monkey. *Philosophical Transactions of the Royal Society of London B*, **298**, 85–95.

Niemeyer, P. (1958). The transventricular amygdalohippocampectomy in temporal lobe epilepsy. In *Temporal lobe epilepsy*, (ed. M. Baldwin and P. Bailey), pp. 461–82. Charles C Thomas, Springfield, IL.

Nyberg, L., McIntosh, A. R., Houle, S., Nilsson, L. G., and Tulving, E. (1996). Activation of medial temporal structures during episodic memory retrieval. *Nature*, **380**, 715–17.

Oxbury, J. and Oxbury, S. (1986). Memory impairment following hippocampal damage in early childhood. *Journal of Neurology, Neurosurgery, and Psychiatry*, **49**, 729.

Oxbury, J. and Oxbury, S. (1989). Neuropsychology: memory and hippocampal pathology. In *The bridge between neurology and psychiatry*, (ed. E. H. Reynolds and M. R. Trimble), pp. 135–50. Churchill Livingstone, Edinburgh.

Oxbury, J. M., Adams, C. B. T., Oxbury, S. M., Carpenter, K., and Renowden, S. A. (1995). En bloc temporal lobectomy v. selective amygdalohippocampectomy as treatments for intracable epilepsy due to hippocampal sclerosis. *Journal of Neurology, Neurosurgery, and Psychiatry*, **59**, 200.

Oxbury, J. M., Matkovic, Z., Oxbury, S. M., Morris, J. H., Hiorns, R. W., and Carpenter, K. (1996). Verbal and non-verbal memory correlates with hippocampal sub-field neuron density. *Journal of Neurology, Neurosurgery, and Psychiatry*, **60**, 115.

Oxbury, S. (1997). Assessment for surgery. In *The clinical psychologists' handbook of epilepsy: assessment and management*, (ed. C. Cull and L. Goldstein), pp. 57–76. Routledge, London.

Oxbury, S., Oxbury, J., Renowden, S., Squier, M., and Carpenter, K. (1997). Severe amnesia: an unusual late complication after temporal lobectomy. *Neuropsychologia*, **35**, 975–88.

Palmini, A. L., Gloor, P., and Jones-Gotman, M. (1992). Pure amnestic seizures in temporal lobe epilepsy. Definition, clinical symptomatology, and functional anatomical considerations. *Brain*, **115**, 749–69.

Penfield, W. and Jasper, H. (1954). *Epilepsy and the functional anatomy of the human brain*. Little, Brown and Co., Boston.

Penfield, W. and Mathieson, G. (1974). Memory: autopsy findings and comments on the role of the hippocampus in experiential recall. *Archives of Neurology*, **31**, 145–54.

Penfield, W. and Milner, B. (1958). Memory deficit produced by bilateral lesions in the hippocampal zone. *Archives of Neurology and Psychiatry*, **79**, 475–97.

Rausch, R. and Babb, T. L. (1987). Evidence for memory specialization within the mesial temporal lobe in man. In *Fundamental mechanisms in human brain function*, (ed. J. Engel), pp. 103–9. Raven Press, New York.

Rausch, R., Babb, T. L., and Brown, W. J. (1985). A case of amnestic syndrome following selective amygdalohippocampectomy. *Journal of Clinical and Experimental Neuropsychology*, **7**, 643.

Renowden, S. A., Matkovic, Z., Adams, C. B. T., Carpenter, K., Oxbury, S., Molyneux, A. J. *et al.* (1995). Selective amygdalohippocampectomy for hippocampal sclerosis: postoperative MR appearances. *American Journal of Neuroradiology*, **16**, 1855–61.

Sagar, H. J. and Oxbury, J. M. (1987). Hippocampal neuron loss in temporal lobe epilepsy: correlation with early childhood convulsions. *Annals of Neurology*, **22**, 334–40.

Saling, M. M., Berkovic, S. F., O'Shea, M. F., Kalnins, R. M., Darby, D. G., and Bladin, P. F. (1993). Lateralisation of verbal memory and unilateral hippocampal sclerosis: evidence of task-specific effects. *Journal of Clinical and Experimental Neuropsychology*, **15**, 608–18.

Saling, M. M., O'Shea, M. F., and Berkovic, S. F. (1995). Verbal memory in temporal lobe epilepsy: cognitive influences on task-specific effects. *Epilepsia*, **36**, (Suppl. 3), S93.

Sass, K. J., Spencer, D. D., Kim, J. H., Westerveld, M., Novelly, R. A., and Lencz, T. (1990). Verbal memory impairment correlates with hippocampal pyramidal cell density. *Neurology*, **40**, 1694–7.

Sass, K. J., Sass, A., Westerveld, M., Lencz, T., Novelly, R. A., Kim, J. H. *et al.* (1992*a*). Specificity in the correlation of verbal memory and hippocampal neuron loss: dissociation of memory, language, and verbal intellectual ability. *Journal of Clinical and Experimental Neuropsychology*, **14**, 662–72.

Sass, K. J., Sass, A., Westerveld, M., Lencz, T., Rosewater, K. M., Novelly, R. A. *et al.* (1992*b*). Russel's adaptation of the Wechsler Memory Scale as an index of hippocampal pathology. *Journal of Epilepsy*, **5**, 24–30.

Sass, K. J., Westerveld, M., Buchanan, C. P., Spencer, S. S., Kim, J. H., and Spencer, D. D. (1994). Degree of hippocampal neuron loss determines severity of verbal memory decrease after left anteromesiotemporal lobectomy. *Epilepsia*, **35**, 1179–86.

Scoville, W. B. (1954). The limbic lobe in man. *Journal of Neurology, Neurosurgery, and Psychiatry*, **11**, 64–6.

Scoville, W. B. and Milner, B. (1957). Loss of recent memory after bilateral hippocampal lesions. *Journal of Neurology, Neurosurgery, and Psychiatry*, **20**, 11–21.

Smith, M. L. and Milner, B. (1981). The role of the right hippocampus in the recall of spatial location. *Neuropsychologia*, **19**, 781–93.

Warrington, E. K. and Duchen, L. W. (1992). A re-appraisal of a case of persistent global amnesia following right temporal lobectomy: a clinico-pathological study. *Neuropsychologia*, **30**, 437–50.

Wolf, R. L., Ivnik, R. J., Hirschorn, K. A., Sharbrough, F. W., Cascino, G. D., and Marsh, W. R. (1993). Neurocognitive efficiency following left temporal lobectomy: standard versus limited resection. *Journal of Neurosurgery*, **76**, 76–83.

Yasargil, M. G., Teddy, P. J., and Roth, P. (1985). Selective amygdalohippocampectomy: operative anatomy and surgical technique. In *Advances and technical standards in neurosurgery*, Vol. 12, (ed. L. Symon, J. Brihaye, B. Guidetti *et al.*), pp. 93–123. Springer, Vienna.

Zola-Morgan, S., Squire, L. R., and Amaral, D. G. (1986). Human amnesia and the medial temporal region: enduring memory impairment following a bilateral lesion limited to field CA1 of the hippocampus. *Journal of Neuroscience*, **6**, 2950-67.

7

Memory systems in primates: episodic, semantic, and perceptual learning

AMANDA PARKER and DAVID GAFFAN

In the experimental study of memory, much research effort has been focused on investigating contrasts between spared and intact functions, using the logic of dissociation between different measures of memory. The evidence in favour of the concept of memory systems in the brain came in the first place from patients with acquired memory disorder ('organic amnesia'). Memory disorder is often produced as one component of a general loss of mental ability ('dementia'), but in some patients amnesia is a discrete disorder, leaving intact many other cognitive abilities such as reasoning, perception, and intelligence. Relatively pure amnesia of this kind is caused by relatively circumscribed brain damage, as opposed to the diffuse damage which is seen in dementia. Neuropathological analysis of the brain damage responsible for producing discrete amnesia suggests that the critical lesion for producing this disorder is any bilateral interruption of a system of interconnected structures. Evidence for other clearly defined memory systems is less solid as yet, but experimental evidence for a dissociable semantic memory system, and for perceptual learning mechanisms that operate relatively separably from episodic and semantic memory, will also be discussed in this chapter.

7.1 Episodic memory

The proposal that episodic memory formation is critically dependent on the 'Papez' circuit of cortical and subcortical structures has a long history in neuroscience, having been first suggested by Benedek and Juba (1940, 1941). Delay and Brion (1969) expanded the theory by proposing that diencephalic and temporal-lobe amnesia were caused by interrupting this circuit at different points, and evidence supporting this position has been accruing over the past half century. In a recent comprehensive review of human amnesia, Kopelman (1995, p. 159) concluded that 'the balance of the more recent evidence appears to suggest that it is a circuit comprising the hippocampus, entorhinal and perirhinal cortex, the mamillary bodies, mamillo-thalamic tract, and the anterior (rather than the medial dorsal) nucleus of the thalamus, which is critical in memory formation'. This list of structures is almost identical to the circuit proposed by Papez (1937), excepting the inclusion of the rhinal cortices and the exclusion of the cingulate gyrus.

Studies of patients with damage to structures of the Delay–Brion circuit can be difficult to interpret due to damage extending beyond the boundaries of these structures. The functional relationship between brain systems and memory is therefore revealed only imperfectly in such patients. The interpretation of such material has necessarily remained to some extent controversial or open to doubt. For example, the causative lesions are produced by the vagaries of disease and trauma; post-mortem neuropathological analysis does not necessarily reveal the whole extent of functional disorder; and the consequent memory impairments must be assessed against the background of wide individual variation in memory ability, in patients whose pre-morbid memory ability is usually unknown. For these and other reasons, a considerable effort has been devoted to the investigation of experimentally produced amnesia in non-human primates.

The results of early studies were puzzling in that macaque monkeys (*Macaca mulatta* and *M. fascicularis*) appeared to show little impairment in some simple tests of object memory after experimentally produced ablations in the Delay–Brion system. However, more recent experiments, investigating a wider range of memory tasks, have shown that these ablations produce a severe impairment in monkeys' memory for complex spatially organized scenes. These impairments are revealed in a wide variety of tasks, including spatial memory tasks in mazes (Murray *et al.* 1989), memory for the location of hidden food rewards (Gaffan and Harrison 1989), memory for complex naturalistic scenes such as frames from a cinema film (Gaffan 1992), and memory for artificial scenes generated by a formal algorithm on a computer-driven display (object-in-place task, Gaffan 1994*a*). After interruption of the Delay–Brion system, monkeys are not impaired in remembering objects independently of the scenes in which the objects were presented, but they are impaired in scene-specific object memory. In terms of cognitive psychology, the 'episodic memory' in which amnesic patients are severely impaired—that is, memory for specific personally experienced events—is analogous to the monkeys' memory for experienced events involving some specific objects set in a specific background or scene. This type of memory for complex specific events is contrasted with 'semantic memory'—that is, acquired general knowledge about objects, independent of any specific background or any specific discrete event. The experimental and clinical evidence indicates that the Delay–Brion system is specially involved in memory for events, as opposed to general knowledge which is not specific to some discrete event in a particular scene. This discovery leads naturally on to the idea that some other memory system or systems, independent of the Delay–Brion system, might be responsible for the kind of memory which is manifested in general knowledge about objects, independent of any one specific scene.

We have now completed a series of experiments (Fig. 7.1) in which pre- and post-operative performance was compared in monkeys with lesions to structures of the Delay–Brion circuit, using an experimental task designed to test episodic memory in monkeys. In the object-in-place memory task, the correct (rewarded) response in each scene is to a particular object of a pair, which always occupies a particular position in a unique background that has been generated using randomly chosen colours and shapes. In each session, the monkey learns a new list of these unique scenes. In the first experiment (Gaffan 1994*a*), a severe impairment in performance was found in monkeys with fornix transection. The second experiment in the series (Parker and Gaffan 1997*a*) showed a similarity of deficit between a fornix-transected group and a group of monkeys with mamillary-body lesions. Because of the spatial nature of the stimuli used in this experiment, it is possible to integrate these results to some extent with experiments that have tested the deficit caused by mamillary-body lesions in rats. Although there are significant species differences in the connections between structures in the Delay–Brion circuit in primates and rodents (Amaral 1987; Nitsch and Leranth 1994), making direct comparisons difficult, deficits in rats have been found frequently on tasks that require a spatial discrimination.

In the third experiment in this series (Parker and Gaffan 1997*b*), anterior thalamic lesions had a clear effect on object-in-place memory, resulting in a severe memory impairment. This result can be compared with case-study reports of human patients showing that focal lesions of anterior thalamus result in anterograde amnesia (Hankey and Stewart-Wynne 1988; Daum and Ackermann 1994; Kim *et al.* 1994) and with studies using rats, where tasks

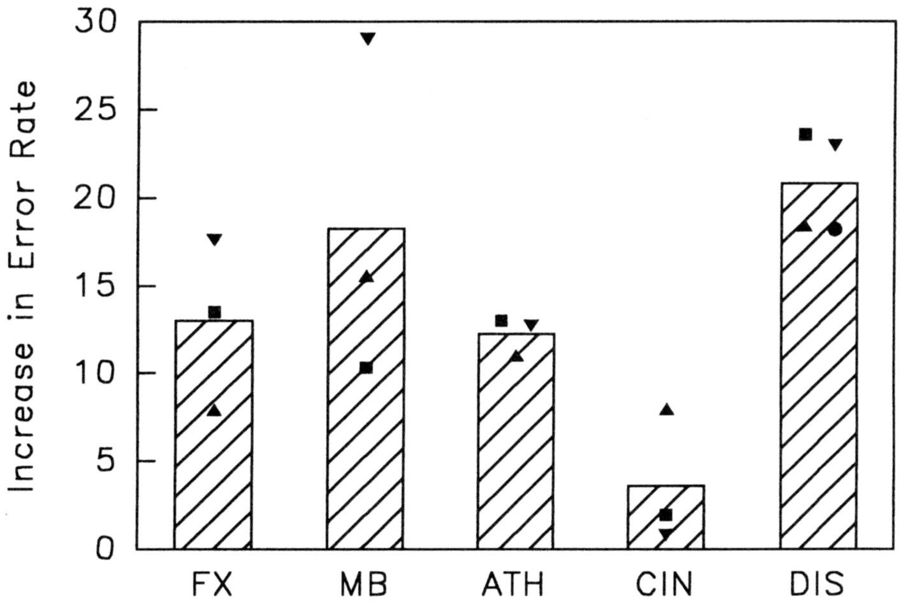

Fig. 7.1 A comparison of the increase in error score for five groups of animals from the object-in-place series of experiments; FX, fornix transection; MB, mamillary nuclei lesion; ANT, anterior thalamic lesion; CIN, cingulate cortex ablation; DIS, perirhinal / fornix disconnection.

having a spatial component have shown large deficits after anterior thalamic lesions, whereas object recognition memory has not shown such a substantial impairment (Aggleton *et al.* 1995*a*, *b*). In contrast to the impairment observed in the anterior thalamus-lesioned animals, a group of monkeys with cingulate cortex lesions was not significantly impaired. This lack of deficit compares well with the lack of reported cases of human amnesia following discrete cingulate cortex damage—the patient reported by Valenstein *et al.* (1987) had retrosplenial cortex damage, but there was a possibility of damage to both the cingulum bundle and the fornix. The results also are in accord with the lack of effect of cingulate cortex lesions in rat studies where the cingulum bundle has not been damaged (Neave *et al.* 1994; Aggleton *et al.* 1995*b*). These studies are in contrast to a series of experiments by Sutherland and his colleagues, who posit an important role for posterior cingulate cortex in spatial memory in the rat (Sutherland *et al.* 1988; Sutherland and Hoesing 1993). This issue is clearly not yet fully resolved, but the fact that the retrosplenial cortex has reciprocal connections with anterior thalamic nuclei, subiculum, and presubiculum certainly suggests some role in memory (Devinsky and Luciano 1993).

The performance of the animals in this series of experiments can be directly compared, as they followed the same experimental regime. As Fig. 7.1 illustrates, the mean increase in error score caused by anterior thalamic (12.2 per cent), fornix (13.0 per cent), and mamillary-body lesions (18.3 per cent) is very similar. The mean increase in error score seen after cingulate lesion (3.6 per cent) does not fit this pattern, suggesting that the cingulate gyrus is not a critical part of this circuit. Analysis of variance among these group means shows a statistically significant main effect. The equivalence of impairment in fornix, mamillary-body, and anterior thalamic lesioned monkeys in these studies strongly suggests that these structures form part of a single functional memory system. However, the lack of an impairment following cingulate ablation raises questions about the inclusion of the cingulate cortex as part of the circuit involved in episodic memory.

The pattern of thalamic degeneration observed in the cingulate-lesioned animals may begin to answer this question. The main focus of the degeneration was the centre of the AV nucleus, with a gradation to less degeneration in all directions. In all cases except one, nucleus AD was acellular, suggesting that the cingulum bundle had been damaged (Aggleton, personal communication). The area of undegenerated anterior thalamus was principally the AM nucleus, which projects to the inferior convexity of the frontal lobe and to the lower bank of the principal sulcus (Goldman-Rakic and Porrino 1985). One possible interpretation of these results is that connections are needed in the object-in-place task with the frontal lobe, for controlled reaching towards a specific target. As these connections are intact in the cingulate-lesioned animals, they are still able to do this task. Although we have been stressing the importance of the Delay–Brion system in integrating memorial representations of objects and space, the system is also important in the relationships of environmental stimuli to the disposition of the person or animal (limbs, head, and eyes) (Gaffan 1987). This distinction can be compared with the distinction between egocentric and allocentric processing. It could well be the case that monkeys with lesions in nuclei AV and AD, or in the cingulum bundle or cingulate cortex, may be impaired in tasks which stress highly the importance of whole-body orientation, and future experiments will investigate the possibility that frontal and subicular connections from the anterior thalamic nuclei play differing roles in episodic memory in primates.

7.2 Semantic memory

Patients with lesions in the neocortex of the anterior temporal lobe, sparing the Delay–Brion system, can show a syndrome which is, in some respects, complementary to the classical amnesic syndrome. Unlike amnesic patients, these patients do not show striking impairments in remembering discrete events, such as the visit of a family member or some particular meal; but, again unlike amnesic patients, they are deficient in general knowledge ('semantic memory') as tested, for example, by the ability to identify and describe a family member or a well-known food item (Hodges *et al.* 1992). The anatomical basis of this type of impairment has been elucidated by experiments with macaque monkeys.

Monkeys with discrete ablation of the perirhinal cortex (a strip of cortex in the anterior temporal lobe, lateral to the rhinal sulcus) show disorders of knowledge about objects. These disorders are revealed in discrimination learning tasks, in which the animal learns for food reward to choose the objects that the experimenter has arbitrarily designated as correct, in preference to other objects that the experimenter has designated as incorrect (Gaffan 1994*b*); a similar disorder is also revealed in the matching-to-sample task with objects, in which the monkey learns to choose the object that is identical to a given sample object (Gaffan and Murray 1992). Both of these impairments occur when the animal has to deal with a large population of objects, requiring an accurate specification of individual objects in order to perform the task correctly: the impairments in the same tasks disappear if only one pair of objects is used repeatedly throughout the experiment (Eacott *et al.* 1994). This kind of impairment was first discovered in experiments with delayed matching (or non-matching) to sample, and with large ablations of the medial temporal lobe, involving not only the perirhinal cortex but also the hippocampus and amygdala (Mishkin 1978). It is now known, however, that damage to the perirhinal cortex alone, sparing the hippocampus and amygdala, produces in these tasks an impairment of almost equal severity to that produced by large medial temporal ablations (Meunier *et al.* 1993). It is also now known that the delay component of delayed matching-to-sample, as tested in early experiments, is not crucial since an impairment is also seen in matching-to-sample with no delay (Eacott *et al.* 1994).

The proposal that the perirhinal cortex is important in knowledge about objects has received support from both monkey lesion and single cell recording experiments. Both Brown *et al.* (1987) and Miller *et al.* (1991) recorded from cells in this area during a visual recognition task and found differences in their responses to previously seen and novel stimuli. Horel *et al.* (1987) showed that both cooling and aspiration lesions of the inferior temporal gyrus, including perirhinal tissue, caused impairments in recognition memory. Gaffan and Murray (1990) tested object discrimination learning and delayed matching-to-sample (DMS) performance in animals with rhinal lesions. They found an impairment both in reacquisition of learned discriminations and DMS performance. More recent studies that have tested object memory in monkeys with lesions limited to perirhinal cortex have found severe impairments. Meunier *et al.* (1993) used a delayed non-matching-to-sample (DNMS) task, and found large post-operative deficits. Gaffan (1994*b*) found that perirhinal ablation caused impairments in DNMS and discrimination learning with complex naturalistic scenes.

7.3 Dissociations between episodic and semantic memory

The memory impairment produced by discrete perirhinal cortex ablation in the monkey is qualitatively dissimilar from that which follows discrete interruption of the Delay–Brion system, by fornix transection, for example. Monkeys with fornix transection are severely impaired in memory for the spatial organization of scenes, and only mildly impaired in matching-to-sample with objects; whereas monkeys with perirhinal cortex ablations show the opposite pattern (Gaffan 1994*b*). Thus, there is clear evidence for at least two distinct specialized memory systems in the primate temporal lobe, and the functions of these discrete anatomical structures correspond, at least in part, to the discrete cognitive functions of episodic memory and object knowledge, or semantic memory.

Why should episodic and semantic memory require separate but interacting systems? The tasks of providing an animal with a representation of objects and of its own position in space are both complex, each necessitating the interaction of a number of different but interrelated subsystems. The nature of the tasks involved requires that one system is not enough—this may well be due to the different computational rules which are necessary for these two types of memory. There is much evidence for the separation of visual processing into dorsal and ventral 'streams' (Ungerleider and Mishkin 1982). The nature of the computational problem that must be solved by the ventral, *object perception and recognition* stream is different from the problem that must be solved by the dorsal, *position in space* stream. In the first of these, the computational problem is concerned with the closed edges of objects and the details of what is inside these edges. Marr (1982) proposed that grouping rules solve the computational problem of grouping together the features that belong to the same 'thing'. This has similarities with the *Gestalt* principle of closure. In contrast, the dorsal stream has to solve the computational problem of the animal's position in, and interaction with, space, and the relative positions of objects compared to this position.

Experimental and anatomical evidence suggest that the perirhinal cortex supplies information about objects to the hippocampusfornix system: therefore one should expect that disconnection of the perirhinal cortex from the fornix would impair object-in-place memory. An experiment by Gaffan and Parker (1996) tested this hypothesis by training animals on the object-in-place memory task, and then making crossed unilateral lesions of the fornix and perirhinal cortex, combined with partial forebrain commisurotomy (involving sectioning the body and splenium of the corpus callosum) to prevent intrahemispheric transfer of visual information between the hemispheres. Post-operatively all the animals showed a severe impairment in object-in-place learning. This impairment was similar in severity to those that have been seen in earlier studies of the object-in-place memory task after bilateral lesions in either the fornix, mamillary bodies, or the anterior nuclei of the thalamus (Fig. 7.1).

The perirhinal cortex and the subiculum of the hippocampus are connected reciprocally within each hemisphere (Amaral and Insausti 1990) and, in addition, can exchange information indirectly by projections to and from the entorhinal cortex (Insausti *et al.* 1987; Witter and Amaral 1991). The majority of the fibres that project in the fornix to the mamillary bodies and anterior thalamus arise from cells of the subiculum and/or hippocampus (Amaral and Insausti 1990). Thus, in the normal brain, visual information can flow from the perirhinal cortex via the subiculum and fornix into the mamillary bodies and anterior thalamus. This information flow was prevented by the surgical disconnection carried out by Gaffan and Parker (1996). The effect of this disconnection shows that normal performance of the object-in-place memory task depends on information flow from the perirhinal cortex into the fornix, and thence to the mamillary bodies and anterior thalamic nuclei.

The perirhinal cortex and the fornix can function independently of each other in some memory tasks. This is shown by the dissociated effects of bilateral lesions in these two structures. For example, monkeys with bilateral fornix transection were impaired in a serial spatial discrimination learning task in which one of two locations (left and right) contained food; but monkeys with bilateral perirhinal cortex ablation were not impaired in this task (Gaffan 1994*b*). Therefore the fornix has a function in some spatial memory tasks that does not depend on the perirhinal cortex. On the other hand, the same monkeys with bilateral perirhinal cortex ablations were more severely impaired than the fornix-transected monkeys in visual delayed matching-to-sample with naturalistic pictures (Gaffan 1994*b*). Furthermore, lesions restricted to the perirhinal cortex produced severe impairments in delayed non-matching-to-sample with visual objects (Meunier *et al.* 1993), but fornix transection produced only mild impairments in several experiments using delayed matching-to-sample or non-matching-to-sample with visual objects.

Therefore, the perirhinal cortex has a function in some visual delayed matching-to-sample tasks that does not depend on the fornix. These dissociations show that the perirhinal cortex and the fornix are not parts of a single memory system.

In the monkey, the Delay–Brion circuit is essential not only for the object-in-place task but also for spatial memory tasks of various kinds. The object-in-place task does not overtly require the monkey to remember the spatial organization of the scenes in the task, but memory for spatial organization of the scenes enhances performance by reducing interference in memory among scenes (Gaffan 1994*a*). Therefore, all these tasks that rely on the fornix for normal performance in the monkey, overtly or covertly require the animal to remember the spatial arrangement of scenes. Memory for spatial organization plays an analogous role in human episodic memory (Gaffan 1994*a*), and increased susceptibility to interference among different scenes or contexts may therefore underlie the effects of fornix transection on human episodic memory (McMackin *et al.* 1995). Ablations restricted to the perirhinal cortex, on the other hand, impair trial-unique matching or non-matching to sample (Meunier *et al.* 1993; Gaffan 1994*b*), but lesions of both perirhinal and entorhinal cortex did not impair matching to sample with a restricted set of stimuli that were used repeatedly within each session (Eacott *et al.* 1994). Eacott *et al.* argued that this pattern of spared and impaired memory performance reflected the role of the perirhinal cortex in identifying multiple individual objects.

To summarize this section, we draw three conclusions:

1. The fornix but not the perirhinal cortex is essential for tasks such as the simple spatial learning task of Gaffan (1994*b*), in which the monkey needs to remember the spatial arrangement of a scene but not the location of multiple individual objects.
2. The perirhinal cortex but not the fornix is essential for tasks such as trial-unique matching to sample with objects, in which the monkey needs to remember multiple individual objects but not their spatial arrangement.
3. Information flow from the perirhinal cortex into the subiculum and fornix is essential for tasks such as the object-in-place task, in which the monkey needs to remember spatial arrangements of multiple individual objects.

7.4 Perceptual learning

Both episodic and semantic memory can be seen as the products of associative learning, in which improvement in performance is attributed to the acquisition of an association between some stimulus that acts as a retrieval cue and some separate event with which that stimulus is correlated in time. Perceptual learning, by contrast, is said to occur when an improvement in performance cannot be attributed to any such association formed to a stimulus, but results instead from an improvement in the perceptual processing of the stimulus itself. One way to demonstrate such an improvement is by physiological measurement of the neuronal activity in sensory pathways. For example, monkeys given extensive practice in a tactual discrimination, in which one particular digit of one hand was always used to make the discrimination, showed an expanded representation of that digit in the somatosensory cortex (Recanzone *et al.* 1992), and human Braille readers have a similar expanded somatosensory representation of the digit used for reading (Pascualleone and Torres 1993). Perceptual learning can also be demonstrated by behavioural measures. For example, stimuli that have benefited from a perceptual learning process support unusually rapid learning in a subsequent associative learning task, presumably because of their enhanced discriminability (Gibson and Walk 1956). The connection between these two approaches to the study of perceptual learning, the physiological and the psychological, has rarely been explored. In a full review of psychological treatments of perceptual learning, Hall (1991) made no mention of any physiological measurements.

McLaren *et al.* (1989) put forward an explanation of perceptual learning in terms of associative learning. The associative learning that takes part during perceptual learning, according to this view, is not the acquisition of associations between a stimulus and some separate event, but the acquisition of associations among the elements or features of the stimulus itself. According to this account, when an animal repeatedly perceives two different stimuli, A and B, the elements of A become associated with each other, the elements of B become associated with each other, elements common to A and B receive more latent inhibition than elements present in only one of the stimuli, and inhibitory associations are formed between elements that are present in one of the stimuli but not in the other. Each of these three associative changes that are intrinsic to the stimuli A and B has the effect that the stimuli will support more rapid extrinsic differential associative learning when, in a subsequent phase, they are associated with different events, such as A with food and B with no food, as compared with a control pair of stimuli, C and D, which had not benefited from perceptual learning. Thus, perceptual learning is explained as a product of a particular example of associative learning—that is, the formation of associations between the elements of stimuli.

The account of McLaren *et al.* is particularly plausible as an explanation of perceptual learning with complex stimuli, such as the extra-maze cues in a spatial learning experiment with rats (Rodrigo *et al.* 1994). Intuitively, the stimuli to which a rat is exposed in the arm of an open radial maze contain many independent elements that can enter into association with each other. The purpose of the first of a recent series of experiments (Gaffan 1996) was to measure perceptual learning in the monkey with similarly complex stimuli, composed of multiple independent elements. The stimuli were artificially generated complex background scenes, as discussed earlier. Unlike the experiments using this task discussed above, each monkey had the same 20 scenes each day, while the determination of correct and incorrect objects by the experimenter changed randomly from day to day. If the monkey's learning proficiency improved from day to day when the same scenes were used every day, this improvement could not be attributed to the extrinsic associations of the foreground objects with food and no food, which changed randomly from day to day. Instead the improvement would be attributable to perceptual learning about the scenes, which, according to McLaren *et al.*, consists of the acquisition of associations among features of the scenes. To check that this improvement was specific to the particular scenes that the animals had experienced, rather than some general improvement in the strategy of learning, the set of scenes that each animal learned about was changed every 4 days. A further experiment along similar lines (Experiment 1b) was designed to test whether experience with particular individual scenes could lead to improvement specific to those individual scenes, as opposed to the improvement in a whole set of scenes, as measured in Experiment 1a.

The results of Experiment 1a (Fig. 7.2) showed that the monkeys improved their within-day learning rate substantially when the same set of scenes was used for four successive days. One might have predicted that a between-day improvement would be seen, particularly with scenes in which the animal's initial preference on any day was for the object that happened to be correct on that day, but there was no sign of a difference in the between-day improvement according to the animal's initial preference (Fig. 7.2*b*). Furthermore, it is not possible to explain these results as simply an example of learning-set formation (learning the strategy appropriate to the task), since the improvement was specific to the specific sets of scenes, returning to baseline on the first day with each successive new set (Fig. 7.2*a*). Thus, this experiment showed perceptual

---

Fig. 7.2 Results from Gaffan 1996, Experiment 1a. In each daily session the monkeys learned to choose one of two unique objects in each of a list of 20 unique scenes. Choice accuracy on the first block of trials was necessarily at chance (50 per cent correct) and the proficiency of within-day learning is measured, in all three panels of the figure, by choice accuracy in the remaining seven trial blocks of each day. (a)The average of the three monkeys' proficiency in within-day learning over a series of 20 days in which five sets of scenes were presented for four successive days each, the correct object in each scene being newly determined at random at the beginning of each daily session. The change to a new set of scenes is shown by the gap in the line of the graph, and it can be seen that learning proficiency improved with experience with each new set of scenes, reverting to a lower baseline of proficiency whenever a new set was introduced. (b) The effect of the monkeys' preference between objects in a scene, as expressed by choices on trial block 1 when no other information was available to guide choice. The hollow triangles show, for the three monkeys on average and for the five sets of scenes on average, the within-day learning proficiency for scenes in which the first-trial choice on that day happened to be correct, and the filled triangles show the proficiency for the scenes in which it happened to be wrong. Not surprisingly, proficiency as measured here was higher (fewer errors) for the scenes in which the first choice happened to be correct; but the perceptual learning effect of improvement across the 4 days within a set was seen in both types of scene. (c) The results from individual monkeys in open symbols,

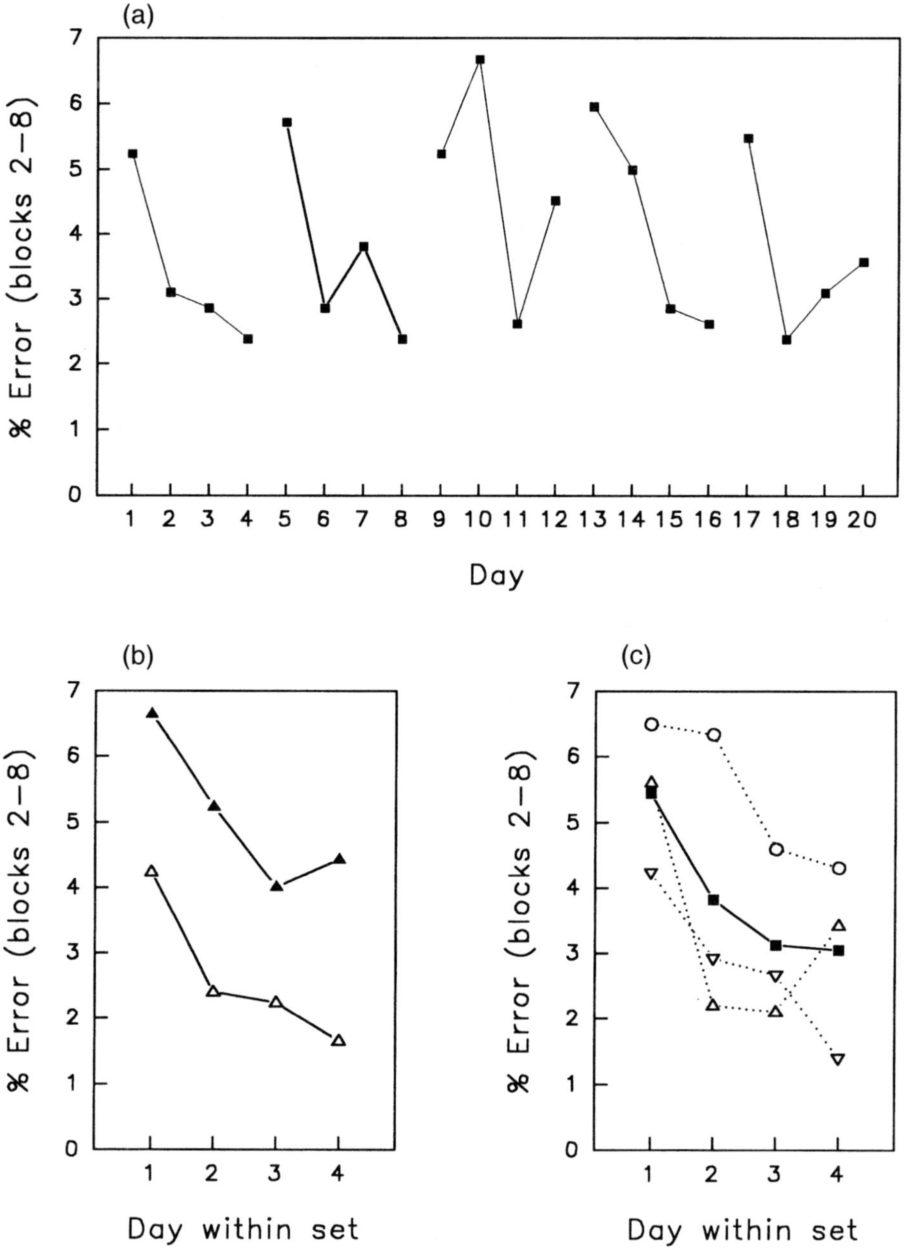

averaged across five sets of scenes and averaged across scenes with a correct first-trial choice and scenes with an incorrect first-trial choice (circle, S1; inverted triangle, S2; triangle, S3; filled square, group average). It can be seen that all three individuals showed, on average, a trend of improvement in within-day learning proficiency across the 4 days with any set of scenes. (Data from Gaffan 1996.)

learning according to the usual criterion for perceptual learning, a stimulus-specific enhancement in the rate of subsequent associative learning.

The procedure used in Experiment 1 was derived from several previous experiments in which monkeys were exposed repeatedly to the same stimuli each day, even though only within-day memories were specifically relevant to task performance. Monkeys perform at high levels when the same set of stimuli is used each day, in spite of the fact that specific memories from one day are made irrelevant to the next day's performance. For example, monkeys learned a recognition memory task where a constant set of pictures was used in each daily session and each picture appeared twice in each session; the first appearance of any picture in any session was not rewarded but the second appearance was rewarded (Gaffan 1977). Specific memory of having seen the picture on previous days is not relevant to this task, and on the basis of interference theory, memory from previous days might even be expected to interfere with the relevant memory task of determining whether a picture has or has not been seen today. Nevertheless, normal monkeys performed virtually perfectly in this task. Todd and Mackintosh (1990) have pointed out that such a task pits memory interference against perceptual learning, suggesting that the advantage derived from perceptual learning outweighs any disadvantage arising from interference in memory between days.

These results from complex scenes in Experiments 1a and 1b fit well with the associative theory of perceptual learning (McLaren *et al.* 1989). The two objects within a scene, which have to be differentiated as predictors of food reward or its absence within a session, are each represented by a complex of features, including the features of the position within the background that each object always occupies. The three types of association that are formed among the elements of stimuli, according to the theory of McLaren *et al.,* could thus be formed among the features of the two objects within any scene, and would then facilitate within-day learning in the same scene on subsequent days. However, the account of McLaren *et al.* is less intuitively attractive if applied to perceptual learning with simple stimuli. Experiment 2 therefore explored monkeys' perceptual learning with colours. Within each day the animals learned which of two colours was rewarded that day. As in Experiment 1, the reward associations of the stimuli could not explain between-day improvement when the same colours were used every day, since the reward associations changed from day to day.

The results of Experiment 2 (Fig. 7.3) show an even more powerful perceptual learning effect than in Experiment 1. Monkeys trained with repeated daily reversals between a pair of colours, similar to the random reversals used in Experiment 1, showed a gradual improvement in the rate of within-day learning. In order to reconcile the results of Experiment 2 with the psychological associative theory of perceptual learning (McLaren *et al.* 1989), one has to make some rather artificial assumptions. The reason for this is that colours are not, intuitively, composed of separate elements. Certainly, a coloured square may be thought of as a combination between shape features and a colour feature, but associations with the shape features of the coloured squares used in Experiment 2 cannot explain the colour-specific improvement, because the shape features are common to all the stimuli in the experiment. For example, if the shape features decline in associability due to latent inhibition, as specified by the associative theory, the consequent enhancement of within-day learning should transfer to a new colour on day 33 because the shape features do not change. The colours themselves (almost pure reds, greens, or blues) have to be composed of elements if the associative theory of perceptual learning (McLaren *et al.* 1989) is to explain these data. One could, of course, declare that the perception of a colour consists of the simultaneous activation of many colour-sensitive elements, perhaps corresponding to different cells in the visual cortex, but this is a physiological theory rather than one appealing to the intuitive notion of a complex stimulus as consisting of elements such as its shape and colour. If one is to construct a physiological theory of perceptual learning, one might as well therefore begin with the direct physiological evidence.

Extensive experience with a class of stimuli results in expansion of the cortical representation of those stimuli, as discussed earlier. Perceptual learning appears to result from an expanded cortical representation of repeatedly

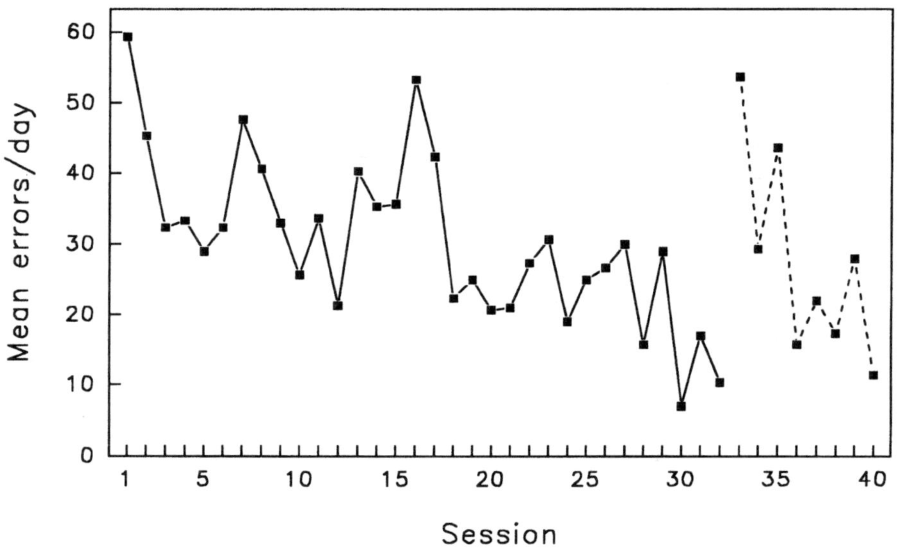

Fig 7.3 Results from Gaffan (1996) Experiment 2. Days 1–32, one monkey became expert at within-day discrimination learning between almost pure red colours, a second between almost pure greens, and a third between almost pure blues. Days 33–40, each monkey was switched to another monkey's colours. The increase in errors between day 32 and day 33 shows that some of the improvement in days 1–32 was specific to the particular colours with which each monkey became expert. (Data from Gaffan 1996.)

perceived stimuli. It is reasonable to predict, on the basis of Experiment 2, that a monkey with extensive training in almost pure red colours (for example) should show an increase in the number of cortical cells responding to those colours, as compared to almost pure blues or greens. This prediction has not, to our knowledge, been specifically tested, but it is simply an extrapolation of the findings of similar experiments on auditory and tactual stimuli (Recanzone *et al.* 1992, 1993) and visual patterns. The monkey's visual cortex shows an increase in the number of cells responding differentially to the particular patterns with which the monkey has been trained (Sakai *et al.* 1994). The increased responsiveness of the visual cortex to patterns with which the monkey has been trained is an expansion of the cortical representation of those patterns, even though the cells are not spatially organized into a map like the map of the monkey's hand in the somatosensory experiments (Recanzone 1992). Colour discrimination in the monkey depends on the temporal lobe visual association cortex (Heywood *et al.* 1995) in which an expanded representation of trained monochromatic patterns has been observed (Sakai *et al.* 1994).

In the light of this physiological evidence for expanded cortical representation of stimuli that a subject has perceived repeatedly, the results of Experiment 2 can be explained plausibly by assuming an expanded cortical representation of the trained colours, and, if so, there is no need for an artificial explanation in terms of associations between hypothetical elements of colours. But if the expanded-representation hypothesis is accepted for Experiment 2, parsimony demands the same explanation for Experiment 1, that is, an expanded cortical representation of the particular stimuli with which an animal has been trained; this explanation renders otiose the psychological hypothesis of associations among stimulus elements as the explanation of perceptual learning (McLaren *et al.* 1989).

7.5 Conclusions

The model of multiple memory systems that we have presented in this chapter and elsewhere stresses the flexibility with which different functional types of memory can be adapted to different tasks. This allows for some redundancy, and means that damage to one system can often be compensated for to some extent. Figure 7.4 illustrates the information flow between some of the anatomical regions involved primarily in visual processing. The crucial point that the results of our experiments illustrate is that each of these areas *can* have independent access to behavioural output, as well as combined output through episodic memory. For example, TE sends information about visual qualities of objects to the perirhinal cortex, and can also influence behaviour through its direct connections with the striatum. Unravelling the effects of lesions to separate regions is therefore a complex process requiring very specifically designed tasks.

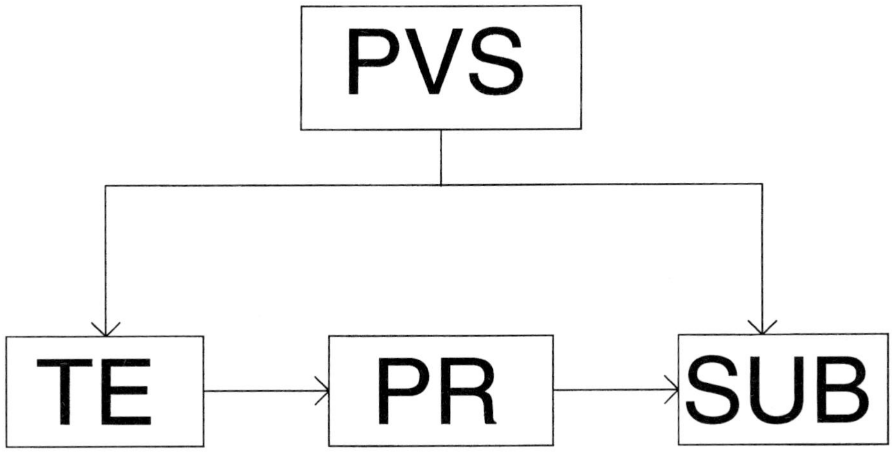

Fig. 7.4 Flow of visual information through some anatomical areas involved in object and spatial processing; PVS, posterior visual system; TE, area TE of von Bonin and Bailey (1947); PR, perirhinal cortex; SUB, subiculum.

The functional relationships between perceptual learning and associative learning are of potentially great importance. It may be that understanding of the physiological basis of perceptual learning can be extended into a physiological explanation of associative learning, a development opposite in direction but similar in ambition to the explanation of perceptual learning by associative learning offered by McLaren *et al.* (1989). Learning that an event A is associated with an event B may consist neurally of an expanded cortical representation of the complex event A-with-B, the same change as that underlying perceptual learning with complex stimuli. Together with the discussion of specialized memory systems, which was put forward earlier, such a hypothesis would go far towards meeting the demand (Vanderwolf and Cain 1994) for a neurobiological, as opposed to psychological, approach to the study of memory.

References

Aggleton, J. P., Neave, N., Nagle, S., and Hunt, P. R. (1995*a*). A comparison of the effects of anterior thalamic, mamillary body and fornix lesion on reinforced spatial alternation. *Behavioural Brain Research*, **68**, 91–101.

Aggleton, J. P., Neave, N., Nagle, S., and Sahgal, A. (1995*b*). A comparison of the effects of medial prefrontal, cingulate cortex, and cingulum bundle lesions on tests of spatial memory: evidence of a double dissociation between frontal and cingulum bundle contributions. *Journal of Neuroscience*, **15**, 7270–81.

Amaral, D. G. (1987). Memory: anatomical organization of candidate brain regions. In *Handbook of physiology—the nervous system, V*, (ed. V. B. Mountcastle), pp. 211–94. American Physiological Assocation, Bethesda, MD.
Amaral, D. G. and Instausi, R. (1990). Hippocampal Formation. In *The human nervous system*, (ed. G. Paxinos), pp. 711–55. Academic Press, London.
Benedek, L. and Juba, A. (1940). Weitere Beiträge zur Frage des anatomischen Substrates des Korsakowchen Symptomen Komplexes. *Archive für Psychiatrie und Nervenkrankheiten*, **112,** 505–16.
Benedek, L. and Juba, A. (1941). Über das anatomische Substrat des Korsakowschen Syndromes. Schweizerisches *Archiv für Psychiatrie und Nervenkrankheiten*, **46**, 174–84.
Brown, M. W., Wilson, F. A. W., and Riches, I. P. (1987). Neuronal evidence that inferomedial temporal cortex is more important than hippocampus in certain processes underlying recognition memory. *Brain Research*, **409**, 158–62.
Daum, I. and Ackermann, H. (1994). Frontal-type memory impairment associated with thalamic damage. *International Journal of Neuroscience*, **77**, 187–98.
Delay, J. and Brion, S. (1969). *Le Syndrome de Korsakoff*. Masson, Paris.
Devinsky, O. and Luciano, D. (1993). The contribution of cingulate cortex to human behavior. In *Neurobiology of cingulate cortex and limbic thalamus*, (ed. B. A. Vogt and M. Gabriel), pp. 528–56. Birkhauser, Boston.
Eacott, M. J., Gaffan, D., and Murray, E. A. (1994). Preserved recognition memory for small sets, and impaired stimulus identification for large sets, following rhinal cortex ablation in monkeys. *European Journal of Neuroscience*, **6**, 1466–78.
Gaffan, D. (1977). Monkeys' recognition memory for complex pictures and the effect of fornix transection. *Quarterly Journal of Experimental Psychology*, **29**, 505–14.
Gaffan, D. (1987). Amnesia, personal memory and the hippocampus: experimental neuropsychological studies in monkeys. In *Cognitive neurochemistry*, (ed. S. M. Stahl, S. D. Iversen, and E. C. Goodman), pp. 46–56. Oxford University Press, Oxford.
Gaffan, D. (1992). Amnesia for complex naturalistic scenes and for objects following fornix transection in the Rhesus monkey. *European Journal of Neuroscience*, **4,** 381–8.
Gaffan, D. (1994*a*). Scene-specific memory for objects: a model of episodic memory impairment in monkeys with fornix transection. *Journal of Cognitive Neuroscience*, **6,** 305–20.
Gaffan, D. (1994*b*). Dissociated effects of perirhinal cortex ablation, fornix transection and amygdalectomy: evidence for multiple memory systems in the primate temporal lobe. *Experimental Brain Research*, **99,** 411–22.
Gaffan, D. (1996). Associative and perceptual learning and the concept of memory systems. *Cognitive Brain Research*, **5**, 69–80.
Gaffan, D. and Gaffan, E. A. (1991). Amnesia in man following transection of the fornix: a review. *Brain*, **114,** 2611–18.
Gaffan, D. and Harrison, S. (1989). Place memory and scene memory: effects of fornix transection in the monkey. *Experimental Brain Research*, **74,** 202–12.
Gaffan D. and Murray E. A. (1990). Amygdalar interaction with the mediodorsal nucleus of the thalamus and the ventromedial prefrontal cortex in stimulus–reward associative learning in the monkey. *Journal of Neuroscience*, **10,** 3479–93.
Gaffan, D. and Murray, E. A. (1992). Monkeys *(Macaca fascicularis)* with rhinal cortex ablations succeed in object discrimination learning despite 24-hr intertrial intervals and fail at matching to sample despite double sample presentations. *Behavioral Neuroscience*, **106,** 30–8.
Gaffan, D. and Parker, A. (1996) Interaction of perirhinal cortex and the fornix–fimbria in primate memory: memory for objects and object-in-place memory. *Journal of Neuroscience*, **16**, 5864–9.

Gibson, E. J. and Walk, R. D. (1956). The effect of prolonged exposure to visually presented patterns on learning to discriminate them. *Journal of Comparative Physiological Psychology*, **49**, 239–42.

Goldman–Rakic, P. S. and Porrino, L. J. (1985). The primate mediodorsal (MD) nucleus and its projections to the frontal lobe. *Journal of Comparative Neurology*, **242**, 535–60.

Hall, G. (1991). *Perceptual and associative learning*. Oxford University Press, Oxford.

Hankey, G. L. and Stewart–Wynne, E. G. (1988). Amnesia following thalamic hemorrhage. Another stroke syndrome. *Stroke*, **19**, 776–8.

Heywood, C. A., Gaffan, D., and Cowey, A. (1995). Cerebral achromatopsia in monkeys. *European Journal of Neuroscience*, **7**, 1064–73.

Hodges, J. R., Patterson, K., Oxbury, S., and Funnell, E. (1992). Semantic dementia: progressive fluent aphasia with temporal lobe atrophy. *Brain*, **115**, 1783–806.

Horel, J. A., Pytko–Joiner, D. E., Voytko, M. L., and Salsbury, K. (1987). The performance of visual tasks while segments of the inferotemporal cortex are suppressed by cold. *Behavioural Brain Research*, **23**, 29–42.

Insausti, R., Amaral, D. G., and Cowan, W. M. (1987). The entorhinal cortex of the monkey: II. Cortical afferents. *Journal of Comparative Neurology*, **264**, 356–95.

Kim, M. H., Hong, S. B., and Roh, J. K. (1994). Amnesia syndrome following left thalamic infarction. *Journal of Korean Medical Science*, **9**, 427–31.

Kopelman, M. D. (1995). The Korsakoff syndrome. *British Journal of Psychiatry*, **166**, 154–73.

McLaren, I. P. L., Kaye, H., and Mackintosh, N. J. (1989). An associative theory of the representation of stimuli: applications to perceptual learning and latent inhibition. In *Parallel distributed processing: implications for psychology and neuroscience*, (ed. R. G. M. Morris), pp. 102–30. Oxford University Press, Oxford.

McMackin, D., Cockburn, J., Anslow, P., and Gaffan, D. (1995). Correlation of fornix damage with memory impairment in six cases of colloid cyst removal. *Acta Neurochirurgica*, **135**, 12–18.

Mair, W. G. P., Warrington, E. K., and Weiskrantz, L. (1979). Memory disorder in Korsakoff's psychosis: a neuropathological and neuropsychological investigation of two cases. *Brain*, **102**, 749–83.

Marr, D. (1982). *Vision*. Freeman, San Francisco.

Meunier, M., Bachevalier, J., Mishkin, M., and Murray, E. A. (1993). Effects on visual recognition of combined and separate ablations of the entorhinal and perirhinal cortex in rhesus monkeys. *Journal of Neuroscience*, **13**, 5418–32.

Miller, E. K., Lin, L., and Desimone, R. (1991). A neural mechanism for working and recognition memory in inferior temporal cortex. *Science*, **254**, 1377–9.

Mishkin, M. (1978). Memory in monkeys severely impaired by combined but not by separate removal of amygdala and hippocampus. *Nature*, **273**, 297–8.

Murray, E. A., Davidson, M., Gaffan, D., Olton, D. S., and Suomi, S. J. (1989). Effects of fornix transection and cingulate cortical ablation on spatial memory in Rhesus monkeys. *Experimental Brain Research*, **74**, 173–86.

Neave, N., Lloyd, S., Sahgal, A., and Aggleton, J. P. (1994). Lack of effect of lesions in the anterior cingulate cortex and retrosplenial cortex on certain tests of spatial memory in the rat. *Behavioural Brain Research*, **65**, 89–101.

Nitsch, R. and Leranth, C. (1994). Substance P-containing hypothalamic afferents to the monkey hippocampus: an immunocytochemical, tracing and coexistence study. *Experimental Brain Research*, **101**, 231–40.

Papez, J. W. (1937). A proposed mechanism of emotion. *Archive of Neurological Psychiatry*, **38**, 725–43.

Parker, A. and Gaffan, D. (1997*a*). Mamillary body lesions in monkeys impair object-in-place memory: functional unity of the fornix–mamillary system. *Journal of Cognitive Neuroscience*, **9**, 512–21.

Parker, A. and Gaffan, D. (1997*b*). The effect of anterior thalamic and cingulate cortex lesions on object-in-place memory in monkeys. *Neuropsychologia*, **35**, 1093–102.

Pascualleone, A. and Torres, F. (1993). Plasticity of the sensorimotor cortex representation of the reading finger in Braille readers. *Brain*, **116**, 39–52.

Recanzone, G. H., Merzenich, M. M., Jenkins, W. M., Grajski, K. A., and Dinse, H. R. (1992). Topographic reorganization of the hand representation in cortical area 3b of owl monkeys trained in a frequency-discrimination task. *Journal of Neurophysiology*, **67**, 1031–56.

Recanzone, G. H., Schreiner, C. E., and Merzenich, M. M. (1993). Plasticity in the frequency representation of primary auditory cortex following discrimination training in adult owl monkeys. *Journal of Neuroscience*, **13**, 87–103.

Rodrigo, T., Chamizo, V. D., McLaren, I. P. L., and Mackintosh, N. J. (1994). Effects of pre-exposure to the same or different pattern of extra-maze cues on subsequent extra-maze discrimination. *Quarterly Journal of Experimental Psychology*, **47B**, 15–26.

Sakai, K., Naya, Y., and Miyashita, Y. (1994). Neuronal tuning and associative mechanisms in form representation. *Learning and Memory*, **1**, 83–105.

Sutherland, R. J. and Hoesing, J. M. (1993). Posterior cingulate cortex and spatial memory. In *Neurobiology of cingulate cortex and limbic thalamus*, (ed. B. A.Vogt and M. Gabriel), pp. 462–6. Birkhauser, Boston.

Sutherland, R. J., Wishaw, I. Q., and Kolb, B. (1988). Contributions of cingulate cortex to two forms of spatial learning and memory. *Journal of Neuroscience*, **8**, 1863–72.

Todd, I. A. and Mackintosh, N. J. (1990). Evidence for perceptual learning in pigeons' recognition memory for pictures. *Quarterly Journal of Experimental Psychology*, **42B**, 385–400.

Ungerleider, L. G. and Mishkin, M. (1982). Two cortical visual systems. In *Advances in the analysis of visual behavior*, (ed. D. J. Ingle, M. A. Goodale, and R. J. W. Mansfield), pp. 549–86. MIT Press, Cambridge, Mass.

Valenstein, E., Bowers, D., Verfaellie, M., Heilman, K. M., Day, A., and Watson, R. T. (1987). Retrosplenial amnesia. *Brain*, **110**, 1631–46.

Vanderwolf, C. H. and Cain, D. P. (1994). The behavioral neurobiology of learning and memory: a conceptual reorientation. *Brain Research Reviews*, **19**, 264–97.

Von Bonin, G. and Bailey, P. (1947). *The neocortex of* Macaca mulatta. University of Illinois, Urbana, IL.

Witter, M. P. and Amaral, D. G. (1991). Entorhinal cortex of the monkey: V. Projections to the dentate gyrus, hippocampus and subicular complex. *Journal of Comparative Neurology*, **307**, 437–59.

8

Interhemispheric transfer following partial commissurotomy in humans and monkeys

MADELINE J. EACOTT

The corpus callosum is the largest fibre tract in the human brain. In humans it has been estimated to contain 200 million fibres (Gazzaniga and LeDoux 1978). The size and prominent position of the corpus callosum in the brain led to it being one of the earliest structures to be investigated; as early as the second century ad, Galen claimed that it served to suspend the cerebral hemispheres from the skull. While much progress has been made since that time in our understanding of the role that the corpus callosum plays in the transfer of information between the two cerebral hemispheres, there are still gaps in our knowledge. This chapter will attempt to review what has been learnt about interhemispheric communication in the monkey, where the corpus callosum and anterior commissure between them contain about 53 million fibres (La Mantia and Rakic 1990), and compare this with what is known about the role of the corpus callosum and anterior commissure in humans.

8.1 The anatomy of the forebrain commissures

Evidence that the corpus callosum served more than simply a structural role in suspending the hemispheres from the skull came in 1890 when Mott and Schaeffer suggested that the axons of the corpus callosum had cell bodies in one hemisphere and their terminals in the other, and therefore formed a bridge between the hemispheres. While this view was roundly criticized at the time by Ranson (1895) who believed that the callosal fibres arose from the thalamus, the idea of the corpus callosum as an interhemispheric pathway soon gained widespread acceptance. The type of interhemispheric connections made by the corpus callosum was clarified by Sherrington (1889), who made lesions of the motor cortex in both dogs and monkeys. By tracing the path of degeneration that followed such lesions, Sherrington was able to identify the paths of the fibre tracts that originated in the lesioned area. He traced degeneration to points in the ipsilateral hemisphere and, by way of the corpus callosum, to many points in the contralateral hemisphere. Interestingly, both homotopic and heterotopic points in the contralateral hemisphere were represented, indicating that the corpus callosum does not simply interconnect symmetrical points across the midline. Typically the corpus callosum connects both homotopic regions and areas on the contralateral hemisphere that are symmetrically opposite those areas to which the originating area is connected in the ipsilateral hemisphere (Mettler 1935). Moreover, fibres are arranged within the corpus callosum in such a way that, in general, they connect regions by the shortest possible route (Curtis and Bard 1939). The important implication of this simple geography is that the corpus callosum is not a unitary structure but different subsections of it interconnect different brain regions. As Curtis and Bard showed, lesions of the medial and ventral prefrontal regions resulted in degeneration in the anterior parts of the corpus callosum, in the dorsal parts of the genu. The central portion of the callosum appears to carry fibres connecting the sensory motor areas, while the posterior section, the splenium, connects the occipital and temporal lobes (Pandya and Seltzer 1986). However, despite this principle of segregation, there is still some overlap within the corpus callosum of fibres that originate from different areas (Seltzer and Pandya 1973; Pandya and Seltzer 1986). For example, fibres originating from the caudal inferior parietal lobule and the medial parietal lobule pass through the same region of the corpus callosum, at the anterior limit of the splenium (Pandya and Seltzer 1986). Similar overlap of fibres can be seen for fibres originating in the frontal lobe (Barbas and Pandya 1984) and the occipital lobe (Tieman *et al.* 1977).

8.2 Behavioural effects of forebrain commissurotomy: the early studies

The above studies serve only to clarify the anatomical role of the corpus callosum and reveal nothing of its function in the brain. Indeed, evidence as to the role it played in the brain was much harder to come by. Despite some historic attempts to explain the effects of brain damage by disconnection of the cerebral hemispheres (discussed by Trevarthen 1990), in 1944 Akelaitis was still able to claim that sectioning the corpus callosum for clinical purposes in humans had no adverse behavioural effects. However, subsequent follow-up studies of the patients of Akelaitis revealed that they did indeed have some deficits which had previously gone undetected, and in any case may well have had incomplete section of the commissures (Goldstein and Joynt 1969). The failure to note deficits which existed in these patients illustrates the importance of knowing where to look when searching for neuropsychological deficits. The important signpost in this search came from the ground-breaking work of Sperry and Myers on cats (Myers and Sperry 1953; Myers 1955, 1956; Sperry *et al.* 1956). Using optic chiasma section and monocular viewing to lateralize visual input to one hemisphere, Myers and Sperry demonstrated that visual information could only be transferred to the other hemisphere when the corpus callosum was intact. When the corpus callosum was surgically sectioned, each hemisphere appeared to be unaware of the visual information in the other. Thus the corpus callosum was the conduit for the interhemispheric transfer of visual information. These early findings were soon replicated using the monkey (Downer 1958; Sperry 1958) and the chimpanzee (Black and Myers 1964).

Downer, for example, found that pattern and colour discriminations learned by monkeys following optic chiasma section and when viewing with one eye were only transferred to the other eye if the interhemispheric commissures were intact. In fact, in both the monkey and the chimpanzee both the corpus callosum and the anterior commissure have to be sectioned in order to prevent interhemispheric transfer of information, while in the cat section of the anterior commissure was unnecessary. In monkeys it has been shown that the anterior commissure carries interhemispheric fibres between many areas that play a role in visual learning, including the ventral temporal pole, rostral inferotemporal cortex, and the superior temporal and parahippocampal gyri (Sunderland 1940; McCulloch and Garol 1941; Pandya and Seltzer 1986). In this respect, the cat is different from the monkey in its interhemispheric connections, and the possibility of interspecies differences must remain an important caveat in studies of interhemispheric communication.

Bearing in mind the possibility of species differences, one can ask to what extent the evidence of the effects of human commissurotomy is in agreement with the evidence that has come from the monkey. The evidence in humans comes from two major sources: first, patients who have undergone surgery to disconnect the cerebral hemispheres, often, although not invariably, as a cure for intractable epilepsy; and, secondly, patients in whom the corpus callosum has failed to develop normally—a condition called agenesis of the corpus callosum (see Chapter 9, this volume). While agenesis of the corpus callosum is often associated with other brain deformities and mental retardation (Loeser and Alvord 1968; Chiarello 1980), this is not invariably the case, and patients may have normal or above average IQs (Loeser and Alvord 1968; Dennis 1976; Chiarello 1980). However, it has been pointed out that because agenesis of the corpus callosum cannot be detected by any routine medical test, it is likely that there are many cases of agenesis of the corpus callosum in the population who, because they have no other neurological deficits, have failed to come to the attention of clinicians.

While the corpus callosum is absent in cases of agenesis, the anterior commissure is often still intact (Loeser and Alvord 1968; Chiarello 1980) and in some cases is enlarged. Indeed, in these cases callosal fibres may be incorporated into the anterior commissure (Geschwind 1974). It is therefore not surprising to find that, while evidence of hemispheric disconnection may be seen (Lassonde *et al.* 1995), interhemispheric communication can still occur in these acallosal patients. For example, some patients with agenesis of the corpus callosum can read words presented to either visual field (Ettlinger *et al.* 1972), or match material presented to different hemispheres (Saul and Sperry 1968; Ettlinger *et al.* 1972)—tasks that require interhemispheric transfer of information. However, Ettlinger *et al.* (1972) described acallosal patients who, although they could cross-match hue, saturation, and patterns between the hemifields, had difficulty making accurate depth and distance judgements. This result seems entirely in agreement with the results from monkeys, where it has been shown that the anterior commissure mediates transfer between the inferior temporal cortices (Pandya *et al.* 1971; Zeki 1973; Gross and Mishkin 1977), whereas the callosal interconnections between the border region of areas 17 and 18 on the two sides are needed in order to make stereoscopic depth judgements (Hamilton and Vermeire 1986).

The other source of knowledge about the effects of human hemispheric disconnnection is provided by patients in whom the corpus callosum and, normally, the anterior commissure have been surgically sectioned. Following such surgery, patients typically develop what has become known as the 'split-brain syndrome' (Bogen 1985). For example, Gazzaniga (1970) found that stimuli presented to the left visual field, and thus the right hemisphere, could not be reported verbally by split-brain patients, whereas those presented to the left hemisphere could. However, other forms of responding, for example pointing to objects or semantic associates with the hand contralateral to the hemisphere that received the visual information, demonstrated that both hemispheres could perceive and identify the objects. The conclusion from these examples is that the interhemispheric transfer of visual information relies on the integrity of the forebrain commissures, and they highlight the basic similarity between the findings in humans and monkeys (Downer 1958; Hamilton and Gazzaniga 1964). However, these conclusions were questioned when the apparent integration of visual information presented to the two hemispheres of split-brain patients was demonstrated (Sergent 1987, 1990). These findings suggested that in more naturalistic situations, where both hemispheres receive information and a unified response needs to be produced, the patients were capable of doing so, presumably by subcortical transfer of information. Interestingly, while the patients appeared to be able to produce unified responses based on information contained in both hemispheres, they were unable to report verbally the information that was directed to the right hemisphere. Thus complete information about what had been presented to the right hemisphere was clearly not available to the left hemisphere. However, subsequent attempts to replicate these findings in different (Seymour *et al.* 1994) or even the same (Corballis and Trudel 1993) groups of patients have proved largely unsuccessful. Sergent's findings may therefore be effects to be found only in one small group of patients who may be atypical in several respects (see Seymour *et al.* 1994 for a fuller discussion), or may be the result of elaborate strategies adopted by highly sophisticated subjects in order to perform the tasks (Corballis 1994). While it remains a possibility that some limited visual information may be integrated between the hemispheres in at least some split-brain patients, the general picture is of a failure of interhemispheric integration following 'split-brain' surgery, as is seen in the monkey.

The above discussion is based on patients who have complete section of the corpus callosum. However, the brief discussion of the anatomy of the corpus callosum given above makes it clear that different subsections of the corpus callosum interconnect different regions of the brain. For this reason, markedly different effects can be expected from disconnecting only some parts of the cerebral cortex by partial section of the corpus callosum. The following sections review what is known about comparative aspects of partial section in humans and monkeys.

8.3 Effects of partial commissurotomy: the splenium and anterior commissure

The early experiments with cats indicated that section of the entire corpus callosum was not necessary to prevent interhemispheric transfer of visual information (Myers 1959). Section of the posterior section, the splenium, alone was sufficient to prevent interocular transfer of visual discrimination learning in the cat. In fact, there appeared to be some overlap in function as portions of tissue left intact in any part of the splenium allowed transfer to take place, while section of the entire splenium did not. Similar results were soon demonstrated in the monkey, although the posterior half to one-fifth of the corpus callosum had to be sectioned in conjunction with the anterior commissure to prevent interhemispheric transfer of visual learning (Sperry 1958; Gazzaniga 1966; Doty *et al.* 1973; Hamilton and Brody 1973).

Although these results were obtained with visual information lateralized by use of optic chiasma section, Eacott and Gaffan (1989) have shown that section of the splenium and anterior commissure also prevents interhemispheric transfer of visual information in monkeys with *intact* optic chiasma. This result was achieved using visual information lateralized through the natural tendency of monkeys to fixate the centre of stimuli, thus naturally lateralizing each half of a visual stimulus to one hemisphere without the need for section of the optic chiasma. The efficiency of this natural method of lateralization was demonstrated by simply transposing the two halves of the visual stimuli: thus what had previously appeared to the left of the centre now appeared on the right and vice versa. Following this transposition, each half stimulus was effectively lateralized to the opposite hemisphere from that which had been trained to recognize it initially. Monkeys that had learned a two-choice discrimination between visual stimuli composed of two abutting halves, transferred this learning to the transposed stimuli while the splenium and anterior commissure were intact, but showed no such transfer in the absence of the splenium and anterior commissure. This result confirms the importance of these fibre systems in interhemispheric transfer of visual information. This new method of lateralizing visual stimuli allows both hemispheres to receive information simultaneously about a stimulus, while avoiding the hemianopia in each eye that is produced by optic chiasma section, and the potential problems raised by incomplete or asymmetric section of the optic chiasma. However, perhaps more importantly, it also demonstrates the role of the commissures in interhemispheric communication when both hemispheres are receiving a normal sensory input, just as would occur naturally in the intact brain.

Using the more conventional method of lateralizing visual input through section of the optic chiasma, it has also been shown that the splenium, alone or in conjunction with the anterior commissure, is sufficient to support interhemispheric transfer of visual information after section of the remainder of the corpus callosum (Doty *et al.* 1994; Lewine *et al.* 1994). In this simple situation, in the monkey at least, the splenium and the anterior commissure appear to be equivalent in their ability to subserve interhemispheric transfer of information, despite the fact that the splenium contains 5–10 times as many visual fibres as the anterior commissure (Ringo *et al.* 1991). For example, no differences between the two have been noted in the transfer of colour or pattern information (Downer 1962; Hamilton and Vermiere 1986), nor of direction of movement (Hamilton 1982), although the anterior commissure may have been marginally worse at transferring orientation information (Hamilton and Vermeire 1986). However, more recently it has been shown that the splenium may be more efficient than the anterior commissure in integrating bilateral engrams (Lewine *et al.* 1994) and the anterior commissure may be less able than the splenium to integrate binocularly disparate images (Ringo *et al.* 1991). The basis for these apparent differences is not yet fully understood.

In humans a similar distinction between the splenium of the corpus callosum and the remaining portions can be drawn. None of the typical symptoms associated with a failure of interhemispheric transfer of visual information was found in two patients who had undergone surgical section of only the anterior portions of the corpus callosum and the anterior commissure, leaving the splenium and the body of the corpus callosum intact (Gordon *et al.* 1971). These patients could report verbally words and objects presented to their left visual field (right hemisphere), and after visual presentation of an object to one hemisphere could retrieve it using tactile cues alone with the ipsilateral hand, a task requiring interhemispheric transfer of visual information. This suggests that the splenium mediates transfer of visual information in humans, as well as in the monkey. However, the role that the anterior commissure plays in interhemispheric transfer is less clear in humans. Note that while the anterior commissure does not mediate transfer of visual information in the cat, it is in many ways equivalent to the corpus callosum in the transfer of visual information in the monkey. There are reports of successful transfer of visual information in commissurotomy patients in whom the anterior commissure has been left intact (Gazzaniga and LeDoux 1978; Risse *et al.* 1978). However, subsequent studies have failed to find such transfer in similar patients (McKeever *et al.* 1981; Holtzman 1984). Failure of transfer in patients who are known to have had brain pathology, as is the case with all 'split-brain' patients, could plausibly be attributed to damage to a critical, but not commissural, structure. However, where one sees apparent interhemispheric transfer one must bear in mind the possibility that the patients are using an, as yet undetected, cross-cueing strategy. Thus there are reasons for treating with caution both the reports of transfer of information by way of the anterior commissure and reports of an absence of transfer. It is not yet clear, therefore, whether the anterior commissure can mediate the interhemispheric transfer of visual information in humans as it does in monkeys. However, the fact that in humans the anterior commissure may vary markedly in its size among subjects (Demeter *et al.* 1988) may explain some of this behavioural variability.

8.4 Effects of partial commissurotomy: the trunk of the corpus callosum

The most striking effects of split-brain surgery can be attributed to the failure of interhemispheric transfer of visual information, and these effects, as we have seen, are mediated by the posterior sections of the corpus callosum—the splenium—and possibly the anterior commissure. We need therefore to determine the function, or functions, of the remaining portions of the corpus callosum.

When intact monkeys learn a tactile discrimination with one hand, the discrimination can be performed using either hand (Ebner and Myers 1962; Ettlinger and Morton 1963; Hunter *et al.* 1975). Following callosal section, the intermanual transfer of somatosensory discrimination habits no longer occurs (Glickstein and Sperry 1960; Ebner and Myers 1962; Ettlinger and Morton 1963; Teng and Sperry 1966; Hunter *et al.* 1975). Therefore one can conclude that the interhemispheric transfer of somatosensory information is subserved by the corpus callosum. However, section of only the posterior central portion of the corpus callosum—the trunk or body of the corpus callosum—is necessary to produce this effect in monkeys (Myers and Ebner 1976). Section of the anterior portions of the corpus callosum or of the splenium and anterior commissure have no effect on transfer of this sort of information. Equally, if the posterior body alone is left intact, while the other parts of the corpus callosum and anterior commissure are sectioned, good intermanual transfer of tactile learning is seen, although at slightly lower levels than is seen in the intact animal (Hunter *et al.* 1975). There is good agreement therefore that transfer of somatosensory information can be localized to the posterior trunk or body of the corpus callosum in the monkey.

The trunk of the corpus callosum appears to play a very similar role in humans. A patient of Geffen *et al.* (1980) failed an interhemispheric tactile matching task following a lesion extending only 30 mm within the somatosensory region of the trunk of the corpus callosum. However, another patient with a similar lesion could perform the task. Both these patients had surgery to remove a ventricular tumour which had led to neurological symptoms, and therefore it remains a possibility that they had other neurological damage which may explain the variation.

For this reason, the case described by Dimond *et al.* (1977) may be instructive. This patient did not exhibit any neurological symptoms prior to the surgical section of the trunk of the corpus callosum to remove an angioma, suffering only from a severe headache, and therefore it is likely that there was no pre-existing damage to brain structures. Moreover, it was possible to test the patient on the same task both before and after surgery. Intermanual transfer of tactile information was severely diminished following surgery, but the effect was relatively short-lived, intermanual transfer returning to pre-operative levels within 20 days. Although the initial deficit may have been caused by bruising and oedema around the area of surgery, a possible alternative explanation of this recovery is that the information about the shape of the objects could be recoded into visual information. Transfer of this visual information could then take place over the intact splenium and anterior commissure. The recoded visual information would then have to be mapped back on to somatosensory structures in the receiving hemisphere. If this were the case, the 'recovery' seen would represent only a change in strategy rather than any functional recovery in the ability to transfer somatosensory information between the hemispheres. Indeed, it was noted that the patient was slower to perform the task when interhemispheric transfer was required than when the task was intrahemispheric. This slowing when interhemispheric transfer was necessary could indicate that complex interhemispheric strategies were in use. In support of this view, a study of a small group of patients (Geffen *et al.* 1985) confirmed the importance of the trunk of the corpus callosum in the interhemispheric transfer of tactile information, but again suggested that the splenium may play some role in transfer. Patients in whom only the splenium was intact, showed a level of interhemispheric transfer of tactile information which was intermediate between that shown by those in whom the posterior body was intact and those in whom the entire corpus callosum had been sectioned. Again, the information transferred by the splenial route may have been the tactile information itself or this information recoded into a visual form. However, the importance of the trunk of the corpus callosum in interhemispheric transfer of somatosensory information is not in question. For example, Bentin *et al.* (1984) examined six patients in whom the various portions of the trunk had been sectioned for removal of a tumour. Three of these patients exhibited deficits in interhemispheric transfer of tactile information and in all three the lesion had included the posterior region of the trunk, just the region implicated in such transfer in monkeys by Myers and Ebner (1976).

8.5 Effects of partial commissurotomy: the anterior corpus callosum

Very little evidence is available concerning the information transferred via the anterior portions of the corpus callosum in humans or in monkeys, and most of the existing evidence is negative, that is evidence of transfer that remains unaffected by section of the anterior corpus callosum. Some of these studies have already been mentioned as throwing light on the functions of other portions of the corpus callosum. For example, section of the anterior portions of the corpus callosum, the rostrum and genu, have no effect of the transfer of visual information in monkeys (Sullivan and Hamilton 1973) or humans (Gordon *et al.* 1971). Similarly, section of these portions did not affect adversely transfer of somatosensory discriminations in either monkeys (Myers and Ebner 1976) or humans (Geffen *et al.* 1985).

An early study by Noble (1973) addressed the question of what information might transfer between the cerebral hemispheres by way of the anterior corpus callosum. He investigated the interhemispheric transfer not only of individual visual discriminations, but also of 'learning sets', acquired sets of abstract rules that allow all visual discriminations to be learned more quickly (Harlow 1949). Noble lateralized the input of visual information by way of optic chiasma section and monocular viewing, and taught monkeys a set of visual discriminations. Transfer was tested by examining learning of novel discriminations when viewing with the other eye, thus testing the ability of the untrained hemisphere. Transfer was demonstrated if the learning of new discriminations was quicker with the untrained hemisphere than it was in the initial stages of training for the previously trained hemisphere. As the discriminations were novel, the faster rate of learning could not be attributed to the transfer of information specific to each visual discrimination: neither hemisphere had any knowledge of the individual discriminations used. However, faster learning could plausibly be attributed to interhemispheric transfer of the principles or abstract rules of discrimination learning, in other words the learning set. As might be expected, monkeys with section of the entire corpus callosum and anterior commissure showed no interocular transfer of either individual discriminations or of the learning set. The untrained hemisphere gained no benefit from the experience of the other hemisphere with similar discriminations. Monkeys with partial section of the corpus callosum, in which either the splenium or the anterior commissure remained intact, showed good interocular transfer of individual problems, as would be expected, but also showed good performance with novel discriminations, showing that the untrained hemisphere had access to information about the general rules or principles governing discrimination learning. This finding, as Noble points out, does not imply that the between-problem learning of the abstract rule had transferred between the hemispheres via the posterior portions of the corpus callosum or the anterior commissure, as transfer of individual problems would be sufficient to allow the untrained hemisphere to build up learning set independently of the trained hemisphere. However, when the anterior portions of the corpus callosum alone remained intact, no interhemispheric transfer of individual visual discriminations was seen, but learning set, as indicated by faster learning of novel discriminations, was seen. This finding implies that the abstract rules constituting the learning set were transferred across the anterior half to one-third of the corpus callosum. A study by Hamilton and Vermeire (1986) came to a similar conclusion after studying the transfer of a 'reversal learning set' in the absence of transfer of any of the individual problems on which the learning set was based.

Further clues as to the functions of the anterior portions of the corpus callosum come from studies that attempt to look at the interhemispheric integration of information, rather than straightforward transfer. In this type of experiment the two hemispheres each receive information that has to be compared in order to complete the task. The method used to achieve simultaneous yet different input to the two hemispheres was devised initially by Trevarthen (1962), and uses optic chiasma section and polarized filters over each of the eyes. The stimuli for each eye are lit by differently polarized light and thus can be seen by only one eye. Using this paradigm, Sperry and Green (1964) found no integration of pattern information presented to opposite hemispheres when the entire corpus callosum, anterior commissure, and optic chiasma were sectioned. Monkeys failed to perform at above-chance levels even after 2000 trials, demonstrating the successful lateralization of the stimuli. However, the same monkeys could perform the task successfully when both elements of the problem were presented to one hemisphere, eliminating the need for interhemispheric communication. In this way, interhemispheric integration appeared to be similar to interhemispheric transfer of visual information in the monkey, just as it appears to be in humans (Seymour *et al.* 1994).

For example Hamilton *et al.* (1968) showed that visual integration in the monkey was possible when either the posterior third of the corpus callosum or the anterior commissure were intact. However, in one animal the anterior two-thirds of the corpus callosum were left intact and some integration between the hemispheres was seen. When the remaining parts of the corpus callosum were sectioned the performance of this animals returned to chance. This demonstrates that the previously above-chance performance had resulted from transfer of some information across the anterior parts of the corpus callosum, rather than from unilaterally available cues or transfer via the peripheral pathways. However, the performance of this animal, while clearly above chance, was still markedly worse than that seen in monkeys in which the splenium and anterior commissure were intact. As interhemispheric transfer of visual discrimination learning does not take place following section of the splenium and anterior commissure, the results imply that some non-visual information was transferred that allowed comparison of the stimuli, but which was much less reliable than visual information.

A similar interpretation may be made of some findings with cats (Voneida and Robinson 1970). The cats were trained to make same/different judgements about visual stimuli. When the optic chiasma and posterior two-thirds of the corpus callosum were sectioned, the cats could only make accurate judgements when all the information was presented to one hemisphere. When interhemispheric transfer of the information was necessary, there was a permanent deficit. However, in this condition some of the cats still performed slightly above chance on the interhemispheric comparison task, despite showing no interhemispheric transfer of visual learning. When the remaining anterior third of the corpus callosum was sectioned in one animal who had shown this above-chance performance, the performance dropped to chance. Again, this implies that some information was transferring across the anterior portions of the corpus callosum but, as there was no transfer of visual discrimination learning, it is unlikely that this information was visual. It is possible that the clue to the nature of the information that was transferring via the anterior corpus callosum can be found in the previously described work of Noble (1973) and Hamilton and Vermiere (1986) which suggested that an abstract rule or strategy could be transferred across these portions of the corpus callosum. Voneida and Robinson (1970) used only two pairs of discriminanda in their same/different judgement task, and trained their cats to criterion on them before surgery; so both hemispheres had experience of the stimuli that were used in the task. It is possible therefore that some learned association of the particular stimuli could be transferred via the intact anterior portions and this was sufficient to allow the receiving hemisphere to draw conclusions about the stimulus that had been presented to the other hemisphere. This possibility could, of course, be tested by teaching the principle of same/different judgements before surgery with a different set of stimuli from those which are used to test integration post-operatively. Such a procedure would prevent the two hemispheres from jointly developing the associations about the stimuli, and therefore transfer of such associations could not provide a clue as to the stimuli being viewed by the other hemisphere.

There is, however, further evidence that the anterior portions of the corpus callosum may transfer information about associations of visual stimuli (Eacott and Gaffan 1990). In this study monkeys were taught a visualmotor conditional discrimination task. Each discrimination problem consisted of a pair of visual stimuli, which were presented to the monkey on a television screen. There were two possible responses to the appearance of a visual stimulus on the screen. The monkey could make a tap repeatedly on the stimulus or 'hold' it, defined as touching the stimulus for a period of 1 second. Within a pair of visual stimuli, rewards could be earned by tapping one of the stimuli and holding the other. The monkey's task was to learn which response was associated with which stimulus. Under the assumption that control of the hand is from the contralateral hemisphere, interhemispheric transfer of this learning was tested by looking for intermanual transfer of the discrimination habit. It was discovered that section of the entire corpus callosum and anterior commissure prevented intermanual transfer of this visualmotor conditional learning. This finding demonstrated both that control of the responding hand was indeed from the contralateral hemisphere and that interhemispheric transfer of this learning was dependent on some part of the corpus callosum and anterior commissure. However, those monkeys with section of the posterior half of the corpus callosum and anterior commissure, leaving the anterior half of the corpus callosum intact, showed good intermanual transfer of this learning. Thus the results of this study show that the anterior portions of the corpus callosum can mediate interhemispheric transfer of some information that allows this task to be performed.

However, it is not entirely clear from this result whether the information that was transferred by this pathway was the association of the stimulus with the response, as was suggested by the previous discussion. A patient reported by Preilowski (1972) had section of the anterior half of the corpus callosum and was reported to be poor at a task designed to require bimanual co-ordination. The relative failure of this patient in the task was interpreted as a failure of interhemispheric integration of 'corollary outflow', that is information about the responses of the other hand. In the experiment of Eacott and Gaffan (1990) interhemispheric transfer of such information across the anterior corpus callosum could result in independent learning of the discriminations by both hemispheres, allowing apparent intermanual transfer to be seen. It is difficult to distinguish between this possibility and the transfer of the associative learning itself and, indeed, both may be transferred across the anterior section of the corpus callosum.

While there is very little evidence as to the information that may be transferred across the human anterior corpus callosum, the limited evidence available supports the view that it may subserve the interhemispheric transfer of associations of stimuli. Sidtis *et al.* (1981) report the case of a patient who underwent staged section of the corpus callosum for the relief of epilepsy. After section of the posterior corpus callosum, the patient showed no evidence of interhemispheric transfer or integration of sensory information. However, with encouragement, the patient could give semantic information about words or pictures that had been presented to the right hemisphere. For example, when presented with the word 'knight' to the right hemisphere, the patient reported a series of appropriate images which led him to guess the correct word. The sensory information itself had clearly not been transferred, but it is possible that the associations of the words and pictures shown, or the concepts that they represented, had been transferred into the verbal left hemisphere, allowing this patient to identify them. Following later complete section of the corpus callosum, this ability disappeared, demonstrating that it was indeed mediated by formerly intact commissural connections, rather than by some peripheral means.

8.6 Conclusions

The results of this highly selective overview of the effects of partial section of the corpus callosum and anterior commissure show a high degree of concordance between the results obtained from monkeys and from humans. Certainly, there is good agreement in the effects of section of the splenium and the trunk of the corpus callosum. While a great deal less is understood about the anterior portions of the corpus callosum, the limited evidence does not suggest any substantial difference between the functions of the corpus callosum in humans and in monkeys.

References

Akelaitis, A. J. (1944). A study of gnosis, praxis and language following section of the corpus callosum and anterior commissure. *Journal of Neurosurgery*, **1**, 94–102.

Barbas, H. and Pandya, D. N. (1984). Topography of commissural fibres of the prefrontal cortex. *Experimental Brain Research*, **55**, 187–91.

Bentin, S., Sahar, A., and Moscovitch, M. (1984). Intermanual information transfer in patients with lesions in the trunk of the corpus callosum. *Neuropsychologia*, **22**, 601–11.

Black, P. and Myers, R. E. (1964). Visual functions of the forebrain commissures in the chimpanzee. *Science*, **146**, 799800.

Bogen, J. E. (1985). Split-brain syndromes. In *Handbook of clinical neurology*, Vol. 45, (ed. P. J. Vinken, G. W, Bruyn, and H. L. Klawans), pp. 99–106. Elsevier, Amsterdam.

Chiarello, C. (1980). A house divided? Cognitive functioning with callosal agenesis. *Brain and Language*, **11**, 128–58.

Corballis, M. C. (1994). Split decisions: problems in the interpretation of results from commissurotomized subjects. *Behavioural Brain Research*, **64**, 163–72.

Corballis, M. C. and Trudel, C. I. (1993). Role of the forebrain commissures in interhemispheric integration. *Neuropsychologia*, **7**, 306–24.

Curtis, J. H. and Bard, P. (1939). Intercortical connections of the corpus callosum as indicated by evoked potentials. *American Journal of Physiology*, **126**, 473–9.

Demeter, S., Ringo, J. L., and Doty, R. W. (1988). Morphometric analysis of the human corpus callosum and anterior commissure. *Human Neurobiology*, **6**, 219–26.

Dennis, M. (1976). Impaired sensory and motor differentiation with corpus callosum agenesis: a lack of callosal inhibition during ontogeny. *Neuropsychologia*, **14**, 455–69.

Dimond, S. J., Scammel, R. E., Brouwers, E. Y., and Weeks, R. (1977). Functions of the centre section (trunk) of the corpus callosum in man. *Brain*, **100**, 453–562.

Doty, R. W., Negrão, N., and Yamaga, K. (1973). The unilateral engram. *Acta Neurobiologiae Experimentalis*, **33**, 711–28.

Doty, R. W., Ringo, J. L., and Lewine, J. D. (1994). Interhemispheric sharing of visual memory in macaques. *Behavioural Brain Research*, **64**, 79–84.

Downer, J. L (1958). Role of the corpus callosum in transfer of training in *Macaca mulatta*. *Federation Proceedings*, **17**, 37.

Downer, J. L (1962). Interhemispheric integration in the visual system. In *Interhemispheric relations and cerebral dominance*, (ed. V. B. Mountcastle), pp. 87–100. Johns Hopkins Press, Baltimore.

Eacott, M. J. and Gaffan, D. (1989). Interhemispheric transfer of visual learning in monkeys with intact optic chiasm. *Experimental Brain Research*, **74**, 348–52.

Eacott, M. J. and Gaffan, D. (1990). Interhemispheric transfer of visuomotor learning *via* the anterior corpus callosum of monkeys. *Behavioural Brain Research*, **38**, 109–16.

Ebner, F. F. and Myers, R. E. (1962). Direct and transcallosal induction of touch memories in the monkey. *Science*, **138**, 51–2.

Ettlinger, G. and Morton, H. B. (1963). Callosal section: its effects on performance of a bimanual skill. *Science*, **139**, 485–6.

Ettlinger, G., Blakemore, C. B., Milner, A. D., and Wilson, J. (1972). Agenesis of the corpus callosum: a behavioural investigation. *Brain*, **95**, 327–46.

Gazzaniga, M. S. (1966). Interhemispheric communication of learning. *Neuropsychologia*, **4**, 183–9.

Gazzaniga, M. S. (1970). *The bisected brain*. Appleton–Century–Crofts, NewYork.

Gazzaniga, M. S. and LeDoux, J. E. (1978). *The integrated mind.* Plenum Press, London.
Geffen, G., Walsh, A., Simpson, D., and Jeeves, M. A. (1980). Comparison of the effects of transcortical and transcallosal removal of intraventricular tumours. *Brain*, **103**, 773–88.
Geffen, G., Nilsson, J., and Quinn, K. (1985). The effect of lesions of the corpus callosum on finger localisation. Neuropsychologia, **23**, 497–514.
Geschwind, N. (1974). Late changes in the nervous system: an overview. In *Plasticity and recovery of function in the central nervous system*, (ed. D. G. Stein, J. J. Rosen, and N. Butters), pp. 467–508. Academic Press, New York.
Glickstein, M. and Sperry, R. W. (1960). Intermanual somesthetic transfer in split-brain rhesus monkeys. *Journal of Comparative and Physiological Psychology*, **53**, 322–7.
Goldstein, M. N. and Joynt, R. J. (1969). Longterm follow-up of a callosal sectioned patient. *Achives of Neurology*, **20**, 96–104.
Gordon, H. W., Bogen, J. E., and Sperry, R. W. (1971). Absence of deconnection syndrome in two patients with partial section of the neocommissures. *Brain*, **94**, 327–36.
Gross, C. G. and Mishkin, M. (1977). The neural basis of stimulus equivalence across retinal translation. In *Lateralization in the nervous system*, (ed. S. Harnad, R. W. Doty, L. Goldstein, J. Jaynes, and G. Krauthamer), pp. 109–22. Academic Press, New York.
Hamilton, C. R. (1982). Mechanisms of interocular transfer. In *Analysis of visual behavior,* (ed. D. J. Ingle, M. A. Goodale, and R. J. W. Mansfield), pp. 693–717. MIT Press, Cambridge, MA.
Hamilton, C. R. and Brody, B. A. (1973). Separation of visual functions within the corpus callosum of monkeys. *Brain Research*, **49**, 185–9.
Hamilton, C. R and Gazzaniga, M. S. (1964). Generalisation of learning of colour and brightness discriminations following brain bisection. *Nature*, **201**, 220.
Hamilton, C. R. and Vermeire, B. A. (1986). Localization of visual function with partially split-brain monkeys. In *Two hemispheres—one brain. Functions of the corpus callosum*, (ed. F. Lepore, M. Ptito, and H. H. Jasper), pp. 315–33. Alan R. Liss, New York.
Hamilton, C. R., Hillyard, S. A., and Sperry, R. W. (1968). Interhemispheric comparison of color in split-brain monkeys. *Experimental Neurology*, **21**, 486–94.
Harlow, H. (1949). The formation of learning sets. *Psychological Review*, **56**, 51–65.
Holtzman, J. D. (1984). Interaction between cortical and subcortical visual areas: Evidence from human commissurotomy patients. *Vision Research*, **24**, 801–13.
Hunter, M., Ettlinger, G., and Maccabe, J. J. (1975). Intermanual transfer in the monkey as a function of the amount of callosal sparing. *Brain Research*, **93**, 223–40.
LaMantia, A. S. and Rakic, P. (1990). Cytological and quantitative characteristics of four cerebral commissures in the rhesus monkey. *Journal of Comparative Neurology*, **291**, 520–37.
Lassonde, M., Sauerwein, H. C., and Lepore, F. (1995). Extent and limits of callosal plasticity: Presence of disconnection symptoms in callosal agenesis. *Neuropsychologia*, **33**, 989–1007.
Loeser, J. D. and Alvord, E. C. (1968). Agenesis of the corpus callosum. *Brain*, **91**, 553–70.
Lewine, J. D., Doty, R. W., Astur, R. S., and Provencal, S. L. (1994). Role of forebrain commissures in bihemispheric mnemonic integration in macaques. *Journal of Neuroscience*, **14**, 2515–30.

McCulloch, W. S. and Garol, H. W. (1941). Cortical origin and distribution of corpus callosum and anterior commissure in the monkey. *Journal of Neurophysiology*, **4**, 555–63.

McKeever, W. F., Sullivan, K. F., Fergusson, S. M., and Royport, M. (1981). Typical cerebral hemisphere disconnection following corpus callosum section despite sparing of anterior commissure. *Neuropsychologia*, **19**, 745–55.

Mettler, F. A. (1935). Corticofugal fiber connections of the cortex of *Macaca mulatta*. The occipital region. *Journal of Comparative Neurology*, **61**, 221–56.

Mott, F. W. and Schaeffer, E. A. (1890). On movements resulting from faradic excitation of the corpus callosum. *Brain*, **13**, 174–7.

Myers, R. E. (1955). Interocular transfer of pattern discrimination in cats following section of crossed optic fibers. *Journal of Comparative and Physiological Psychology*, **48**, 470–3.

Myers, R. E. (1956). Function of the corpus callosum in interocular transfer. *Brain*, **79**, 358–63.

Myers, R. E. (1959). Localization of function in the corpus callosum. *Archives of Neurology*, **1**, 44–7.

Myers, R. E. and Ebner, F. F. (1976). Localisation of function in the corpus callosum: tactile information transfer in *Macaca mulatta*. *Brain Research*, **103**, 455–62.

Myers, R. E and Sperry, R. W. (1953). Interocular transfer of a visual discrimination habit in cats after section of the optic chiasm and corpus callosum. *Anatomical Record*, **115**, 351–2.

Noble, J. (1973). Interocular transfer in the monkey: Rostral corpus callosum mediates transfer of object learning set but not of single problem learning. *Brain Research*, **50**, 147–62.

Pandya, D. N. and Seltzer, B. (1986). The topography of commissural fibres. In *Two hemispheres—one brain. Functions of the corpus callosum* (ed. F. Lepore, M. Ptito, and H. H. Jasper), pp. 47–73. Alan R. Liss, New York.

Pandya, D. N., Karol, E. A., and Heilbronn, D. (1971). The topographical distribution of interhemispheric projections in the corpus callosum of the rhesus monkey. *Brain Research*, **32**, 31–43.

Preilowski, B. F. (1972). Possible contributions of the anterior forebrain commissures to bilateral motor coordination. *Neuropsychologia*, **10**, 179–94.

Ranson, W. B. (1895). On tumors of the corpus callosum. *Brain*, **18**, 532–50.

Ringo, J. L., Doty, R. W., and Demeter, S. (1991). Bi–verus monohemispheric performance in split-brain and partially split-brain macaques. *Experimental Brain Research*, **86**, 1–8.

Risse, G. L., LeDoux, J., Springer, S. P., Wilson, D. H., and Gazzaniga, M. S. (1978). The anterior commissure in man: Functional variation in a multisensory system. *Neuropsychologia*, **16**, 23–31.

Saul, R. E. and Sperry, R. E. (1968). Absence of commissurotomy symptoms with agenesis of the corpus callosum. *Neurology*, **18**, 307.

Seltzer, B. and Pandya, D. N. (1973). The distribution of posterior parietal fibres in the corpus callosum of the rhesus monkey. *Experimental Brain Research*, **49**, 147–50.

Sergent, J. (1987). Subcortical coordination of hemispheric activity in commissurotomized patients. *Brain*, **109**, 357–69.

Sergent, J. (1990). Furtive incursions into bicameral minds: integrative and coordinating role of subcortical structures. *Brain*, **113**, 537–68.

Seymour, S. E., Reuter-Lorenz, P. A., and Gazzaniga, M. S. (1994). The disconnection syndrome. Basic findings reaffirmed. *Brain*, **117**, 105–15.

Sherrington, C. S. (1889). On nerve tracts degenerating secondarily to lesions of the cortex cerebri. *Journal of Physiology*, **10**, 429–32.
Sidtis, J. J., Volpe, B. T., and Holtzman, J. D. (1981). Cognitive interaction after staged callosal section: Evidence for transfer of semantic activation. *Science*, **212**, 344–6.
Sperry, R. W. (1958). Corpus callosum and interhemispheric transfer in the monkey (*Macaca mulatta*). *Anatomical Record*, **131**, 297.
Sperry, R. W. and Green, S. M. (1964). Corpus callosum and perceptual intergration of visual half fields. *Anatomical Record*, **148**, 339.
Sperry, R. W., Stamm, J. S., and Miner, N. (1956). Relearning tests for interocular transfer following division of optic chiasm and corpus callosum in the cat. *Journal of Comparative and Physiological Psychology*, **49**, 529–33.
Sullivan, M. V. and Hamilton, C. R. (1973). Memory establishment *via* the anterior commissure of monkeys. *Physiology and Behavior*, **11**, 873–9.
Sunderland, S. (1940). The distribution of commissural fibres in the corpus callosum in the macaque monkey. *Journal of Neurology and Psychiatry*, **3**, 9–18.
Teng, E. L. and Sperry, R. W. (1966). Intermanual stereognostic size discriminations in split-brain monkeys. *Journal of Comparative and Physiological Psychology*, **62**, 84–9.
Tieman, S. B., Hamilton, C. R., and Meyers, R. C. (1977). Commissural connections of the visual cortical areas in the macaque. *Anatomical Record*, **187**, 731.
Trevarthen, C. B. (1962). Double visual learning in the split-brain monkey. *Science*, **136**, 258.
Trevarthen, C. (1990). Integrative functions of the cerebral commissures. In *Handbook of neuropsychology*, Vol. 4, (ed. F. Boller and J. Grafman), pp. 49–83. Elsevier, Amsterdam.
Voneida, T. J. and Robinson, J. S. (1970). Quantitative differences in performance on abstract discriminations using one or both hemispheres. *Experimental Neurology*, **26**, 72–83.
Zeki, S. (1973). Comparison of the cortical degeneration in the visual regions of the temporal lobe of the monkey following section of the anterior commissure and splenium. *Journal of Comparative Neurology*, **148**, 167–76.

9

Visual integration in callosal agenesis

MALCOLM A. JEEVES

9.1 Introduction

A fresh interest by neuropsychologists in callosal agenesis followed publication of the dramatic findings on surgical split-brain patients by Roger Sperry and his colleagues in the late 1950s and early 1960s (Sperry 1968*a*). From their animal studies with cats and monkeys, and their investigations of a small group of patients who had had their major neocortical commissures sectioned to reduce the spread of epilepsy from one side of the brain to the other, they showed that the major neocortical commissure, the corpus callosum, was essential for the normal transfer, comparison, and sharing of information arriving separately in the two cerebral hemispheres. The question arose: would one observe a similar full-blown disconnection syndrome in people born without the corpus callosum, and if not, why not?

George Ettlinger organized the 1964 CIBA Foundation Symposium on *Functions of the corpus callosum* at which I presented the results from my early studies of acallosal patients. Shortly afterwards, Ettlinger, together with colleagues in London, undertook his own studies of acallosal patients (Ettlinger *et al.* 1972) and speculated about possible compensatory mechanisms that might explain their findings of lack of evidence of the disconnection syndrome.

Early on, it was recognized that because callosal agenesis was frequently associated with other, often undetected, cerebral abnormalities, the task of interpreting the results of neuropsychological studies of these patients was extremely difficult. Soon, however, evidence from post-mortem studies of acallosal brains (for example, Bossy 1970) established that there are instances in which the absence of the corpus callosum appeared to be the only major brain abnormality. Hence the possibility of detailed study of patients with few other cerebral abnormalities, apart from the absent corpus callosum, were undertaken by ourselves and others. Since that time, with the rapid development of brain imaging techniques, the possibility of correlating the results of fine-grained neuropsychological testing with relatively secure knowledge of brain abnormalities has taken important steps forward (for example, the symposium on *Callosal agenesis* held in Québec in 1992: see Lassonde and Jeeves 1994).

In this chapter, I shall limit myself to an aspect of cognitive functioning in callosal agenesis that has received most attention from neuropsychologists; the results of these studies having implications for our understanding of interhemispheric processing generally. The research to be reviewed addresses not only questions about the functioning of the corpus callosum but also of the anterior commissure and subcortical pathways. It also presents some new, as yet unpublished, results specifically studying interhemispheric visual integration in callosal agenesis and for the first time, I believe, offers, very speculatively, a possible role for the Probst bundles. These are groups of cortical neurones found only in acallosal brains, which project abnormally in a longitudinal direction within one hemisphere.

9.2 Interhemispheric processing—transmission speed and transfer capacity

9.2.1 Interhemispheric transmission times

Simple reaction times to a stimulus ipsilateral to the hand making a response have been presumed to measure an 'uncrossed' or short pathway, involving a single hemisphere in stimulus reception and motor execution. Responses to stimuli contralateral to the stimulus are presumed to measure a 'crossed' or long pathway, involving stimulus reception in one hemisphere and motor execution in the other. Poffenberger (1912) showed that in the normal population, the difference between the crossed and uncrossed responses is of the order of 3 ms. A series of studies beginning in the 1960s (Jeeves 1969) demonstrated that in callosal agenesis the interhemispheric transmission time, as measured by the CUD (crossed–uncrossed difference), is lengthened. Reviews by Berlucchi (1978) and Milner and Rugg (1989) have established that the conventional reaction time (RT) techniques for estimating CUD in normal subjects measure non-visual callosal transmission. The main evidence for this is that by manipulating visual stimulus parameters, which have a substantial effect on the absolute values of the RTs, there are nevertheless no detectable effects on the CUDs. In contrast, the evidence suggests that similar reaction time techniques measure visual latencies in acallosal subjects. Milner (1982) and Milner *et al.* (1985) tested two acallosal subjects and demonstrated clear and statistically significant variations in the CUDs measured as the range of stimulus luminance was varied. If the cross–midline transfer was visually encoded, then the lower the stimulus energy, the longer the CUD should be; and this was what they found. Few confirmatory studies are available, but one by Clarke and Zaidel (1989) also found a (non-significant) increase in the CUD with a change in the luminance level of the stimulus. Milner (1994, p. 176) concluded that 'evidence at present suggests that the CUD in acallosals reflects a visually coded relay'. In seeking to address the question of which of the possible routes this might take, he looked to the indirect evidence available from the study of the California split-brain patients, L.B. and N.G., in whom all of the cerebral commissures were cut (Bogen *et al.* 1988). In such cases, the anterior commissure would not be available for mediating crossed RTs, yet the CUDs in these patients have been shown to be not significantly longer than those of some acallosals (Sergent and Myers 1985; Clarke and Zaidel 1989). Reviewing the evidence from these studies, Milner (1994, p.177) concluded that 'On balance there is some evidence for an effect of luminance on CUDs in the predicted direction; and the interpretation of this as arguing for a visual relay in these split-brain subjects is bolstered by the finding that three out of four such subjects showed significant stimulus eccentricity effects on the CUD (Clarke and Zaidel, 1989).' He went on, 'It seems inevitable that this visual relay could only be subcortical, since there is no anterior commissure present; and if this can occur in commissurotomized patients, it could also do so in acallosal subjects.'

A series of studies has demonstrated that interhemispheric transmission time can also be measured by recording event-related potentials from symmetrical points on either side of the scalp (Lines *et al.* 1984; Rugg *et al.* 1984, 1985*a*, 1987; Saron and Davidson 1989; Brown and Jeeves 1993, and in preparation; Brown *et al.* 1994). The CUD as measured by use of these techniques averaged between 10 and 15 ms for electrodes placed over occipital regions, and the value varied as a function of stimulus luminance. By comparison, CUDs as estimated by use of centrally placed electrodes, i.e. over sensorimotor cortex, averaged only around 4 ms and these did not vary with stimulus luminance. In acallosals, while it is possible to record the visual event-related potentials (ERPs) in the hemisphere contralateral to the stimulus, it is not possible to detect corresponding deflections in the waveform recorded over the ipsilateral hemisphere (Rugg *et al.* 1985*b*). In their most recent study, Brown and Jeeves (in preparation), in speculating over the possible role of the anterior commissure known to be present in their patients, found that it was not sufficient to mediate the cross-callosal visual P1/N1 components of the ERP. None the less, the appearance of a later positive wave in recordings over both hemispheres in the normals and acallosals (but not visible in a commissurotomy patient) suggests that the anterior commissure is mediating sufficient bihemispheric stimulus information for a P300 to be elicited and recordable over both hemispheres. Thus, while a neural representation of the stimulus (at P1/N1) cannot cross in the absence of the corpus callosum, the anterior commissure may allow interhemispheric transfer of information regarding the meaning and significance of the event. An important caveat to this argument, however, is that it is possible that the P300 recorded over the ipsilateral hemisphere may be a product of volume conduction from the contralateral hemisphere and not neuroelectrically generated in the ipsilateral hemisphere.

A recent study (Jeeves *et al.*, in preparation) of a partial acallosal male in whom the anterior one-third of the corpus callosum has been shown by magnetic resonance imaging (MRI) to be present, revealed an intriguing picture as far as the CUD is concerned. The patient, C.O., a 17-year-old male of normal intelligence, completed 960 RT trials, affording reliable response latency estimates. His CUD averaged 2.5 ms, firmly in the normal range. The absence of any manipulation of stimulus luminance leaves the interpretation of these data, in terms of a sensory or motor transmission, ambiguous. On the one hand, it could support the view (Berlucchi 1978; Milner and Lines 1982) that the RTs were mediated by a motor crossing, passing through the anterior part of the corpus callosum, known to be intact in this patient. On the other hand, other testing with this patient (see below) of the interhemispheric transmission of visual information could indicate that, as suggested by Innocenti *et al.* (1995), the part of the corpus callosum that is present may contain fibres that would normally cross in the posterior parts of the callosum, and in dysgenesis track more posteriorly to interconnect the visual parts of the cortices.

After the initial testing, this patient underwent surgery for the relief of epilepsy attributed to a focus in the left temporal lobe. The surgeon's notes indicated that the location and extent of the temporal lobe surgery would be expected to cause a total or partial visual deafferentation of the anterior commissure, known to be present in this patient. It is of interest therefore that results with this patient post-operatively, when he completed a total of 640 trials, resulted in an overall CUD of 3.25 ms. This again is firmly within the normal range and very similar to his pre-operative testing. The presumed deafferenting of the anterior commissure clearly produced no significant lengthening of the CUD, as might have been expected if the anterior commissure, in the absence of the posterior two-thirds of the corpus callosum, had been involved in the interhemispheric transmission of punctate visual information. Such a finding leaves undetermined whether what is present of the corpus callosum in C.O. carries fibres that cross-connect the visual cortices or that cross-connect motor areas so that, as in normals on this task (Berlucchi 1981), a motor crossing is being measured.

9.2.2 Interhemispheric transmission of visual pattern information in callosal agenesis

It is unlikely, on the basis of the available evidence, that preserved left visual hemifield naming in callosal agenesis is due to bilateral speech mechanisms. It is likewise unlikely in the light of available evidence (see Milner 1994) that an appeal to a greatly increased nasotemporal overlap of retinal projections can provide an adequate explanation for the ability of acallosal subjects to cross-match visually between the two hemispheres. It seems clear from reaction times made to punctate stimulation arriving at one hemiretina that such information has no functional access to ipsilateral brain structures by abnormally decussating optic nerve fibres. It seems even less likely that more complex visual information would have direct bilateral access to allow pattern cross-matching without the need for commissural transmission. Indeed recent evidence has shown that the nasotemporal division at the retina is already rather sharp at the 69th fetal day in the monkey, which is before any appreciable loss of ganglion cells occurs (Lia *et al.* 1988). That certainly argues against the possibility that extensive 'wrongly' projecting optic nerve fibres might be retained in callosal agenesis. It seems probable therefore that some kind of non-callosal commissural transmission of visual information must be taking place in callosal agenesis.

As in the case of reaction time studies, then, we can ask where such cross-over might plausibly occur. Here the major candidate, much canvassed by some researchers, is the anterior commissure. The evidence from studies in monkeys shows that it plays an important role in interhemispheric visual integration. Although still open to some debate, on balance it seems that the majority of acallosals do possess an anterior commissure (Loeser and Alvord 1968; Lemire *et al.* 1975; Barkovich and Norman 1988). It is even possible that it may be enlarged abnormally in some cases. That was certainly the view taken by Norman Geschwind (1974). On the other hand, we also know that the anterior commissure is smaller in some cases (Rauch and Jinkins 1994; section 9.3). In view of the recent report of a sevenfold range in cross-sectional area of the anterior commissure in normal subjects (Demeter *et al.* 1988), a detailed comparative study would be required to substantiate Geschwind's claim.

Pointing to the likelihood of the anterior commissure as a leading candidate has been the complexity of the visual information that apparently can be transmitted in acallosal subjects. Materials used by experimenters in the past have included simple words, figural drawings, and geometric patterns. In the monkey, the anterior commissure heavily connects the anterior two-thirds of the two temporal lobes, including the inferior neocortical areas, most intimately implicated in pattern processing (Jouandet and Gazzaniga 1979; Pandya and Seltzer 1986; Demeter *et al.* 1990).

However, evidence from the study of the surgical split-brain patients, surprisingly, does not point to the anterior commissure as having a significant role for visual functions in normal people. McKeever *et al.* (1981) and Holtzman (1984) demonstrated little superiority in visual integration when it is spared than when it is cut. Moreover, it is a very small structure with an average cross-sectional area of only 1 per cent that of the corpus callosum. Aside from this evidence, there is an important possibility of a different role for the anterior commissure in the acallosal brain. Indirect embryological evidence suggests that the anterior commissure might draw upon a far wider cortical territory than in the normal brain. The anterior commissure develops earlier than the corpus callosum, appearing around the ninth/tenth week of fetal life (Auroux and Roussel 1967); at this time it appears that the anterior commissure supplies a very widespread range of neocortical areas. If the corpus callosum develops normally, however, these 'exuberant' connections retract and by the fourth month of fetal life, the range of the anterior commissure is much restricted while callosal connections are beginning to occupy the vacated territory. It could be, therefore, that with the failure of growth of the corpus callosum, the exuberant projections of the anterior commissure are maintained and do not withdraw. Such a wider linking of cortical areas remains a possibility regardless of whether the anterior commissure appears to be physically enlarged in callosal agenesis.

A further alternative is one that I proposed during the 1964 conference organized by George Ettlinger (Jeeves 1965), that mesencephalic commissures could be playing an important role in visual integration in callosal agenesis. The candidates here would include the collicular commissure, the posterior commissure, and the massa intermedia. Certainly in those acallosals who lack both the anterior commissure and the corpus callosum, any successful cross-visual integration must, of necessity, depend on subcortical pathways. The evidence from animal work certainly would point to the superior colliculus as the prime candidate, since it possesses visually responsive commissural neurones, though at present there is little evidence that subcortical visual structures, including the superior colliculus, can carry form analysis (Goldberg and Robinson 1978). With these alternatives in mind, I shall review briefly the evidence from the studies of acallosal patients, first when given visuoperceptual tasks employing lateralized stimuli.

Visual processing of lateralized stimuli within and between fields

Ettlinger and his collaborators (Ettlinger *et al.* 1972) reported that an acallosal subject they studied could match bilaterally presented patterns and colours. We have observed that the same applies to words. Lassonde (1986) has reported that the acallosals she studied did not differ in terms of error rates from normal controls on a task of cross-matching visual patterns. Martin (1985) also reported that an acallosal patient performed well at identifying words and abstract shapes presented unilaterally to either visual hemifield. On the other hand, the patient performed poorly at *localizing* stimuli within a spatial frame in his right visual field as compared with his left visual field. Martin cited arguments that the inferior temporal region in the monkey is involved in visual pattern recognition but not in spatial functions (Ungerleider and Mishkin 1982). Extending this argument, he proposed therefore that the patient's anterior commissure could successfully carry pattern information, but not spatial information. Hence the right hemifield would show worse results than the left hemifield on the assumption that in this patient the right hemisphere is, as normally, dominant in the performance of visuospatial tasks. Jeeves and Milner (1987) sought to generalize Martin's results, but found that their two patients performed as well on right visual field localization as on left visual field localization, despite the use of a task carefully modelled on that devised by Martin. They were able to exclude the possibility that their two patients had abnormal cerebral dominance for spatial perception (Jeeves and Milner 1987). Other studies by Holtzman *et al.* (1981) on callosotomized patients indicated that spatial information can be transferred by non-callosal commissures even though such information may not reach awareness. The most likely explanation is that the intertectal commissure was mediating the spatial interaction that we observed in our acallosal subjects, this being particularly likely given what we know about the spatial coding that takes place in the superior colliculus (Sparks and May 1990). Martin may therefore have been right in his supposition that the anterior commissure does not transmit spatial information, albeit for the wrong reasons.

To explore further any possible limitations on the transmission capacity of residual commissures in agenesis, we have recently developed a set of visual tasks that can be administered easily using a PC. In each case we require our subjects to make same–different judgements when two patterns appear. The two patterns might appear either within a visual hemifield (up/down) or one in each visual field (left/right), using four different positions on the screen spaced as a square. The visual stimuli used were:

(1) rectangular blocks of uniform visual texture, each of which were either yellow or light blue;
(2) rectangular blocks of white light, varying in apparent brightness and visual texture; and
(3) the letters A and B, one in upper case and the other in lower case.

In developing these tasks and the computerized means of their easy administration, we gave them first to normal subjects and then as a pilot study to two acallosals we had studied previously (M.M. and J.D.) in California. We then gave them to two patients in Australia on whom we have published a series of reports, extending in one instance over a 30-year period (P.H., Jeeves 1965; and D.C.).

Of the California patients, M.M. was a 14-year-old, right-handed adolescent male with agenesis of the corpus callosum confirmed by MRI scan. The MRI revealed that the anterior commissure was present. From the neuroradiological data so far available, the best judgement that can be made is that M.M. has no Probst bundles. The second patient, J.D., was a left-handed 19-year-old with complete agenesis of the corpus callosum confirmed by MRI. The anterior commissure was clearly visible on the MRI, and the neuroradiological reports indicated evidence for the presence of Probst bundles. Of the Australian patients, P.H. was first tested in 1960 when he was 5 years old. His neurological status, based on ventriculograms, pneumoencephalograms, computed tomography (CT) scans, and MRI is characterized by total agenesis of the corpus callosum, an intact anterior commissure, and the absence of Probst bundles. The second Australian patient, D.C., was born in 1981. Based on ultrasound as a neonate and MRIs when he was 10 years old, the best assessment of his neurological status is a total agenesis of the corpus callosum, an anterior commissure present but possibly of reduced size, and Probst bundles clearly visible and present.

For each task, the dependent measures were response latency in milliseconds, and accuracy as percentage error. A unilateral score was computed for each subject by taking the mean of the left visual field (LVF) and right visual field (RVF) presentations, and a bilateral score was computed by taking the mean of symmetrical or diagonal presentations. The histograms in Fig. 9.1 summarize the results for each task based on percentage errors and response latencies.

Since the primary purpose of these studies was to compare performance when responding to pairs of stimuli presented unilaterally within one visual field with performance when the same stimuli appeared bilaterally in two visual fields, the analysis here concentrates on those comparisons. A full report of the patients' results and those of their respective control groups will appear elsewhere. Here I focus particularly on those aspects of the patients' performance which may shed additional light on the nature and extent of compromised interhemispheric information transmission in callosal agenesis, and the extent to which selective compensatory mechanisms may, in some cases, reduce this.

All four patients, M.M., J.D., P.H., and D.C., completed between 300 and 600 trials on each of the three tasks administered. Overall, the patterns of their performance confirmed earlier reports indicating that on unilateral presentations their performance fell normally within the range of their matched controls, while their performance under the bilateral presentation conditions was worse than that of their controls. Another aspect of the results of earlier studies, such as those of Lassonde (1986), was evident here: whereas the performance of the patients as measured in terms of errors made under the bilateral presentation condition approximated that of their controls, when assessed in terms of speed of performance they were markedly worse than their controls.

The data summarized in the histograms in Fig. 9.1 are presented to allow ready comparisons between the two patients with neuroradiologically verified presence of Probst bundles (D.C. and J.D.) and the two patients without (P.H. and M.M.). Since, fortuitously, the IQs of the two pairs of patients, P.H. and M.M, lacking the Probst bundles, and J.D. and D.C. with the Probst bundles, are rather similar, this reduces the likelihood that any observed differences in performance are attributable to differences in cognitive level. As Fig. 9.1 indicates, the profile of responses of these four patients on the three tasks reveal differences in performance between the two pairs of subjects. In each instance in Fig. 9.1, the data are presented first in terms of percentage errors made under the unilateral and bilateral presentation conditions and then in terms of response latencies under the same two conditions.

On the colour task, P.H. and M.M., whilst making few errors under the unilateral presentation conditions, made a large number of errors under the bilateral conditions, their performances approaching chance level. In contrast, D.C. and J.D. made few errors whether they were performing under the unilateral or bilateral presentation conditions. The relative performances of each patient in terms of response latencies showed that all four were slower on the bilateral than the unilateral condition. P.H. overall was very much slower than the other three patients. On the brightness/texture task, P.H. and M.M. made many more errors under both unilateral and bilateral presentation conditions than either D.C. or J.D.; P.H. and M.M. also were slower in responding than D.C. and J.D., again P.H. markedly so. On the letter matching task, whether in terms of errors or latencies, P.H. was by far the

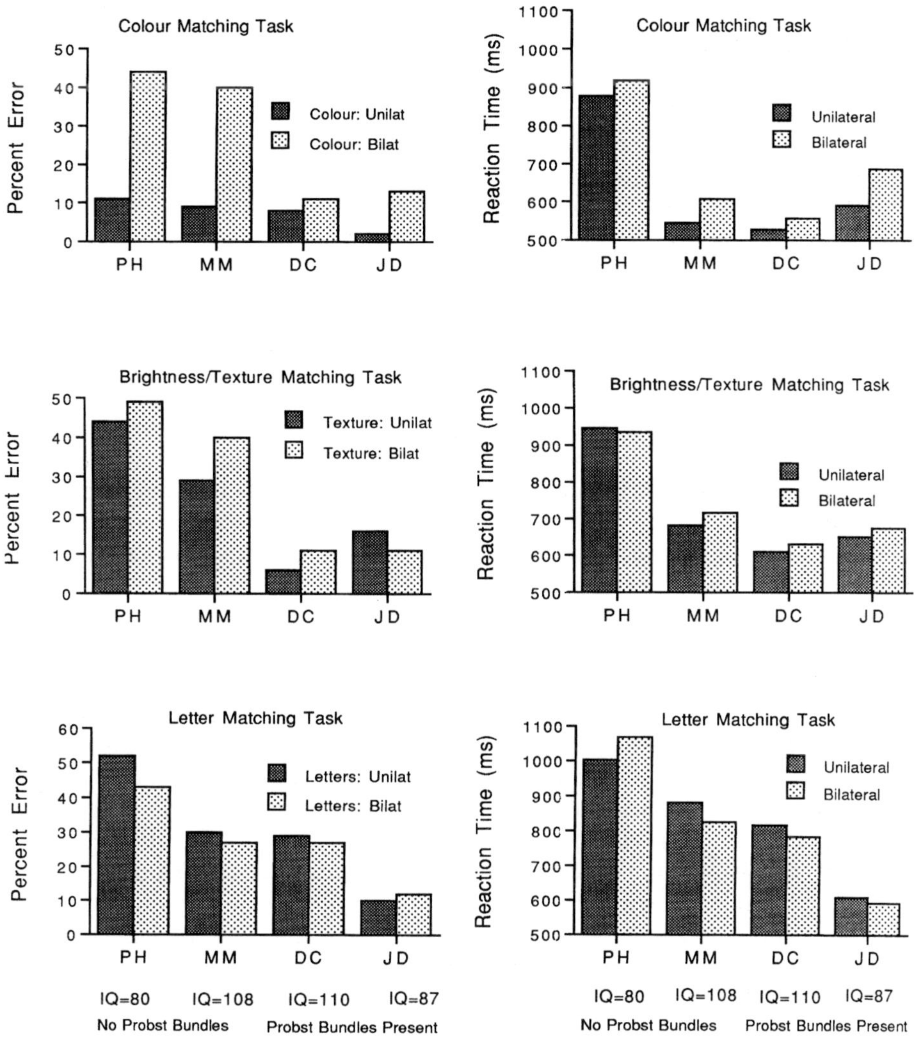

Fig. 9.1 Performance of four acallosal subjects on three tests of visual matching. Results are presented as percentage errors (left) and as reaction time in milliseconds (right). Patients PH and MM have no radiographic evidence of the presence of Probst bundles, whereas DC and JD have clear MRI evidence of the presence of these structures (see text). In each case, scores are shown separately for unilateral (within-hemifield) and for bilateral (cross-hemifield) matching.

worst performer. M.M. performed in a way similar to D.C., whereas J.D. was clearly the best performer.

Taking performance on all three tasks together, it appears that whether assessed in terms of errors made or latencies in responding, the two patients

P.H. and M.M., lacking Probst bundles, made more errors and were slower than the two patients D.C. and J.D. *with* Probst bundles. That P.H. and M.M. were closely matched with D.C. and J.D. on IQ reduces the likelihood that such differences can be attributed solely to differences in general matching ability.

As regards performance on specific tasks, the most striking feature of the performances of P.H. and M.M., and that which most clearly differentiates them from D.C. and J.D., is their performance in terms of errors made under the bilateral presentation condition on the colour matching task. I shall speculate later on whether this suggests a putative function for the Probst bundles which enable D.C. and J.D., under these bilateral matching conditions on the colour task, to perform well, whereas P.H. and M.M., lacking Probst bundles, perform very poorly. We may further speculate that the presence of Probst bundles in both D.C. and J.D. may have been a contributory factor to their overall pattern of superior performance to P.H. and M.M., whether measured in terms of errors made or response latencies. This applied across all three tasks; most clearly so on the colour matching task, but also in terms of percentage error on the brightness/texture matching task, and marginally so whether in terms of percentage errors or response latencies on the letter matching task.

Perceptual integration at the visual midline

One of the striking features of the performance of the classical Californian split-brain patients is their inability to integrate the two halves of chimeric stimuli meeting at the vertical meridian. When the subject is fixating at a point on the vertical meridian, each hemisphere receives different stimulus inputs. Levy *et al.* (1972) presented to their patients, amongst other things, faces, nonsense shapes, pictures of common objects, patterns of crosses and squares, and words. Under all the conditions, patients tended to give a single response on those trials where there was competitive information in the two halves of the chimera. The investigators also reported that the non-responding hemisphere gave no evidence that it had any perception of what had happened. They reported that if the right hemisphere, for example, responded, there was no indication, either by word or facial expression, that the left hemisphere in any way challenged the choice made and, likewise, if the left hemisphere responded, nothing the patient did suggested a disagreement by the right hemisphere. If the patients were asked to describe the stimulus they saw, then the left hemisphere percept was described. The reason for this is that in these classical split-brain patients, the right hemisphere cannot speak. Even so, the right hemisphere could certainly hear what the left hemisphere was describing and presumably if this disagreed with some percept that it had, one might have expected some puzzlement or head shaking or other indication that the right hemisphere disagreed with the judgement made. The authors concluded that their observations indicated that double perceptions did not occur in the majority of cases. It seems that, for whatever reason, the non-responding hemisphere failed to use the sensory information that it was perfectly well able to process.

When Levy *et al.* used faces to make up their chimeric figures, they found a strong right hemisphere dominance using a pointing response to an array lying on the table in front in free vision. The right hemisphere dominance was also found in tasks requiring the matching of nonsense shapes and the other stimuli mentioned earlier. They concluded, 'Where the task needs no more than visual recognition, a visual encoding ensues, mediated by the right hemisphere, and based on the form properties of the stimulus as such, rather than on separate feature analysis' (Levy *et al.* 1972, p. 75). We have carried out a limited number of studies to examine the performance of congenitally acallosal patients with chimeric stimuli (Jeeves 1979; Milner and Jeeves 1979). The most striking feature of these studies on three adult acallosals was that they were unaware of the chimeric nature of the stimuli; in this case, faces. One of the patients, K.C., performed very much like Levy *et al.*'s split-brain patients when the right hand was pointing to the full face pictures in free view, whereas her performance with the left hand matched that of the normal controls. The male, K.T., also performed like Levy's patients with the right hand, but when pointing with the left hand, there was no difference between the sides of the face selected. P.H., discussed above, performed significantly worse than either of the others, making 30 per cent errors, and on the remaining trials there was no difference in the likelihood of the left or right halves of the chimeric figure being selected, either with the right hand or the left hand.

The failure of the acallosals to detect the chimeric nature of the faces and their readiness to complete across the midline finds some support from the data gathered in the recent studies of P.H. and D.C. described above. We note (see Fig. 9.2a, b, c) a marked tendency for P.H. to make 'same' responses, resulting in a preponderance of errors on bilateral no-match trials on all three tasks. This would be consistent with his completing across the midline so that he 'sees' a pattern by filling in the second half-field, thus matching the one present in the first half-field. This tendency is much more evident in P.H. than D.C., who at times shows a response bias to make 'different' responses. In the other two patients, M.M. and J.D., the clearest evidence for a tendency to complete across the midline is in the performance of M.M. on the brightness/texture task (Fig. 9.2b) where his performance is very similar to that of P.H.

This raises the question of whether in some of the acallosals there are interhemispheric processes in the visual system still functional, allowing veridical comparisons of the two visual fields, thus reducing the tendency to complete across the midline. Since P.H., M.M., D.C., and J.D. are all reported to have the anterior commissure, the absence or presence of this structure cannot in itself provide an adequate explanation for observed differences. One alternative hypothesis worth considering is that when Probst bundles are present, as in the cases of D.C. and J.D., cross-field comparisons are facilitated. A variant of this would be that, where Probst bundles are present *together with* the hippocampal commissures, the latter could act as a 'sling'

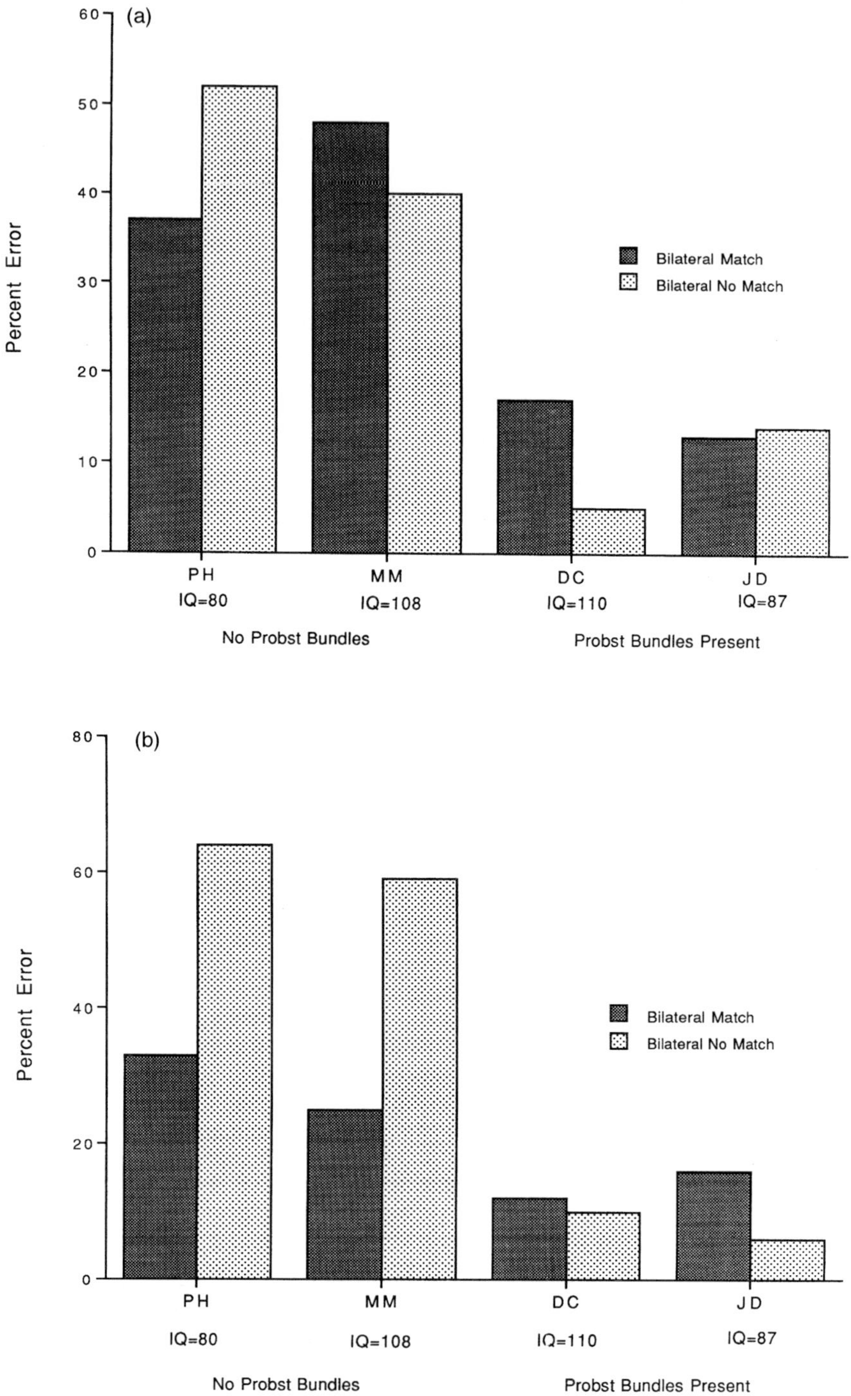
(a)
Percent Error
60
50
40
30
20
10
0
Bilateral Match
Bilateral No Match
PH
IQ=80
MM
IQ=108
DC
IQ=110
JD
IQ=87
No Probst Bundles
Probst Bundles Present
(b)
Percent Error
80
60
40
20
0
Bilateral Match
Bilateral No Match
PH
IQ=80
MM
IQ=108
DC
IQ=110
JD
IQ=87
No Probst Bundles
Probst Bundles Present

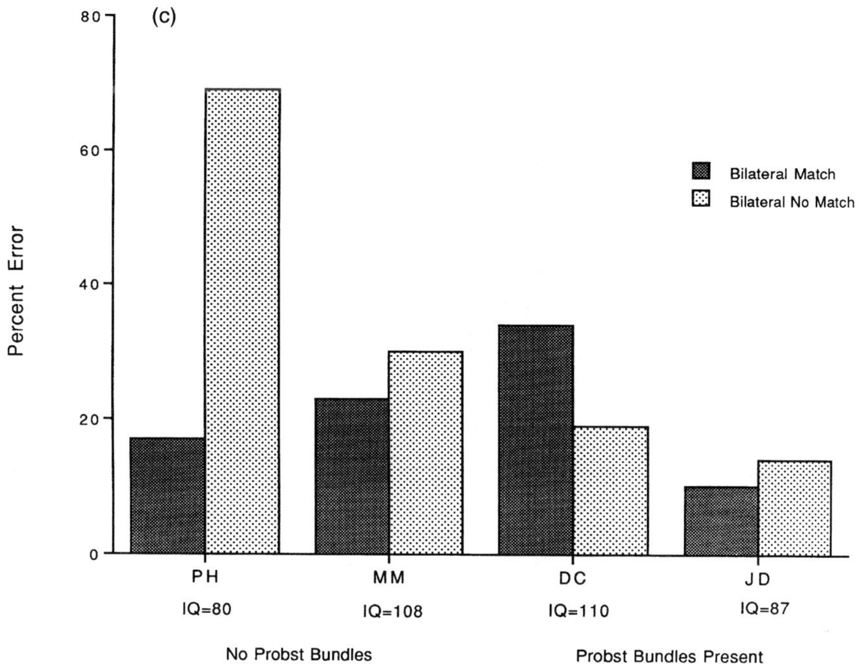

Fig. 9.2 Performance of the four acallosal patients (see Fig. 9.1) on bilateral matching of (a) colours, (b) brightness/textures, and (c) upper/lower case letters. Percentage error scores are presented separately for 'match' (same stimuli) trials and 'no-match' (different stimuli) trials.

or 'bridge' to enable selected fibres in Probst bundles to cross to the other hemisphere, thus affording additional interhemispheric transfer not available when Probst bundles are absent, as in P.H. and M.M.

9.3 Compensatory mechanisms

Mindful of the convincing demonstration by Roger Sperry and his co-workers of the major part played by the forebrain commissures in the normal integration of activity between the two cerebral hemispheres and in the transferring of information from one hemisphere to the other (Sperry 1968*a*), the question naturally arises as to how it is possible that people born without the corpus callosum are able to function, in at least some cases, seemingly normally. It is worth remembering that on brief social interactions, even the surgical split-brain patients appear to be normal; in general their deficits become evident only with the use of sophisticated neuropsychological experimentation. Presumably if they have acquired strategies to cope with everyday life, then this must be expected to have happened even more so in the case of callosal agenesis. Acallosals, after all, unlike the adult surgical patients, have had a lifetime in which to develop neural and behavioural compensatory mechanisms.

From time to time, starting with Sperry's (1968*b*) discovery of bilateral language representation in an acallosal patient he studied using the amytal test, the possibility of generalized representation of functions bilaterally in callosal agenesis has been discussed. As mentioned earlier, others have speculated about a possibly enhanced involvement of the anterior commissure where present, as well as of a role for subcortical pathways (Jeeves 1965; Jeeves and Milner 1987). Another candidate is an enhanced development of ipsilateral sensory and motor pathways. Finally, there remains the possibility, raised above, of a role for Probst bundles, evident in some acallosals.

Bearing in mind the general neuropsychological profile outlined earlier in this chapter, we may now address briefly a number of questions regarding compensatory mechanisms in interhemispheric visual processing. If other pathways do take over from the absent callosal pathways, then which are they, and how might they achieve their compensatory role? What about Probst's bundles: is there any evidence to suggest that they might have a role to play?

9.3.1 The role of the anterior commissure and of subcortical pathways

The possibility for a major role of the anterior commissure in callosal agenesis when it is present remains a candidate for compensation that is still in serious contention today. An early case report by Geschwind (1974) claimed there was a significantly larger anterior commissure in a callosal agenesis patient he studied. A recent study by Fischer *et al.* (1992) of two boys with callosal agenesis reported that in one of them, an MRI scan, while confirming the callosal agenesis, also demonstrated an enlarged anterior commissure. They claimed that their results support the hypothesis that hypertrophy of the anterior commissure is an important mechanism of functional compensation in agenesis of the corpus callosum. Although they may be right in this particular case, nevertheless the work by Rauch and Jinkins (1994), also based on MRI studies, makes it quite clear that although 10 per cent of their agenesis cases did indeed show an enlarged anterior commissure, equally, 10 per cent of the cases showed a smaller than normal structure. Animal data are consistent with these human data. Thus Wahlsten and Osaki's (1994) study of acallosal mice indicated that absence of the corpus callosum did not correlate with expansion in the sizes of the hippocampal and anterior commissures. Furthermore, they reported that, in mice at least, putative callosal axons which failed to cross to the opposite hemisphere generally do not re-route through the anterior commissure. If the same applies in humans, it may curb enthusiasm for attributing too great a compensatory role to the anterior commissure in the absence of the corpus callosum.

Milner (1994), after a critical review of the relevant literature and assessment of the roles of the anterior commissure and subcortical pathways, comes down clearly in favour of the importance of subcortical pathways rather than the anterior commissure. His paper was based entirely on studies of vision. At the same time, Lepore *et al.* (1994) add a further observation that, in general, compensatory mechanisms are better for those modalities which are more bilaterally organized, for example, temperature and audition, than for those that project mainly to contralateral cortical structures, for example, touch and vision.

As indicated, the evidence from animal studies tends not to support the suggestion that callosal fibres are re-routed through the anterior commissure in the absence of the corpus callosum. Nevertheless, such evidence as there is would support the view that if they do, then they may exhibit normal topography. This finding would also be important when considering cases of partial dysgenesis of the corpus callosum, so that the fibres that remain may not simply cross-connect cortical areas which had been demonstrated to be linked through that part of the callosum in animal studies of the topography of commissure fibres (e.g. Pandya and Seltzer 1986) or through studies of the neuropsychological consequences of surgical callosal section in adults, but rather that the fibres that remain may cross-connect widely separated areas of the two cerebral cortices and in this way follow the normal topography of callosal connections.

As regards the specific possible compensatory functions of the anterior commissure, it may be important to distinguish between the transmission of egocentric spatial information as compared with the carrying of object-based information. The former would seem a much more unlikely role for the anterior commissure in view of the termination pattern of fibres passing through it, a territory that includes the anterior temporal but not the occipital or parietal lobes. This likely restriction of the anterior commissure's role receives support from the work of Martin (1985), mentioned earlier. But given that his results were not replicated in other acallosal subjects by Jeeves and Milner (1987), Milner (1994) suggests that the intertectal commissure is typically able to mediate such spatial integration, via the egocentric spatial coding known to exist within the superior colliculus. Certainly our results cannot be explained on Martin's view (Martin 1985) that visual spatial integration can only be achieved via the corpus callosum.

The evidence concerning the abilities of acallosals on tasks requiring midline stereopsis have been interpreted as further support for a compensatory role for the anterior commissure in such tasks. The animal evidence, such as the work of Cowey (1985) and Hamilton and Vermier (1986) with monkeys, and Timney and co-workers (Timney *et al.* 1985; Timney and Lansdown 1988) with cats, supports this contention. At the same time, the work of Sergent (1986, 1990) is consistent with Milner's argument that more visual information is transferred subcortically than had previously been suspected.

That some form of interhemispheric communication takes place in the absence of the cerebral commissures is now reasonably well established. The evidence suggests that this includes low-level visual perceptual information (Trevarthen and Sperry 1973) as well as higher-level linguistic and non-linguistic information (Sperry *et al.* 1979; Sauerwein and Lassonde 1983; Johnson 1984; Myers and Sperry 1985; Cronin-Golomb 1986; Sergent 1990). It is noteworthy that in these studies the stimulus set sizes were small and usually the stimuli could be verbalized. Such a scenario immediately raises the possibility that any comparisons that were achieved were performed by cross-cueing rather than by subcortical visual transfer.

Although I have concentrated in this chapter almost exclusively on total callosal agenesis, there is an aspect of partial callosal dysgenesis which is important in considering possible compensatory mechanisms. Recent evidence on animals has shown that when only a small remnant of the callosum is present, the fibres in that remnant may show the apparently normal topography to be expected of fibres when the whole of the callosum is present. This may help to explain why it is that in dysgenesis, as compared with agenesis, many of the features of the neuropsychological profile well documented in total agenesis are not in evidence. The likelihood then is that the remnant of the callosum which is present contains fibres with the normal widespread topographic linkage of the two cerebral hemispheres, albeit with drastically reduced numbers of fibres in each case. That, on the face of it, may be sufficient to handle many tasks involving hemispheric interactions, but may reveal deficits when the load placed on those, by the nature of the task given, reaches a certain maximum. There is already some evidence suggesting that this might be the case.

9.3.2 The role of Probst bundles and the hippocampal commissures

A final possible compensatory mechanism is the formation of Probst's bundles. Hitherto there is, to the best of my knowledge, no evidence to suggest that these aberrant fibres actually have any functional importance. A report by Wahlsten and Ozaki (1994), based on studies of cortical axon trajectories and growth cone morphologies in fetuses of acallosal mice, gives some hints of the possible importance of Probst's bundles. They established that at the time of emergence, the growth rate of corpus callosum axons in the four cortical regions (frontal, parietal, temporal, and occipital) were normal in the acallosal strain studied. The corpus callosum axons arrived at the midplane on schedule but then often looped back to form the longitudinal Probst bundle. They found that the probability of joining the Probst bundle was highest for axons originating in the frontal cortex, which arrive at the midplane first, and lowest for occipital axons, which arrive last. They also found that once a few corpus callosum axons found a path to the other side, via the hippocampal commissure, those that arrived later then crossed relatively smoothly. Wahlsten and Ozaki further discovered that some Probst bundle axons managed to traverse the midline in this same manner. However, when no corpus callosum axons crossed, almost all of them entered the Probst bundle and eventually left it within a few hours to proceed into the ipsilateral white matter, never turning back towards the midplane. They also reported that growth cones approaching the midplane ipsilaterally and those that had crossed the midline and entered contralateral white matter, as well as corpus callosum axons in the Probst bundle, exhibited a normal range of size and complexity. Wahlsten and Ozaki (1994) believe that their results demonstrate that the problem with callosal agenesis resides *not* in the cells of origin of the axons or the growth cones themselves, but in the substrates of axon guidance at the mid-sagittal plane.

An important point for present purposes is Wahlsten and Ozaki's discovery that the corpus callosum axons in the Probst bundle did in fact express a normal range of size and complexity. The possibility therefore remains that the neurones were still physiologically functional. With this possibility in mind, we can speculate that the discovery that our total acallosals *with* Probst bundles were able to perform well on some bilateral matching tasks, for example the colour task, whereas other total acallosals, apparently similar in all other aspects, but lacking the Probst bundle, performed at chance level in the crossed condition of presentation (but at a very high level in the unilateral condition), may be the first (if indirect) evidence of a functional role for the Probst bundles. It is for this reason that I raised the question of whether the axons in the Probst bundle *within* a hemisphere may in fact become physiologically functional and take forward information from the parietal and occipital regions to more anterior parts of each hemisphere where, if there is an anterior commissure present, a route might be available to convey this information—via the Probst bundle on the *opposite* side—to the corresponding occipito-temporal regions on that side. This at least is a plausible explanation of the findings reported earlier in this chapter on colour matching in acallosals with and without the Probst bundles. Of course, having made this case, I hasten to qualify it with the reminder that an alternative explanation could invoke a role for the hippocampal commissure when present, either in its own right or as a 'bridge' for the passage of fibres in Probst bundles or other unspecified pathways linking cortical areas in the two hemispheres.

9.3.3 Longitudinal studies of compensatory mechanisms

Whatever compensatory mechanisms develop in callosal agenesis, we may reasonably expect that some of them may increase in their efficacy in the course of early normal development. The results from relevant studies extending over periods as long as several decades are few and far between. Such hints as there are, however, suggest that at least some deficits in interhemispheric processing in acallosals are not reduced with the passage of the years and in the course of normal maturational development. By way of example, we may consider studies that have been carried out on the patient P.H. described earlier. I noted that the basic timing of differences between crossed and uncrossed responses to a punctate light source measured at intervals over a 30-year period remained unchanged at about 20 ms. When midline processing was examined in 1964, by standard optometric procedures, P.H. showed evidence of a deficit. This was still evident 13 years later, when he was tested using the chimeric figures, a finding reinforced when he was tested on midline stereopsis, using a haploscope, a further 10 years later. Thus the subtle midline deficits appear to have remained relatively constant over upwards of a 30-year period.

9.4 Hemispheric interactions in callosal agenesis

It has been natural, following Sperry's pioneering work (1968*a*), that the focus of study of the major forebrain commissures has been on the transfer of coded information between the two cerebral hemispheres. However, when considering the functional consequences of the absence of the corpus callosum from before birth, it is prudent to consider not only information transfer functions of the callosum but other functions of a more general kind that have been discussed from time to time.

9.4.1 Inhibition

In 1961, Richard Jung, having listened to a series of presentations on cerebral asymmetries, commented that most, if not all, of the findings that were reported could only have come about as a result of an inhibitory role for the forebrain commissures (Jung 1962). This has been reiterated in different contexts by others since then. Berlucchi and Antonini (1990) pointed out that local inhibitory neurones are activated by callosal input. Maureen Dennis (1976, 1981), after her study of two acallosals, argued that the course of normal development involves the progressive suppression of uncrossed sensory and motor projections. On her view, the acquisition of fine distal motor control requires the progressive inhibition of motor pathways, other than crossed pyramidal ones. In her 1981 study, she developed this point, arguing that callosal agenesis patients showed an inability to suppress the ipsilateral component of an auditory stimulus when there is spectral temporal overlap of the stimuli presented. A similar theme was taken up by Preilowski (1972), who argued for an important inhibitory role for the callosum, noting that if this was reduced it resulted in the lowered quality and speed of performance that he had demonstrated in split-brain patients when they performed a bimanual co-ordination task. Zaidel (1976, 1986) suggested that the efficient performance of certain tasks depends on a unique hemispheric processing style and that this may at times be inhibited by the other hemisphere. Zaidel (1986) discussed callosal dynamics and argued that the corpus callosum is a complex dynamic channel, both facilitatory and inhibitory. Our own work on bimanual co-ordination in callosal agenesis (Silver and Jeeves, 1994; Moes *et al.* 1995) further develops the arguments put forward by Preilowski and lends support for an important inhibitory role in callosal functioning.

9.4.2 Facilitation

Lassonde has emphasized repeatedly the need to take account of facilitatory influences through the corpus callosum. The absence of this in acallosals has effects both *intra*hemispheric as well as *inter*hemispheric (Lassonde 1986). Lassonde found that in a task requiring acallosals and matched-IQ normal subjects to make a same/different judgement of pairs of visual stimuli (letters, numbers, colours, and forms) the acallosals were able to effect interhemispheric comparisons and that their accuracy of performance did not differ from that of the matched-IQ controls either intra- or interhemispherically. She found, however, that when she examined the response latencies to carry out these tasks, the acallosals required twice as long as the matched controls. As I have shown from data presented earlier in this chapter, our own studies have added further support to Lassonde's conclusions. She has argued that the corpus callosum participates in the bilateral activation of those regions typically implicated in neural activity required by her tasks. She goes on to point out that in the absence of the corpus callosum, neural activity in the regions concerned may be reduced and hence cause the delayed responsiveness that she observed.

Kuks *et al.* (1987), using the method of quantitative analysis of EEG by means of coherence functions, demonstrated the augmentation of interhemispheric coherence with maturation, observing that others had shown that interhemispheric bioelectric synchrony increases with age in pre-term and full-term neonates. It has also been shown that this continues to increase between 2 and 17 years of age. Kuks *et al.*'s study of two acallosal children, carefully matched according to gestational age with 13 controls, indicated an overall lowering of coherence in both cases, and they argued that this was unlikely to be explained by a difference in the developmental stage of myelination. More recently, Koeda *et al.* (1995) have developed Kuks' work and reported a further study of EEG in acallosal children. They estimated the inter- and intrahemispheric coherence in acallosal children and compared it with normal children in the resting state. They also reported findings from two acallosal adults, at the same time trying to take into account the individual anatomical differences between their patients, such as the presence or absence of the anterior commissure and the posterior commissure, as well as the extent of the dysgenesis of the corpus callosum in the individuals studied. Their expectation was that the interhemispheric coherences would, in general, be lower in acallosals, as had been suggested by the work of Kuks *et al.* (1987). Their results showed a general decrease of interhemispheric coherences in the acallosal subjects for frontal, central, parietal, and occipital regions, with the frontal values being the most marked. Pointing out that the coherence levels as measured are normally associated with the inter-regional coupling, they argued that the interhemispheric coherence decreases observed reflected a defective interhemispheric interaction between the cortical regions in acallosals. They commented further that the higher bilateral (interhemispheric) temporal-lobe coherences shown by the acallosals suggested a possible compensatory mechanism through the anterior commissure. This view, however, was compromised by the fact that the individual interhemispheric coherence levels of the particular patients did not vary clearly in the temporal domain with the presence or absence of the anterior commissure and the posterior portion of the callosal body, known to connect postero-temporal regions of the right and left hemispheres. They did, however, argue that the specificity of the interhemispheric alterations observed corresponded to individual anatomical differences in interhemispheric commissures, suggesting an essential role of the commissures in interhemispheric synchronization.

They also found that the *intra*hemispheric coherences discriminated between the acallosal subjects and their matched controls. As regards the left hemisphere, the majority of the intrahemispheric coherences did not differ between the acallosals and the normals. However, within the right hemisphere, the values were lower in the acallosals for pairs of derivations, including the right temporal area. They believe that these intrahemispheric coherence data reflect reduced connectivity within the right hemisphere specific to acallosal subjects.

Bearing in mind the data reported earlier in this chapter, when comparing patients with and without Probst bundles, we may speculate that if the techniques used by Koeda *et al.* were applied to patients with and without Probst bundles, we might expect increased hemispheric coherence levels in those acallosals with Probst bundles, both inter- and intrahemispherically, as compared with those without. We might also expect this to apply more evidently between the frontal/occipital/parietal areas and less between temporal areas, assuming that the anterior commissure is present.

References

Auroux, M. and Roussel, C. (1967). Relations néocorticales assurées par la commissure blanche anterieure chez le foetus humain. *Comptes Rendus de l'Association des Anatomistes,* **137,** 152–9.

Barkovich, A. J. and Norman, D. (1988). Anomalies of the corpus callosum: correlation with further anomalies of the brain. *American Journal of Roentgenology*, **151**, 171–9.

Berlucchi, G. (1978). Interhemispheric integration of simple visuomotor responses. In *Brain mechanisms and perceptual awareness*, (ed. P. A. Buser and A. Rougeul-Buser), pp. 83–94. Raven Press, New York.

Berlucchi, G. (1981). Recent advances in the analysis of the neural substrates of interhemispheric communication. In *Brain mechanisms and perceptual awareness*, (ed. O. Pompeiano and C. Ajmone Marsan), pp. 133–52. Raven Press, New York.

Berlucchi, G. and Antonini, A. (1990). The role of the corpus callosum in the representation of the visual field in cortical areas. In *Brain circuits and functions of the mind. Essays in honour of Roger W. Sperry*, (ed. C. Trevarthen), pp. 129–39. Cambridge University Press, Cambridge.

Bogen, J. E., Schultz, D. H., and Vogel, P. J. (1988). Completeness of callosotomy shown by magnetic resonance imaging in the long term. *Archives of Neurology*, **45**, 1203–5.

Bossy, J. G. (1970). Morphological study of a case of complete, isolated, and asymptomatic agenesis of the corpus callosum. *Archives of Anatomy, Histology and Embryology*, **53**, 289–340.

Brown, W. S. and Jeeves, M. A. (1993). Bilateral visual field processing and evoked potential interhemispheric transmission time. *Neuropsychologia*, **31**, 1267–81.

Brown, W. S. and Jeeves, M. A. (in preparation). Bilateral field advantage and evoked potential interhemispheric transmission in commissurotomy and acallosal individuals.

Brown, W. S., Larson, E. B., and Jeeves, M. A. (1994). Directional asymmetries in interhemispheric transmission time: evidence from visual evoked potentials. *Neuropsychologia*, **32**, 439–48.

Clarke, J. M. and Zaidel, E. (1989). Simple reaction times to lateralized light flashes. Varieties of interhemispheric communication routes. *Brain*, **112**, 849–70.

Cowey, A. (1985). Disturbances of stereopsis by brain damage. In *Brain mechanisms and spatial vision*, (ed. D. Ingle), pp. 259–78. NATO Advanced Study Institute Series. D. Martinus Nijhoff, The Hague.

Cronin-Golomb, A. (1986). Subcortical transfer of cognitive information in subjects with complete forebrain commissurotomy. *Cortex*, **22**, 499–519.

Demeter, S., Ringo, J. L., and Doty, R. W. (1988). Morphometric analysis of the human corpus callosum and anterior commissure. *Human Neurobiology*, **6**, 219–26.

Demeter, S., Rosene, D. L, and Van Hoesen, G. W. (1990). Fields of origin and pathways of the interhemispheric commissures in the temporal lobe of macaques. *Journal of Comparative Neurology*, **302**, 29–53.

Dennis, M. (1976). Impaired sensory and motor differentiation with corpus callosum agenesis: a lack of callosal inhibition during ontogeny. *Neuropsychologia*, **14**, 455–69.

Dennis, M. (1981). Language in a congenitally acallosal brain. *Brain and Language*, **12**, 33–53.

Ettlinger, G., Blakemore, C. B., Milner, A. D., and Wilson, J. (1972). Agenesis of the corpus callosum: a behavioural investigation. *Brain*, **95**, 327–46.

Fischer, M., Ryan, S. B., and Dobyns, W. B. (1992). Mechanisms of interhemispheric transfer and patterns of cognitive function in acallosal patients of normal intelligence. *Archives of Neurology*, **49**, 271–7.

Geschwind, N. (1974). Late changes in the nervous system: an overview. In *Plasticity and recovery of function in the central nervous system*, (D. G. Stein, J. J. Rosen, and N. Butters), pp. 467–508. Academic Press, New York.

Goldberg, M. E. and Robinson, D. L. (1978). The superior colliculus. In *Handbook of Behavioral Neurobiology*, Vol. 1. *Sensory Processing*, pp. 119–65. Plenum, New York.

Hamilton, C. R. and Vermeire, B. A. (1986). Localization of visual functions with partially split-brain monkeys. In *Two hemispheres—one brain: functions of the corpus callosum*, (ed. F. Lepore, M. Ptito, and H. H. Jasper), pp. 315–33. Liss, New York.

Holtzman, J. D. (1984). Interactions between cortical and subcortical visual areas: evidence from human commissurotomy patients. *Vision Research*, **24**, 801–13.

Holtzman, J. D., Sidtis, J. J., Volpe, B. T., Wilson, D. H., and Gazzaniga, M. S. (1981). Dissociation of spatial information for stimulus localization and the control of attention. *Brain*, **104**, 861–72.

Innocenti, G. M., Aggoun-Zouaoui, D., and Lehmann, P. (1995). Cellular aspects of callosal connections and their development. *Neuropsychologia*, **33**, 961–87.

Jeeves, M. A. (1965). Psychological studies of three cases of congenital agenesis of the corpus callosum. In *Functions of the corpus callosum*, CIBA Foundation Study Groups, Vol. 20, (ed. E. G. Ettlinger), pp. 73–94. Churchill, London.

Jeeves, M. A. (1969). A comparison of interhemispheric transmission times in acallosals and normals. *Psychonomic Science*, **16**, 245–6.

Jeeves, M. A. (1979). Some limits to interhemispheric integration in cases of callosal agenesis and partial commissurotomy. In *Structure and function of the cerebral commissures*, (ed. I. S. Russell, M. W. van Hof, and G. M. Berlucchi), pp. 449–74. Macmillan, London.

Jeeves, M. A. and Milner, A. D. (1987). Specificity and plasticity in interhemispheric integration: evidence from callosal agenesis. In *The duality and unity of the brain*, (ed. D. Ottoson), pp. 416–41. Macmillan, London.

Jeeves, M. A., Milner, A. D., and Moes, P. (in preparation). Effects of lateralized temporal lobe surgery on a partial acallosal.

Johnson, L. E. (1984). Vocal responses to left visual stimuli following forebrain commis surotomy. *Neuropsychologia*, **22**, 153–66.

Jouandet, M. L. and Gazzaniga, M. S. (1979). Cortical field of origin of the anterior commissure of the rhesus monkey. *Experimental Neurology*, **66**, 381–97.

Jung, R. (1962). In *Interhemispheric relations and cerebral dominance*, (V. B. Mountcastle), pp. 274–5. Johns Hopkins Press, Baltimore.

Koeda, T., Knyazeva, M., Njiokiktjen, C., Joukman, E. J., De Sonneville, L., and Vildavsky, V. (1995). The EEG in acallosal children. Coherence values in the resting state: left hemisphere compensatory mechanism? *Electroencephalography and Clinical Neurophysiology*, **95**, 397–407.

Kuks, J. B. M., Vos, J. E., and O'Brien, M. J. (1987). Coherence patterns of the infant sleep EEG in absence of the corpus callosum. *Electroencephalography and Clinical Neurophysiology*, **66**, 8–14.

Lassonde, M. (1986). The facilitatory influence of the corpus callosum on intrahemispheric processing. In *Two hemispheres—one brain: functions of the corpus callosum*, (ed. F. Lepore, M. Ptito, and H. H. Jasper), pp. 385–401. Liss, New York.

Lassonde, M. and Jeeves, M. A. (1994). *Callosal agenesis: a natural split brain?* Plenum Press, New York.

Lemire, R. J., Loeser, J. D., Leech, R. W., and Alvord, E. C. (1975). *Normal and abnormal development of the human nervous system*. Harper and Row, Hagerstown, MD.

Lepore, F., Lassonde, M., Poirier, P., Schiavetto, A., and Veillette, N. (1994). Midline sensory integration in callosal agenesis. In *Callosal agenesis: a natural split brain?*, (ed. M. Lassonde and M. A. Jeeves), pp. 155–69. Plenum Press, New York.

Levy, J., Trevarthen, C., and Sperry, R. W. (1972). Perception of bilateral chimeric figures following hemispheric deconnexion. *Brain*, **95**, 61–78.

Lia, B., Snider, C. J., and Chalupa, L. M. (1988). The nasotemporal division of the retinal ganglion cell decussation pattern in the fetal rhesus monkey. *Society for Neuroscience Abstracts*, **14**, 458.

Lines, C. R., Rugg, M. D., and Milner, A. D. (1984). The effect of stimulus intensity on visual evoked potential estimates of interhemispheric transmission time. *Experimental Brain Research*, **57**, 89–98.

Loeser, J. D. and Alvord, E. C. (1968). Clinicopathololological correlations in agenesis of the corpus callosum. *Neurology*, **18**, 745–56.

McKeever, W. F., Sullivan, K. F., Ferguson, S. M., and Rayport, M. (1981). Typical cerebral hemisphere disconnection deficits following corpus callosum section despite sparing of the anterior commissure. *Neuropsychologia*, **19**, 745–55.

Martin, A. (1985). A qualitative limitation on visual transfer *via* the anterior commissure. *Brain*, **108**, 43–63.

Milner, A. D. (1982). Simple reaction times to lateralised visual stimuli in a case of callosal agenesis. *Neuropsychologia*, **20**, 411–19.

Milner, A. D. (1994). Visual integration in callosal agenesis. In *Callosal agenesis: a natural split brain?*, (ed. M. Lassonde and M. A. Jeeves), pp. 171–83. Plenum Press, New York.

Milner, A. D. and Jeeves, M. A. (1979). A review of behavioural studies of agenesis of the corpus callosum. In *Structure and function of the cerebral commissures*, (ed. I. S. Russell, M. W. van Hof, and G. M. Berlucchi), pp. 428–48. Macmillan, London.

Milner, A. D. and Lines, C. R. (1982). Interhemispheric pathways in simple reaction time to lateralised light flash. *Neuropsychologia*, **20,** 171–9.

Milner, A. D. and Rugg, M. D. (1989). Interhemispheric transmission times. In *Developments in clinical and experimental neuropsychology*, (ed. J. R. Crawford and D. M. Parker), pp. 99–112. Plenum Press, New York.

Milner, A. D., Jeeves, M. A., Silver, P. H., Lines, C. R., and Wilson, J. (1985). Reaction times to lateralised visual stimuli in callosal agenesis: stimulus and response factors. *Neuropsychologia*, **23**, 323–3l.

Moes, P., Jeeves, M. A., and Cook, K. (1995). Bimanual coordination with aging: implications for interhemispheric transfer. *Developmental Neuropsychology*, **11**, 23–40.

Myers, J. J. and Sperry, R. W. (1985). Interhemispheric communication after section of the forebrain commissures. *Cortex*, **21**, 249–60.

Pandya, D. N. and Seltzer, B. (1986). The topography of commissural fibers. In *Two hemispheres—one brain: functions of the corpus callosum*, (ed. F. Lepore, M. Ptito, and H. H. Jasper), pp. 47–73. Liss, New York.

Poffenberger, A. T. (1912). Reaction time to retinal stimulation with special reference to time lost in conduction through nerve centers. *Archives of Psychology (NY)*, **23**, 1–73.

Preilowski, B. F. P. (1972). Possible contributions of the anterior forebrain commissures to bilateral motor coordination. *Neuropsychologia*, **10**, 267–7.

Rauch, R. A. and Jinkins, J. R. (1994). Magnetic resonance imaging of corpus callosum dysgenesis. In *Callosal agenesis: a natural split brain*, (ed. M. Lassonde and M. A. Jeeves), pp. 83–95. Plenum Press, New York.

Rugg, M. D., Lines, C. R., and Milner, A. D. (1984). Visual evoked potentials to lateralized visual stimuli and the measurement of interhemispheric transmission time. *Neuropsychologia*, **22**, 215–25.

Rugg, M. D., Lines, C. R., and Milner, A. D. (1985*a*). Further investigation of visual evoked potentials elicited by lateralized stimuli: effects of stimulus eccentricity and reference site. *Electroencephalography and Clinical Neurophysiology*, **62**, 81–7.

Rugg, M. D., Milner, A. D., and Lines, C. R. (1985*b*). Visual evoked potentials to lateralised stimuli in two cases of callosal agenesis. *Journal of Neurology, Neurosurgery and Psychiatry*, **48**, 367–73.

Rugg, M. D., Milner, A. D., Lines, C. R., and Phalp, R. (1987). Modulation of visual event-related potentials by spatial and non-spatial visual selective attention. *Neuropsychologia*, **25**, 85–96.

Saron, C. D. and Davidson, R. J. (1989). Visual evoked potential measures of interhemispheric transfer time in humans. *Behavioral Neuroscience*, **103**, 1115–38.

Sauerwein, H. and Lassonde, M. C. (1983). Intra- and interhemispheric processing of visual information in callosal agenesis. *Neuropsychologia*, **21**, 167–71.

Sergent, J. (1986). Subcortical coordination of hemisphere activity in commissurotomized patients. *Brain*, **109**, 357–69.

Sergent, J. (1990). Furtive incursions into bicameral minds. *Brain*, **113**, 537–68.
Sergent, J. and Myers, J. J. (1985). Manual, blowing, and verbal simple reactions to lateralized flashes of light in commissurotomized patients. *Perception and Psychophysics*, **37**, 571–8.
Silver, P. H. and Jeeves, M. A. (1994). Motor coordination in callosal agenesis. In *Callosal agenesis: a natural split brain?*, (ed. M. Lassonde and M. A. Jeeves), pp. 207–19. Plenum Press, New York.
Sparks, D. L. and May, L. E. (1990). Signal transformations required for the generation of saccadic eye movements. *Annual Review of Neuroscience*, **13**, 309–36.
Sperry, R. W. (1968*a*). Hemisphere deconnection and unity in conscious awareness. *American Psychologist*, **23**, 723–33.
Sperry, R. W. (1968*b*). Plasticity of neural maturation. *Developmental Biology, Suppl.*, **2**, 306–27.
Sperry, R. W., Zaidel, E., and Zaidel, D. (1979). Self recognition and social awareness in the disconnected minor hemisphere. *Neuropsychologia*, **17**, 153–66.
Timney, B. and Lansdown, G. (1988). Binocular depth perception, visual acuity and visual fields in cats following neonatal section of the optic chiasm. *Experimental Brain Research*, **74**, 272–8.
Timney, B., Elberger, A. J., and Vandewater, M. L. (1985). Binocular depth perception in the cat following early corpus callosum section. *Experimental Brain Research*, **60**, 19–26.
Trevarthen, C. and Sperry, R. W. (1973). Perceptual unity of the ambient visual field in human commissurotomy patients. *Brain*, **96**, 547–70.
Ungerleider, L. G. and Mishkin, M. (1982). Two cortical visual systems. In *Advances in the analysis of visual behavior*, (ed. D. J. Ingle, M. A. Goodale, and R. J. W. Mansfield), pp. 549–86. MIT Press, Cambridge, Mass.
Wahlsten, D. and Ozaki, H. S. (1994). Defects of the fetal forebrain in acallosal mice. In *Callosal agenesis: a natural split brain?*, (ed. M. Lassonde and M. A. Jeeves), pp. 125–33. Plenum Press, New York.
Zaidel, E. (1976). Language, dichotic listening and the disconnected hemispheres. In *Conferences on human brain function*, (ed. D. O. Walter, L. Rogers, and J. M. Finzi-Fried), pp. 103–10. Brain Information Service/BRI Publications Office, UCLA.
Zaidel, E. (1986). Callosal dynamics and right hemisphere language. In *Two hemispheres—one brain: functions of the corpus callosum*, (ed. F. Lepore, M. Ptito, and H. H. Jasper), pp. 435–95. Alan Liss, New York.

10

Towards a unified view of cerebral hemispheric specializations in vertebrates

PETER F. MacNEILAGE

10.1 Introduction

This paper can be regarded as a sequel to George Ettlinger's 1984 paper; 'Humans, apes and monkeys: the changing neuropsychological viewpoint'. He noted that in 1963 'there was no evidence for cerebral functional asymmetry in any nonhuman animal' (pp. 689–90). He then reviewed a number of findings of functional asymmetries in other primates, reported in the following 20 years and concluded that while 'it might be prudent not to assert that cerebral hemispheric specialization is homologous in man and in monkey . . . the likelihood of such an eventual outcome has increased enormously' (p. 691). The time for prudence on this matter has now passed. I will contend that there is not only homology across vertebrate taxa for a number of individual specializations, but there is probably some evolutionary continuity in relationships between specializations. Unfortunately, in the space available, I will not be able to spell out some of the individual arguments underlying these contentions in detail, though I intend to do so in the future.

10.2 Hemispheric specializations for vocalization and limb use: a left hemisphere motor specialization?

It has been known for a long time that there is a left hemisphere specialization for song production in some songbirds (reviewed by Arnold and Bottjer 1985) and for vocal reception in non-human primates (Petersen *et al.* 1978; Heffner and Heffner 1984; Hauser and Andersson 1993). The primate specialization is presumably productive as well as receptive. Paul R. MacNeilage (1996) has shown that rhesus monkeys tend to open the right side of the mouth more than the left when making 'coo' sounds, just as right-handed humans do when speaking (e.g. Graves *et al.* 1990).

The first post-1984 evidence that this specialization was more widely distributed in vertebrates was provided by Ehret (1987) who showed that female mice are more responsive to the ultrasonic distress calls of their infants when input was available to the right ear than when it was available to the left. Holman and Hutchinson (1991) have found left-sided hypothalamic control of ultrasonic vocal control during sexual interactions in Mongolian gerbils.

Most recently, Bauer (1993) has found that damage to the left hemisphere of frogs affects their vocal communication, but that right hemisphere damage does not. There may be a left hemisphere vocal communication specialization in all vertebrate taxa that make more than negligible use of vocal communication.

Perhaps the most important development bearing on the phylogeny of human cerebral specializations since 1984 is the realization that handedness exists in non-human primates. Lateralized hand use has suddenly become our best directly observable behavioural datum on the phylogeny of asymmetries of cerebral function in primates. In 1987, my colleagues and I reviewed 45 studies of primate handedness and concluded that, contrary to the existing consensus, other primates do show instances of handedness (MacNeilage *et al.* 1987). Ettlinger (with others) was politely sceptical of this conclusion, as is indicated in the title of his peer response to our paper: 'How nice if really were so' (Ettlinger 1987). However, since 1987 at least as many more studies have confirmed this conclusion (Ward and Hopkins 1993; MacNeilage 1997*a*). The basic outline of these findings will be given in the following paragraphs.

More than 15 studies, most from Ward's laboratory (reviewed by Ward *et al.* 1993), have shown a left-hand preference for prehension in prosimians (see also Masataka 1989; Mason *et al.* 1995). The fact that one of the most momentous adaptations of the earliest prosimians—the first primates—was for unimanual predation, which is necessarily an asymmetrical act, led my colleagues, Lindblom and Studdert-Kennedy, and I (MacNeilage *et al.* 1987) to suggest that the origin of this left handedness was in a visuospatiomotor specialization of the left hand–right hemisphere system. We also suggested that a complementary right side–left hemisphere postural control specialization arose at this time because of the postural demands of unimanual predation from the vertical clinging posture typical of early prosimians.

Instances of left-hand preferences in monkeys and apes have also been reported in tasks that are visuospatially demanding, such as catching goldfish by squirrel monkeys (King and Landau 1993) and adjusting the position of clear Plexiglas screens in baboons and gorillas (Fagot and Vauclair 1988*a*,*b*). However, the dominant finding in monkeys and apes is a human-like right handedness. Two common conditions across subsets of these studies are a demand for manipulation and the presence of upright posture (some key studies are Masataka 1990; Hopkins 1993, 1995; Hopkins *et al.* 1993; Diamond and McGrew 1994; Hopkins and Bard 1995). Thus left handedness and right handedness for different purposes may have a tendency to co-occur in monkeys and apes, and the co-occurrence is shown directly in a study of stumptail macaques, who tended to reach for food rewards with the left hand, but performed manipulative acts on puzzle boxes with their right hands (Beck and Barton 1972). The trend toward right-hand preferences in monkeys and apes can be interpreted in the following way: 'With the abandonment of vertical clinging, more omnivory and more invasive foraging and manual food processing in many higher primates, the right side of the body, with its greater physical strength and its postural heritage of on-line control may have become the operative side' (MacNeilage 1997*a*).

In earlier papers (MacNeilage 1991, 1993) I presented a posture-related scenario for the evolution of the left hemisphere vocal communication specialization in non-human primates as well as for unimanual predation. (The term 'posture' here refers to the relative arrangement of body parts whether the animal is stationary or in action.) It began with the supposition that whole-body postural communication was presumably an important part of the repertoire of the earliest primates. Vocal and facial communicative gestures were presumably linked with postural displays. As the new arboreal habitat of the earliest primates involved new and relatively extreme postural demands, the putative left hemisphere postural controller may have been called upon for communicative actions. However, the accumulating evidence that there is a left hemisphere specialization for vocal communication in other major vertebrate taxa seems to call for a different interpretation. Rather than concluding that the non-human primate communicative specialization was not posturally motivated, I suggest that the communicative specializations in all the various vertebrate taxa may be postural, in the sense that they involve a specialized controller for action of the whole body. Certainly there must be body postural correlates of vocalizations in all vertebrates. They are typically produced in characteristic body configurations. And they involve temporary co-ordination with an otherwise continuously dominant movement complex—- the one that controls respiration. (For a discussion of this state of affairs in frogs, see Schmidt 1992.) From this standpoint, the involvement of a lateralized posture controller for prosimian vocalization may have simply entailed the continued use of a specialization for whole-body postural control already present in mammals ancestral to primates.

Evidence for the basic role of a lateralized body postural mechanism in the evolution of communication comes from an unlikely source—humans. I have argued that footedness is indicative of a contralateral postural control specialization because of the necessity of whole-body postural support for standing unipedal manoeuvres (MacNeilage 1991). In my view, this hemisphere would also tend to be specialized for language. In the traditional view of the evolution of speech lateralization (e.g. Corballis 1983; Kimura 1993), according to which a speech specialization arose from a lateralized manual skill, probably in *Homo habilis*, language control should tend to be in the hemisphere opposite the preferred hand. These two predictions can be differentiated in the 10 per cent of humans who have mixed limb preferences, roughly 5 per cent of whom are right-handed left-footers and 5 per cent are left-handed right-footers (MacNeilage 1991). It has now been shown in four different studies that language lateralization is more closely related to foot preference than to hand preference (Searleman 1980; Maki 1990, summarized in MacNeilage 1991; Day and MacNeilage 1996; Elias and Bryden 1996).

Further evidence for a left hemisphere body postural specialization in primates, including humans, comes from data of laterality in initiation of locomotion. Seltzer *et al.* (1990) conclude from a review of studies revealing a right leading limb preference for locomotor initiation in humans, four species of apes, and one species of prosimian, that such a bias 'may extend across contemporary primate species' (p. 164). They go on to surmise that 'If corresponding neural substrates for this lateralization are found, researchers may infer the origination of the bias in a common ancestor' (p. 164).

The possibility that begins to arise from all these results, namely that 'the left hemisphere mainly controls motor activity' in all vertebrates, has also been suggested by Bianki (1988, p. 147) on the basis of a review of an extremely large body of evidence, mainly on rats, and mainly by Russian researchers. One important basis for this conclusion is studies of selective hemispheric inactivation which show increased activity after right hemisphere inactivation and decreased activity after left hemisphere inactivation. This led to the conclusion 'that it is the left hemisphere that dominates in activating motor function whereas the right hemisphere inhibits it' (Bianki 1988, p. 140). Gunturkun and Hoferichter (1985) also implicate the left hemisphere in motor control in pigeons. They found that section of the left forebrain bundle, which is the main outflow from the forebrain, markedly reduces rates of key pecking, while section of the right forebrain bundle has no such effect.

Bianki (1988) reports a finding of significant right forepaw bias in a study of 302 domestic mice (see also Waters and Denenberg 1994), and reports the finding of Glumov and colleagues of a significant right forepaw bias in a study of 119 cats (Glumov 1984). Tan and his colleagues have also found right paw preferences for cats (Tan *et al.* 1990; Tan and Kutlu 1991) and dogs (Tan 1987). However, there are contrary findings in the literature, leading Bradshaw and Rogers (1993), who have summarized most of these findings, to conclude that the factors involved in non-primate mammalian paw preferences are, as yet, little understood. The nature of the task and the affective state of the animal may be two of these factors.

As to limb preferences in non-mammalian species, a preference for use of the right forelimb has been found in toads (Bisazza *et al.* 1996). The authors conclude that 'pawedness has a long evolutionary history, dating back at least to early tetrapods' (p. 408). However, a left foot preference, often extremely strong, has been repeatedly noted in most species of parrots that have been studied (Bradshaw and Rogers 1993). Despite appearances, this may not be counter-evidence to a left hemisphere motor specialization. In an animal that evolved to have bipedal posture but not forelimbs, and which could have some freedom from postural demands, the left hemisphere may not have been able to directly extend its body motor control specialization beyond its postural support role to concurrent skilled use of the contralateral extremity. In contrast with parrots, domestic chickens prefer to scratch with their right leg (Bradshaw and Rogers 1993), perhaps because this relatively stereotyped operation is less posturally demanding than the complex foot–mouth interaction observed in parrots.

10.3 A right hemisphere specialization for apprehension of the world in situations with survival-related risk?

The most well known specialization of the right hemisphere in humans is for spatial functions (De Renzi 1982). It is perhaps most clearly indicated in the left-sided neglect that often follows right parietal lobe damage in humans. This specialization may also have deep phylogenetic roots. As my colleagues and I have hypothesized (MacNeilage *et al.* 1987), it is probably a factor in the left-hand unimanual predation capability of prosimians. A face recognition capacity of the right hemisphere, presumably related to spatial integration capability, is also apparently common to humans and monkeys (Hamilton and Vermeire 1991). Bradshaw and Rogers (1993) conclude that in birds the left eye–right hemisphere system 'is specialized for processing topographical information; it responds to the changed position of a stimulus and is used to build up a map of the environment and respond to changes in it' (p. 93). In addition, spatial deficits are more likely to follow right than left hemisphere lesions in rats (Crowne *et al.* 1992; King and Corwin 1992).

Although the most clearly documented input-related specialization of the right hemisphere common to various vertebrates can be described as spatial, it is possible that this hemisphere is specialized for processing input in general in the service of apprehension of the external world for purposes most closely related to survival. The present-day human right hemisphere has just the properties needed for this function. It is considered to have a bilateral attentional specialization. Left-sided neglect phenomena in humans have been considered to result from the inability of the left hemisphere to compensate ipsilaterally for a bilateral deficit in right hemisphere attentional control (Mesulam 1981; Posner and Petersen 1990). The human right hemisphere performs better in vigilance tasks (Heilman 1995) and there is evidence that it has a superior depth perception capacity (Carmon and Bechtold 1969).

Most of the evidence for a special role of the right hemisphere for input processing in vertebrates has come from the visual modality. However, further evidence that there is a fundamental right hemisphere input specialization in vertebrates comes from the olfactory domain. A right nostril advantage in the discrimination of odours has been found in humans (Zatorre and Jones-Gotman 1990, 1992) implying a right hemisphere specialization. A similar right nostril discrimination advantage has been shown in the chick (Vallortigara and Andrew 1994). Day *et al.* (1996) have found the lateral cortex of two species of lizards—a region involved in olfaction—to be larger on the right side than on the left.

The capacity of the right hemisphere for what has been called 'global' information processing also seems to fit with the proposed role of this hemisphere for apprehension of the world. A rapid overall judgement of input could often be highly adaptive. The global capacity has been opposed to a 'local' capacity of the left hemisphere. Hellige (1995) has pointed out that this dichotomy is paralleled by two other dichotomies in processing which seem to be related to it: a bias towards efficient use of low versus high visual spatial frequencies, and a tendency to construct co-ordinate versus categorical relationships. The latter distinction, proposed by Kosslyn (1987), is considered to be based on computation of actual spatial relationships in a right hemisphere metrical system versus specifying them in terms of verbal categories such as 'on' or 'above' in a left hemisphere system. These three distinctions can be thought of in terms of the grain of analysis—coarse grained versus fine grained. A difference between the hemispheres in grain of analysis was suggested many years ago by Semmes, who found more specificity in deficits following left hemisphere damage than right hemisphere damage in humans (Semmes 1968). This lesion-based conclusion has been supported recently by Thatcher (1994), who found more widely distributed relations between electroencephalographic patterns in the right hemisphere of 10-year-olds than in the left.

A similarity to the hemispheric differences in processing visual spatial frequencies has been found in humans in the auditory modality. Ivry and Lebby (1993) found that humans were faster and more accurate in judging relatively low frequency sounds presented to the left ear (right hemisphere) than to the right ear, but found the opposite result for higher frequencies.

10.4 A right hemisphere perceptuo-motor specialization?

So far it has been argued that the vertebrate left hemisphere may possess a basic output control specialization, while the right hemisphere may possess a special-purpose input analysis specialization. But input analysis must be in the service of action. If indeed the right hemisphere has a specialization that includes rapid input processing in situations crucial to survival, then the apparent implication is that there is a specialized interhemispheric linkage that enables a left hemisphere motor response to such emergencies. This seems counterintuitive. The hemisphere best suited for immediate response to input is the ipsilateral one. The two observed instances of left limb preference, in prosimians and parrots, may have evolved partly because the right side of the body, controlled by a basic left hemisphere motor specialization, was required for postural purposes. However, the extremely specialized nature of the prosimian left-handed action suggests that a more elaborate evolutionary scenario might have been involved—one that involved a relation between ipsilateral perceptual and motor brain specializations of the right hemisphere. A key observation is that present-day vertical clinging prosimians can make a ballistic prehensile strike movement faster than the eye can see (Bishop 1964). Development of the implications of this fact requires some background.

I consider prosimian left handedness to be of profound significance in the context of vertebrate evolution in general. An arboreal environment makes extreme postural demands on all aspects of an organism's behaviour—for example, resting positions, locomotion, feeding, sexual reproduction, care of the young, fighting, and communication. Two major adaptations of form accompanied this momentous change to a totally arboreal habitat which occurred in ancestral primates—frontal vision and the prehensile hand. These are often thought of as locomotor adaptations, but manual predation, which is thought to have been the feeding mode in the earliest primates, has at least as large a claim on these changes in form (Cartmill 1975). Other, non-arboreal, predators, such as owls, also have frontal vision and prehensile capabilities. For the first time in almost half a billion years of vertebrate evolution the earliest prosimians gave up bilaterally symmetrical oral predation for asymmetrical manual predation. If there was a pre-existing tendency towards a right hemisphere specialization for visual representation in these animals, and if there was a left hemisphere action specialization already engaged by the postural demands of the arboreal habitat, including vertical clinging and leaping, then a specialized use of the left upper limb for ballistic reaching under direct right hemisphere control could have emerged as a crucial feeding adaptation.

The vertical clinging and leaping adaptation of prosimians was abandoned in Anthropoidea. In addition, the other feeding-related developments described earlier began to occur. At this point, the left hand–right hemisphere system presumably lost its predominance in favour of the side linked to the overall body action control specialization, except under circumstances for which it was especially fitted (e.g. goldfish catching). But I have argued that a residue of this left hand–right hemisphere specialization is still manifest in humans (MacNeilage 1991; MacNeilage *et al.* 1991), and is revealed in faster left arm reaction times in standing right-handed humans (Lee 1980). Also, Verfaellie *et al.* (1988) have observed faster left-hand than right-hand response in humans in a reaction time task in which subjects were given short notice as to which hand to respond with. In addition, Kimura and Watson (1989) have reported the unexpected finding that the left hand of right-handed adults is no worse than the right in batting down approaching objects. It seems more likely that these otherwise perplexing left-limb capabilities may be part of a fundamental vertebrate perceptuo-motor capability than that they arose in hominids as part of a default specialization of the right hemisphere after the left hemisphere of *Homo habilis* got involved in manual and linguistic specializations. In addition, there is an increasing consensus (e.g. Donald 1991) that true language did not evolve in *Homo habilis*, or even in *Homo erectus*, but only very recently, say in the past 100 000 years, which would leave very little time for the right hemisphere to develop compensatory activities.

If a right hemisphere specialization for apprehension of the world for basic survival purposes predated primate evolution, then a specialized immediate response capacity of the left side might also have predated primate evolution.

Though I presently know of no good evidence that this is the case, it might be worthwhile to seek it.

10.5 A motor basis for left hemisphere input processing specializations

I have argued that the input processing specialization of the right hemisphere may be associated with an output specialization capable of rapid response. Can we find a mirror image of this type of intrahemispheric linkage in the left hemisphere? Does it have an input specialization linked to its motor output specializations? Chicks have a left hemisphere advantage in visual discrimination which may be related to the control of routine feeding behaviour (Bradshaw and Rogers 1993). Corballis (1991) has recently argued that the evolution of a specialized 'praxic' (purposive movement) capability in hominids for both vocal and manual purposes gave rise to a 'generative assembling device' (GAD) specialized 'for constructing representations . . . from small vocabularies of primitive units' (p. 219). The units relevant to manual function are like a set of primitive forms ('geons') considered to be basic to image understanding by Biederman (1987). The vocal units are phonemes. Corballis considers the GAD to be equally relevant to input and output capabilities. I am sympathetic to the possibility that the evolution of vocal and manual output capabilites could be an important factor in the development of the three left hemispheric input analysis capacities grouped together by Hellige (1995)—local, high spatial frequencies, categorical. Although Corballis sees these developments as only becoming important in hominids, I would expect some related capability to be present in primates which have well-developed capabilities of hand-internal control, and a well-developed right-hand preference. Hopkins (1996) has found evidence of a local processing advantage for hierarchical visual stimuli in chimpanzees in the form of a shorter reaction time for local decisions with right visual field stimuli (left hemisphere) than with left.

10.6 Hemispheric specializations in the domain of affect: complementarity with the other functional specializations

Damasio (1994) has argued forcefully, primarily on neurobiological grounds, that 'Descartes' error' was to separate the cognitive domain from the affective domain—a theme also emphasized by Trevarthen (for example, 1990). In an analysis of both the frontal lobe syndrome, well known since the time of Phineas Gage, and the unilateral neglect syndrome, resulting (most usually) from right hemisphere damage, Damasio concluded that the symptom patterns cannot be understood without joint consideration of cognitive and affective symptomatology. There is a great deal of evidence for deep-seated affective asymmetries in the cerebral hemispheres of vertebrates (Lane and Jennings 1995; Robinson and Downhill 1995; Wittling *et al.* 1995), and many of the observed patterns are quite compatible with the specializations of the hemispheres that have already been described.

It is generally accepted that the right hemisphere has an emotional control specialization (e.g. Bradshaw and Rogers 1993; Hellige 1993). Rogers (1980) has observed right hemisphere dominance for attack in domestic chickens. Denenberg (1981) has observed an increase in mouse killing in rats after left hemispheric damage, which presumably releases right hemisphere propensities. A significant tendency towards more emotional responses to videotapes presented to the right hemisphere than to the left has been found in monkeys by Ifune *et al.* (1984). In what appears to be a related finding, Hatta and Koike (1991) have shown extremely strong left-hand preferences in adult female monkeys in removal of infants from threatening situations, though not in routine acts involving prehension. Most recently, Deckel (1995) has found that in the lizard *Anolis*, in which visual fields do not overlap and visual pathways from the eye are virtually completely crossed, significantly more aggressive behaviours were produced under the guidance of the left eye. A long-standing finding in humans is that with left hemisphere damage, the 'released' right hemisphere seems to produce depression (Robinson and Downhill 1995).

In his review of asymmetries of autonomic activity in a number of species, Wittling (1995) suggests a role of the right hemisphere consistent with the hypothesis, derived from its input processing capabilities, that it is specialized for survival-related purposes:

> The right brain seems to be primarily involved in control of vital functions supporting survival and enabling the organism to cope actively with stress and external challenges. This has been especially suggested by Gerendai's findings (e.g. Gerandai 1987) showing higher mortality rates following damage to the right brain, as well as by human and animal studies revealing a stronger involvement of the right brain in noradrenergic and serotonergic neurotransmitter activity, in the regulation of the stress hormone cortisol, in the control of blood pressure and chronotropic cardiac activity, and in sensitivity to pain-related and noxious stimuli. (Wittling 1995, p.336)

He also concludes that there is evidence for right hemisphere control of 'both upregulation and downregulation of autonomic–physiologic activity'.

It has often been suggested that the two hemispheres have opposite affective roles. Contrasting effects of cortical damage are well known in humans (Corballis 1991). While the effect of left hemisphere damage tends to be depressive, patients with right hemisphere damage are often indifferent to their condition (Damasio 1994) and manic (Robinson and Downhill 1995). In one well-developed line of work, Davidson and Fox and their colleagues asserted that while the right hemisphere is specialized for withdrawal, the left hemisphere is specialized for approach (Davidson 1995; see also Fox 1991). This dichotomy has been shown to exist in human infants as well as adults. Recently, homologous left hemisphere effects have been shown in monkeys (Davidson *et al.* 1992).

Another dichotomy has been suggested by Tucker and Williamson (1984; see also Liotti and Tucker 1995). This dichotomy is consistent with the roles of the two hemispheres proposed here. In their view, the right hemisphere is influenced by a subcortical phasic arousal system mediating noradrenaline increases and supporting the capacity of the hemisphere for making orientation responses to novelty. In contrast, they propose a subcortical tonic activation system supporting motor readiness of the left hemisphere.

An important part of their proposal regarding the motor readiness of left hemisphere is the role of the neurotransmitter dopamine. Dopamine is associated primarily with motor control (Wittling 1995). For example, dopamine deficency in the nigro-striatal system is involved in the symptomatology of Parkinson's disease. A post-mortem study of humans has shown higher levels of dopamine in the left corpus striatum than in the right, presumably correlated with the right-sided action bias of human right-handers (Glick *et al.* 1982). The human left globus pallidus, a component of the corpus striatum, is also larger than the right (Kooistra and Heilman 1988). Work in rats has shown turning preferences contralateral to the side of the brain with higher striatal dopamine levels (Glick and Shapiro 1985). Although turning preferences seem to be subject to strain differences in rats, the generally higher left hemisphere dopamine levels in humans seem to provide evidence for a left hemisphere control system integrating affective and motor lateralities.

10.7 The (somewhat) optional nature of direction of forelimb preference

Vertebrates only have one axial complex, and live in only one world, but they have pairs of limbs. However, the vertebrate morphological plan has never departed markedly from a basic symmetry in limb pairs, and their neural innervation. The thesis advanced here is that the most basic cerebral hemispheric specializations in vertebrates are for the control of the whole body, particularly axial structures (left hemisphere) and apprehension of the whole available world (right hemisphere), together with their associated perceptual or motor specializations and their compatible affective specializations. Although these specializations tend, sometimes, to have strong typical linkages to contralateral limbs, as in right handedness in humans and left handedness in prosimians, there can apparently be some leeway in this regard in some individual members of a species. Some recent studies provide evidence of a degree of independence between handedness and other aspects of hemispheric specialization in non-human primates in particular. Rogers *et al.* (1994) found a left eye preference in all of six small-eared bushbabies—a preference that I would interpret in terms of a right hemisphere input processing specialization—but found that the preference was independent of handedness. Hopkins and Washburn (1994) found that while a group of left-handed monkeys performed better on a task involving delayed response to spatial position, which presumably invoked a right hemisphere specialization, a group of right-handed monkeys did better on a form cue task, which presumably invoked a left hemisphere specialization. In a similar vein, Hopkins and Bennett (1994) found that right-handed monkeys approached and touched novel objects significantly more quickly than left-handed monkeys, suggesting a relation between hand preferences and each of the two poles of the affective approach–avoidance dichotomy of Davidson (1995). The two latter studies suggest that in different monkeys, hand preference may become linked to different cerebral specializations, implying some intraspecies independence between hand and hemisphere despite the presence of population-level handedness asymmetries. Human left-handed right-footers seem to be an example of the exercise of an unusual option in linkage of the preferred limb to the specializations of the hemispheres. There is strong evidence that they usually have a language specialization and the associated postural control specialization in the left hemisphere (Day and MacNeilage 1996), and they probably have the usual human right hemisphere spatial specialization as well.

10.8 Conclusions

In this review of cerebral hemispheric specializations in vertebrates there was not a single case in which a specialization was found to be confined to hominids, unless one wishes to distinguish between language and the non-linguistic vocal communication specialization from which it was probably derived (see MacNeilage 1997*b*). On the contrary, there is one specialization —left limb specialization—which is obviously present in other taxa but not readily observable in humans. In addition, in three cases—specializations for vocal communication, spatial function, and negative affect—a specialization is present in a majority of major vertebrate taxonomic groups. Furthermore, the taxa in which few specializations have been observed have been subject to little enquiry. All in all, the evidence suggests that human-like cerebral hemispheric specializations are extremely frequent elsewhere in the vertebrate phylum, and that the burden of proof may now need to be shouldered by those who assert that these specializations are sporadic (e.g. Hiscock and Kinsbourne 1995).

I have suggested that the basic pattern of cerebral hemispheric specializations in vertebrates may be a left hemisphere motor specialization for routine purposes and a right hemispheric specialization for apprehension of the world for basic survival purposes, and that each hemisphere also has an affective specialization related to its basic functional purpose. Beyond this I have argued that there have arisen complementary intrahemispheric input/output specializations for particular purposes—a left-side rapid response specialization directly linked to the right hemisphere input apprehension specialization, and left hemispheric input analysis specializations relevant to its motor role in chick feeding, advanced primate praxic capabilities, and, in the case of modern hominids, language. This dichotomy has affinities with the view of Goldberg on the differences between the two hemispheres in humans (Goldberg and Costa 1981; Goldberg and Podell 1995), except that in focusing on humans they tend to place more emphasis on cognition. According to Goldberg and Podell (p. 93): 'The right hemisphere appears to be critical for processing novel cognitive situations. The left hemisphere appears to be central to the processes mediated by well routinized representations and strategies.'

How did these hemispheric differences originate? For answers to this question we need much more work on modern representatives of early vertebrate forms. One proposal, by Andrew *et al.* (1982), is that in animals in which the visual fields of the two eyes do not overlap, some lateralized specialization is necessary to avoid conflicting responses from the two hemispheres.

It may be noted that some aspects of the cerebral dichotomies suggested here can be mapped on to various traditional metafunctional dichotomies applied to the hominid cerebral hemispheres—analytic versus synthetic, serial versus parallel (motor control is serial, rapid perceptual apprehension is parallel), rational versus intuitive. However, I am arguing that such dichotomies, are, in the final analysis, rooted directly in particular adaptive behaviours, fundamental to all vertebrates, rather than being selected for, as such, in hominids.

Regardless of the correctness of the detailed proposal, I hope I have convinced all but the most hardened sceptic that there are important phylogenetic bases for human cerebral hemispheric specializations and their relationships. The anthropomorphic approach to other animals has been widely regarded as impeding their understanding (Kennedy 1992). There has been much less interest in the possibility that it might aid in the understanding of humans.

References

Andrew, R. J., Mench, J., and Rainey, C. (1982). Right–left asymmetry of response to visual stimuli in the domestic chick. In *Analysis of visual behavior*, (ed. D. J. Ingle, M. A. Goodale, and R. J. Mansfield), pp. 197–209. MIT Press, Cambridge, MA.

Arnold, A. P. and Bottjer, S. W. (1985). Cerebral lateralization in birds. In *Cerebral lateralization in nonhuman species*, (ed. S. D. Glick), pp. 11–39. Academic Press, Orlando.

Bauer, R. H. (1993). Lateralization of neural control for vocalization by the frog (*Rana pipiens*). *Psychobiology*, **21**, 243–8.

Beck, C. H. M. and Barton, R. L. (1972). Deviation and laterality of hand preference in monkeys. *Cortex*, **8**, 339–63.

Bianki, V. L. (1988). *The right and left hemispheres of the animal brain*. Gordon and Breach, New York.

Biederman, I. (1987). Recognition by components: A theory of human image understanding. *Psychological Review*, **94**, 115–47.

Bisazza, A., Cantalupo, C., Robins, A., Rogers, L. J., and Vallortigara, G. (1996). Right-pawedness in toads. *Nature*, **379**, 408.

Bishop, A. (1964). Use of the hand in lower primates. In *Evolutionary and genetic biology of primates*, Vol. 2, (ed. J. Buettner-Janush), pp. 133–238. Academic Press, New York.

Bradshaw, J. L. and Rogers, L. J. (1993). *The evolution of lateral asymmetries, language, tool use, and intellect*. Academic Press, New York.

Carmon, A. and Bechtold, H. P. (1969). Dominance of the right cerebral hemisphere for stereopsis. *Neuropsychologia*, **7**, 29–39.

Cartmill, M. (1975). *Primate origins*. Burgess, Minneapolis.

Corballis, M. C. (1983). *Human laterality*. Academic Press, New York.

Corballis, M. C. (1991). *The lopsided ape: evolution of the generative mind*. Oxford University Press, Oxford.

Crowne, D. P., Novotny, M. F., Mier, S. E., and Vitols, R. W. (1992). Spatial deficits and their lateralization following unilateral parietal cortex lesions in the rat. *Behavioral Neuroscience*, **106**, 808–19.

Damasio, A. R. (1994). *Descartes' error: emotion, reason and the human brain*. Putnam, New York.

Davidson, R. J. (1995). Cerebral asymmetry, emotion and affective style. In *Brain asymmetry*, (ed. R. J. Davidson and K. Hugdahl), pp. 361–88. MIT Press, Cambridge, MA.

Davidson, R. J., Kalin, N. H., and Shelton, S. E. (1992). Lateralized effects of diazepam on frontal brain electrical asymmetries in rhesus monkey. *Biological Psychiatry*, **32**, 438–51.

Day, L. B. and MacNeilage, P. F. (1996). Postural asymmetries and language lateralization in humans (*Homo sapiens*) *Journal of Comparative Psychology*, **110**, 88–96.

Day, L. B., Wilczynski, W., and Crews, D. (1996). Hemispheric lateralization of the dorsal and lateral cortices in lizards. *Society for Neuroscience Abstracts*, **21**, 432.

Deckel, A. W. (1995). Laterality of agressive responses in *Anolis*. *Journal of Experimental Zoology*, **272**, 194–200.

Denenberg, V. H. (1981). Hemispheric laterality in animals and the effects of early experience. *Behavioral and Brain Sciences*, **4**, 1–49.

De Renzi, E. (1982). *Disorders of space exploration and cognition*. Wiley, New York.

Diamond, A. and McGrew, W. C. (1994). True handedness in the cotton-top tamarin (*Saguinus oedipus*)? *Primates*, **35**, 69–77.

Donald, M. (1991). *Origins of the modern mind: Three stages in the evolution of culture and cognition*. Harvard University Press, Cambridge, MA.

Ehret, G. (1987). Left hemisphere advantage in the mouse brain for recognizing ultrasonic communication calls. *Nature*, **325**, 249–51.

Elias, L. J. and Bryden, M. P. (1996). Footedness is a better predictor of language lateralization than handedness. *Laterality*, in press.

Ettlinger, G. (1984). Humans, apes and monkeys: The changing neuropsychological viewpoint. *Neuropsychologia*, **22**, 685–96.

Ettlinger, G. (1987). Primate handedness: how nice if it really were so. *Behavioral and Brain Sciences*, **10**, 271–3.

Fagot, J. and Vauclair, J. (1988*a*). Handedness and manual specialization in the baboon. *Neuropsychologia*, **26**, 795–804.

Fagot, J. and Vauclair, J. (1988*b*). Handedness and bimanual coordination in the lowland gorilla. *Brain Behavior and Evolution*, **32**, 89–95.

Fox, N. A. (1991). If it's not left, it's right: Electroencephalographic asymmetry and the development of emotion. *American Psychologist*, **46**, 863–72.

Gerendai, I. (1987) Laterality in the neuroendocrine system. In *Duality and unity of the brain*, (ed. D. Ottoson), pp. 17–28. Macmillan, London.

Glick, S. D. and Shapiro, R. M. (1985). Functional and neurochemical mechanisms of cerebral lateralization in rats. In *Cerebral lateralization in nonhuman species*, (ed. S. D. Glick), pp. 158–84. Academic Press, New York.

Glick, S. D., Ross, D. A., and Hough, L. B. (1982). Lateral asymmetry of neural transmitters in human brain. *Brain Research*, **234**, 53–63.

Glumov, G. M. (1984). Asymmetry of the forepaw motor function in cats. *Physiological Journal of the USSR*, **70**, 1332–7.

Goldberg, E. and Costa, L. D. (1981). Hemispheric differences in the acquisition and use of descriptive systems. *Brain and Language*, **14**, 144–73.

Goldberg, E. and Podell, K. (1995). Lateralization in the frontal lobes. In *Epilepsy and the functional anatomy of the frontal lobe*, (ed. H. H. Jasper, S. Riggio, and P. S. Goldman-Rakic), pp. 85–96. Raven Press, New York.

Graves, R., Landis, T., and Goodglass, H. (1990). Asymmetry in mouth opening during different speech tasks. *International Journal of Psychology*, **25**, 179–89.

Gunturkun, O. and Hoferichter, H.-H. (1985). Neglect after section of a left telencephalotectal tract in pigeons. *Behavioral Neuroscience*, **18**, 1–9.

Hamilton, C. R. and Vermeire, B. A. (1991). Functional lateralization in monkeys. In *Cerebral laterality: theory and research*, (ed. F. Kitterle), pp. 19–34. Erlbaum, Hillsdale, NJ.

Hatta, T. and Koike, M. (1991). Left-hand preference in frightened mother monkeys in taking up their babies. *Neuropsychologia*, **29**, 207–9.

Hauser, M. and Andersson, K. (1993). Left hemisphere dominance for processing vocalizations in adult, but not infant, rhesus monkeys: field experiments. *Proceedings of the National Academy of Sciences, USA*, **91**, 3946–8.

Heffner, H. E. and Heffner, R. S. (1984). Temporal lobe lesions and the perception of species-specific vocalizations by macaques. *Science*, **226**, 75–6.

Heilman, K. M. (1995). Attentional asymmetries. In *Brain asymmetry*, (ed. R. J. Davidson and K. Hugdahl), pp. 217–34. MIT Press, Cambridge, MA.

Hellige, J. B. (1993). *Hemispheric asymmetry: What's right and what's left*. MIT Press, Cambridge, MA.

Hellige, J. B. (1995). Hemispheric asymmetry for components of visual information processing. In *Brain asymmetry*, (ed. R. J. Davidson and K. Hugdahl), pp. 99–122. MIT Press, Cambridge, MA.

Hiscock, M. and Kinsbourne, M. (1995). Phylogeny and ontogeny of cerebral lateralization. In *Brain asymmetry*, (ed. R. J. Davidson and K. Hugdahl), pp. 535–78., MIT Press, Cambridge, MA.

Holman, S. D. and Hutchinson, J. B. (1991). Lateralized action of androgen and development of behavior and brain sex differences. *Brain Research Bulletin*, **27**, 261–5.

Hopkins, W. D. (1993). Posture and reaching in chimpanzees (*Pan troglodytes*) and orangutans (*Pongo pygmaeus*). *Journal of Comparative Psychology*, **107**, 162–8.

Hopkins, W. D. (1995). Hand preferences for a coordinated bimanual task in 110 chimpanzees (*Pan troglodytes*): Cross sectional analysis. *Journal of Comparative Psychology*, **109**, 291–7.

Hopkins, W. D. (1996). Hemispheric specialization for local and global processing of heirarchical visual stimuli in chimpanzees. *Neuropsychologia*, in press.

Hopkins, W. D. and Bard, K. (1995). Asymmetries in spontaneous head turning in infant chimpanzeess. *Behavioral Neuroscience*, **109**, 808–12.

Hopkins, W. D. and Bennett, A. J. (1994). Handedness and approach-avoidance behavior in chimpanzees (*Pan*) *Journal of Experimental Psychology: Animal Behavior Processes*, **20**, 413–18.

Hopkins, W. D. and Washburn, D. A. (1994). Do right and left-handed monkeys differ on cognitive measures? *Behavioral Neuroscience*, **108**, 1207–12.

Hopkins, W. D., Bennett, A. J., Bales, S. L., Lee, J., and Ward, J. P. (1993). Behavioral laterality in captive bonobos (*Pan paniscus*). *Journal of Comparative Psychology*, **107**, 403–10.

Ifune, C. K., Vermeire, B. A., and Hamilton, C. R. (1984). Hemispheric differences in split brain monkeys viewing and responding to videotaped recordings. *Behavioral and Neural Biology*, **41**, 231–5.

Ivry, R. B. and Lebby, P. (1993). Hemispheric differences in auditory perception are similar to those found in visual perception. *Psychological Science*, **4**, 41–5.

Kennedy, J. S. (1992). *The new anthropomorphism.* Cambridge University Press, Cambridge.

Kimura, D. (1993). *Neuromotor mechanisms in human communication.* Oxford University Press, Oxford.

Kimura, D. and Watson, N. V. (1989). Right hand superiority for throwing but not for interception. *Neuropsychologia*, **27**, 1399–414.

King, J. E. and Landau, V. I. (1993). Manual preferences in varieties of reaching in squirrel monkeys. In *Primate laterality: current evidence of primate asymmetries*, (ed. J. P. Ward and W. D. Hopkins), pp. 107–24. Springer-Verlag, New York.

King, V. R. and Corwin, J. V. (1992). Spatial deficits and hemispheric asymmetries in the rat following unilateral and bilateral lesions of posterior parietal or medial agranular cortex. *Behavioural Brain Research*, **50**, 53–68.

Kooistra, C. A. and Heilman, K. M. (1988). Motor dominance and lateral asymmetry of the globus pallidus. *Neurology*, **38**, 388–90.

Kosslyn, S. M. (1987). Seeing and imaging in the cerebral hemispheres. *Psychological Review*, **94**, 148–75.

Lane, R. D. and Jennings, J. R. (1995). Hemispheric asymmetry, autonomic asymmetry, and the problem of sudden cardiac death. In *Brain asymmetry*, (ed. R. J. Davidson and K. Hugdahl), pp. 271–304. MIT Press, Cambridge, MA.

Lee, W. A. (1980). Anticipatory control of postural and task muscles during rapid arm flexion. *Journal of Motor Behavior*, **12**, 185–96.

Liotti, M. and Tucker, D. M. (1995). Emotion in asymmetric corticolimbic networks. In *Brain asymmetry*, (ed. R. J. Davidson and K. Hugdahl), pp. 389–424. MIT Press, Cambridge, MA.

MacNeilage, P. F. (1991). The postural origins theory of neurobiological asymmetries in primates. In *The biological foundations of language development*, (ed. N. Krasnegor, D. Rumbaugh, M. G. Studdert-Kennedy, and R. Schiefelbusch), pp. 165–88. Erlbaum, Hillsdale, NJ.

MacNeilage, P. F. (1993). Implication of primate functional asymmetries for the evolution of cerebral hemispheric specializations. In *Primate laterality: current evidence of primate asymmetries*, (ed. J. P. Ward and W. D. Hopkins), pp. 319–41. Springer-Verlag, New York.

MacNeilage, P. F. (1996). Articulatory asymmetry in rhesus monkeys: An indication of brain asymmetries underlying vocal communication. Undergraduate honors thesis, Harvard University.

MacNeilage, P. F. (1997*a*). Evolution of the mechanism of language output: comparative neurobiology of vocal and manual communication. In *Evolution of language*, (ed. J. R. Hurford, M. G. Studdert-Kennedy, and C. Knight), in press.

MacNeilage, P. F. (1997*b*). The frame/content theory of evolution of speech production. *Behavioral and Brain Sciences*, in press.

MacNeilage, P. F., Studdert-Kennedy, M. G., and Lindblom, B. (1987). Primate handedness reconsidered. *Behavioral and Brain Sciences*, **10**, 247–63.

MacNeilage, P. F., Studdert-Kennedy, M. G., and Lindblom, B. (1991). Primate handedness: The other theory, the other hand and the other attitude. *Behavioral and Brain Sciences*, **14**, 344–9.

Maki, S. (1990). An experimental approach to the postural origins theory of neurobiological asymmetries in primates. Unpublished Ph.D. dissertation, University of Texas at Austin.

Masataka, N. (1989). Population level asymmetries of hand preference in lemurs. *Behaviour*, **110**, 1–4.

Masataka, N. (1990). Handedness of capuchin monkeys. *Folia Primatologia*, **55**, 189–92.

Mason, A. M., Wolfe, L. D., and Johnson, J. C. (1995). Hand preference in the Sifaka (*Propithecus verreauxi*) during feeding in captivity. *Primates*, **36**, 275–80.

Mesulam, M.-M. (1981). A cortical network for directed attention and unilateral neglect. *Annals of Neurology*, **10**, 309–15.

Petersen, M., Beecher, B., Zoloth, S., Moody, D., and Stebbins, W. (1978). Neural lateralization of species-specific vocalizations by Japanese macaques (*Macaca fuscata*). *Science*, **202**, 324–7.

Posner, M. I. and Petersen, S. E. (1990). The attention system of the human brain. *Annual Review of Neuroscience*, **13**, 25–42.

Robinson, R. J. and Downhill, J. E. (1995) Lateralization of psychopathology in response to focal brain injury. In *Brain asymmetry*, (ed. R. J. Davidson and K. Hugdahl), pp. 693–712. MIT Press, Cambridge, MA.

Rogers, L. J. (1980). Functional lateralization in the chicken forebrain revealed by cyclohexamide treatment. In *Acta XVI Congressus Ornithologici, Berlin, 1978*, Vol. 1, (ed. R. Nohring), pp. 653–9). Deutsche Ornithologen-Gesellschaft, Berlin.

Rogers, L. J., Ward, J. P., and Stafford, D. (1994). Eye dominance in the small-eared bushbaby *Otolemur garnetti*. *Neuropsychologia*, **32**, 257–64.

Schmidt, R. S. (1992). Neural correlates of frog calling: production by two semi-independent generators. *Behavioural Brain Research*, **50**, 17–30.

Searleman, A. (1980). Subject variables and cerebral organization for language. *Cortex*, **16**, 239–54.

Seltzer, C., Forsythe, C., and Ward, J. P. (1990). Multiple measures of motor lateralization in human primates (*Homo sapiens*). *Journal of Comparative Psychology*, **104**, 159–66.

Semmes, J. (1968). Hemispheric specialization: a possible clue to mechanism. *Neuropsychologia*, **6**, 11–26.

Tan, U. (1987). Paw preferences in dogs. *International Journal of Neuroscience*, **32**, 825–9.

Tan, U. and Kutlu, N. (1991). The distribution of paw preferences in right-, left-, and mixed pawed male and female cats: The role of a female right shift factor in handedness. *International Journal of Neuroscience*, **59**, 219–29.

Tan, U., Yaprak, M., and Kutlu, N. (1990). Paw preferences in cats: Distribution and sex differences. *International Journal of Neuroscience*, **50**, 195–208.

Thatcher, R. W. (1994). Cyclical cortical reorganization: origins of human cognitive development. In *Human behavior and the developing brain*, (ed. G. Dawson and K. W. Fischer), pp. 232–66. Guilford Press, New York.

Trevarthen, C. (1990). Growth and education of the hemispheres. In *Brain circuits and functions of the mind: essays in honour of Roger W. Sperry*, (ed. C.Trevarthen), pp. 334–63. Cambridge University Press, Cambridge.

Tucker, D. and Williamson, P. A. (1984). Asymmetric neural control systems in human self-regulation. *Psychological Review*, **91**, 185–215.

Vallortigara, G. and Andrew, R. J. (1994). Olfactory lateralization in the chick. *Neuropsychologia*, **32**, 417–23.

Verfaellie, M., Bowers, D., and Heilman, K. M. (1988). Hemispheric asymmetries mediating intention but not selective attention. *Neuropsychologia*, **26**, 521–31.

Ward, J. P. and Hopkins, W. D. (ed.) (1993). *Primate laterality: current evidence of primate asymmetries*. Springer-Verlag, New York.

Ward, J. P., Milliken, G., and Stafford, D. K. (1993). Patterns of lateralized behavior in prosimians. In *Primate laterality: current evidence of primate asymmetries*, (ed. J. P. Ward and W. D. Hopkins), pp. 43–74. Springer-Verlag, New York.

Waters, N. S. and Denenberg, V. H. (1994). Analysis of two measures of paw preference in a large population of inbred mice. *Behavioural Brain Research*, **63**, 195–204.

Wittling, W. (1995). Brain asymmetry in the control of autonomic-physiologic activity. In *Brain asymmetry*, (ed. R. J. Davidson and K. Hugdahl), pp. 305–58. MIT Press, Cambridge, MA.

Zattore, R. J. and Jones-Gotman, M. (1990). Right nostril advantage for discrimination of odors. *Perception and Psychophysics*, **47**, 526–31.

Zattore, R. J., Jones-Gotman, M., Evans, A. C., and Meyer, E. (1992). Functional localization and lateralization of human olfactory cortex. *Nature*, **360**, 339–40.

11

Brain mechanisms of apraxia

ULRIKE HALSBAND

11.1 Introduction

Apraxias have been defined as higher-order motor disturbances that are not due to paresis, a primary motor defect (normal strength, reflexes, co-ordination), ataxia, aphasia, or dementia. The basic deficit of an apraxic patient lies in the fact that the production of different natural movements is no longer possible. This can apply to complex manual actions or gestural movements, but also to routine everyday actions, such as dressing oneself or walking. Following acute brain damage, apraxias can appear at least as commonly as paresis or elementary motor disturbances (Freund 1987; Poeck 1989).

At a first glance it appears as if the patient has lost the memory of movements which were highly overlearned and automatized. But like aphasia, apraxia represents not only a condition where previously learned movements are lost, but also where new motor learning is grossly affected. Thereby the question arises of a possible disturbance of the motor (procedural) memory system (Cohen 1984; Squire 1986). On the other hand, it is surprising that movements that cannot be made in accordance with verbal command or imitation, can often be flawlessly produced in other contexts (Geschwind 1975; De Renzi *et al.* 1980). This contextual dependence suggests a problem of retrieval of motor programs. Indeed, one of the fundamental issues in current apraxia research is whether the motor impairments observed in apraxic patients actually result from the disruption of an abstract representation of motor acts (e.g. Bay 1965; Lehmkuhl and Poeck 1981; Roy and Square 1985; Roy *et al.* 1993; Halsband *et al.* 1995; Rizzolatti *et al.* 1996).

Anatomically, apraxias appear as a consequence of damage to the memory and/or motor association areas; these areas comprise a large part of the cortical surface (e.g. Heilman 1979; Freund 1987, 1992; Poeck 1989; Halsband and Freund 1993). Among the various structures involved, lesions in the posterior parietal lobe of the language-dominant hemisphere undoubtedly lead to the most dramatic apraxic disturbances in man. The disturbance of conceptual planning of movement leads to an error-prone control of the primary motor areas. This does not appear as a motor weakness but as a temporal and spatial disintegration of movement. One major problem is that the analysis of apraxic disturbances has until now been characterized mainly through verbal description of the motor deficits. The standardized tests for apraxia use descriptive scales of the severity of apraxia in a similar fashion to those used with aphasics. To date, only a few studies exist which enable a more direct glimpse into the nature of apraxic disturbances.

The asymmetrical disposition of these motor programming systems in the human brain may explain why there is still no adequate model of apraxia in non-human primates (Ettlinger 1969; Poeck 1989). After examining more than 50 monkeys with unilateral or bilateral posterior brain lesions, Ettlinger (1969, p. 296) concluded that 'parietal removals have never, in my experience, been followed by a motor condition resembling apraxia'. Although recent contributions from neurophysiological and brain lesion studies in non-human primates have made substantial progress in the understanding of the functional mechanisms of motor learning and memory, the results have had relatively little impact on current concepts of apraxias, whose study still remains within the domain of clinical neuropsychology.

11.2 Concepts and models of the apraxias

11.2.1 Liepmann's classification re-examined

Steinthal introduced the term apraxia in 1871, but the symptoms had first been described by Hughlings Jackson 5 years earlier (reprinted in Taylor 1932). He pointed out that some aphasic patients were unable to perform voluntary movements, such as protruding the tongue, although there were no signs of weakness in the muscles involved.

Liepmann (1900, 1908) justifiably receives credit for establishing apraxia as a distinct neuropsychological entity. He proposed the classic concept of three different types of apraxia:

(1) *ideomotor* or *ideo-kinetic apraxia*: a disorder in performing single gestures, while the level of ideation is preserved;

(2) *ideational apraxia:* defective performance of a complex sequence of movements with a disruption of the overall plan of action, although the individual elements of the total act are executed correctly; and

(3) *limb-kinetic apraxia*: loss of kinetic memories for the use of a limb.

Although the division of the apraxias into the ideomotor, ideational, and kinetic types is by no means undisputed (e.g. Freund 1992), this terminology is still used in apraxia research owing to the lack of a better typology based on detailed descriptions of the various patterns of disturbance.

The most commonly described form of apraxia is ideomotor apraxia, which can be summarized as a disturbance of the selection of motor elements that constitute a particular movement. It has been proposed that ideomotor apraxia is caused by lesions that either damage visuokinaesthetic engrams for skilled movements stored in the left parietal lobe, or disconnect these engrams from motor association areas (Heilman 1979; Heilman and Rothi 1985). Anatomically, ideomotor apraxia has been associated with damage to the inferior parietal lobe (Brodmann's areas 39 and 40) and with lesions to the superior parietal cortex (Brodmann's areas 5 and 7) (e.g. Faglioni and Basso 1985; Heilman and Rothi 1985). In ideomotor apraxia the patient does not know how to perform a particular motor act. Such patients cannot perform a motor act in response to a verbal command or by imitation. In patients with ideomotor apraxia, imitation of meaningless and novel movements is as faulty as that of symbolic gestures (De Renzi *et al.* 1980; Roy *et al.* 1991; Goldenberg 1995).

There has been much confusion about the term *ideational* apraxia. Liepmann (1908) described it as an 'apraxia of action sequences', whereas others have defined it as a defect in the actual handling of objects (Zangwill 1960; De Renzi *et al.* 1968), or as an impairment in a verbally mediated motor sequence (Heilman 1973). According to Roy and Square (1985), ideational apraxia results from a dysfunction of the conceptual praxis system, which contains three types of abstract information relevant to praxis:

(1) knowledge of objects and tools in terms of their functions;
(2) 'decontextualized' knowledge of action that is independent of objects or tools; and
(3) knowledge about the serial organization of motor sequences.

Ideational apraxia could thus be defined as a deficit of the conception of the movement so that the patient does not know what to do (Freund 1987).

Ideational apraxia is typically seen after lesions in the posterior temporo-parietal region of the dominant hemisphere (De Ajuriaguerra *et al.* 1960; De Renzi and Lucchelli 1988). Platz and Mauritz (1995) directly compared the kinematic abnormalities of patients with ideational and ideomotor apraxia. Subjects were asked to make triangular arm movements in space without visual control. Motion was analysed three-dimensionally before and after kinaesthetic training with a triangular stencil. It was found that patients with ideational apraxia showed signs of impaired motor planning. These patients had major difficulties in selecting the body parts to be moved, and the movement concept and configurational aspects were deficient. Kinaesthetic sensorimotor training was not adequate to reduce these deficits. In contrast, patients with ideomotor apraxia presented with major difficulties in programming movement elements. Submovements were segmented and characterized by irregularities and, in addition, non-requested motor components occurred. Interestingly, these deficits could be reduced by task-specific sensorimotor training.

Liepmann's (1900, 1908) third form of apraxia, which he named limb-kinetic apraxia, appears in complex sequential movements that demand a high degree of skill, temporal co-ordination, and fine accuracy, e.g. the finger movements of a pianist or a typist (Luria 1966; Stuss and Benson 1986). The problem posed by limb-kinetic apraxia lies primarily in the carrying out of correctly conceptualized movements. Kinetic apraxias are usually described as following lesions of the premotor cortex (PMC) and supplementary motor area (SMA) (Freund and Hummelsheim 1985; Freund 1992; Halsband *et al.* 1993).

11.2.2 Constructional apraxia

Constructional apraxia has been defined as a disorder in reproducing visual configurations, in which the spatial aspect of the performance is disrupted. Such symptoms were first described clinically by Strauss (1924), but the term was introduced by Kleist 10 years later (1934). After first considering certain drawing disabilities of neurological patients to be a form of 'optic apraxia' Kleist (1934) later called it *konstruktive optische Apraxie*. Constructional apraxia is characterized by difficulties in putting together simple elements: assembling, drawing, joining, or articulating them to form a single unitary structure. According to Kleist (1934) this particular disorder was to be distinguished from others that were rooted in visuoperceptual difficulties. In the chain of production of voluntary movements, the nature of the defect was argued to be neither visuoperceptive nor motor, but rather to be in the transformation of information from visual perception into the appropriate action.

Ettlinger *et al.* (1957) discussed the difficult relation between visual agnosia and constructional apraxia, which has remained a controversial issue ever since. In this now-classic study, the visuospatial abilities of 10 patients with lesions in the right posterior cortex were carefully examined. Tasks included copying of a bicycle from a model, drawing a map of England, and assembling matchsticks to form a star pattern. The authors gave a detailed analytical account of the characteristic disturbances in spatial perception and manipulative skill. They formulated the relation between visuospatial agnosia and constructional apraxia as follows:

> Although it has been customary to ascribe difficulties in drawing on assembly tasks . . . to special forms of 'apraxia' it is difficult to say how far such disabilities are truly dyspraxic and how far merely secondary to perceptual or ideational disorder. In the majority of our cases . . . constructional . . . disabilities appear to arise principally on a basis of disordered spatial perception . . . At the same time, it would probably be incorrect wholly to exclude a concomitant disorder in the executive aspects of performance. (Ettlinger *et al.* 1957, p. 359)

As a clinician one is confronted with constructional deficits which may differ from each other in many respects, e.g. in the type of movement and the degree of motor dexterity required in achieving the task, and whether the patient's problems involve construction in two or three spatial dimensions. Therefore it is not surprising that many controversies have surrounded the question whether constructional apraxia should be regarded as a separate and single entity or whether it includes distinct types of disorder (e.g. Warrington *et al.* 1966; Benton 1969; Carlesimo *et al.* 1993). Constructional failures can be observed after damage to either the non-dominant or dominant hemisphere. Hécaen and Albert (1978) pointed out that the disorder may result from a breakdown in different underlying neuropsychological mechanisms, depending on the hemisphere damaged. Hypotheses about the underlying deficits in left versus right hemisphere constructional apraxias remain a matter of debate. Although the available evidence is not conclusive, it is reasonable to assume that damage to the dominant (left) hemisphere results in difficulties in the planning of constructive processes, while damage to the non-dominant (right) hemisphere may cause deficits in processing the relevant spatial and configurational sensory information.

This conclusion is in agreement with the most recent findings by Platz and Mauritz (1995) who used quantitative three-dimensional motion analysis and reported difficulties in making use of new visual information relevant for spatially directed action in two patients suffering from constructional apraxia after right brain damage. A promising line for future research would be to compare these findings with comparable kinematic motion analyses of patients suffering from constructional apraxia after *left* brain damage.

11.2.3 Other forms of apraxia

Over the years, a number of different types of apraxia have been suggested, based largely on distinctions of different categories of motor behaviour, including buccofacial apraxia (disturbance of voluntary facial acts), dressing apraxia (difficulties in orienting and correctly disposing clothing with respect to one's own body), apraxia of speech (increase of articulatory errors as the complexity of motor adjustments required of the articulators increases, Darley 1982), and callosal apraxia (disconnection of the speech areas from the motor area).

11.2.4 Models of the neural basis of apraxia

Two influential models of the neural basis of apraxia have been put forward, both of which are still very much in dispute:

(1) Geschwind's (1965) disconnection model; and
(2) Heilman's representational hypothesis (Heilman 1979; Heilman and Rothi 1993).

According to Geschwind (1965) language gives rise to planned motor behaviour through a neural substrate similar to that proposed by Wernicke (1874) to explain language processing. It is well known that Wernicke's area plays a crucial role in language comprehension. It is connected to the premotor areas (PMC) by the arcuate fasciculus, and there are strong connections from the PMC to the primary motor cortex (Chavis and Pandya 1976; Godschalk *et al.* 1984). When a subject is instructed verbally to perform a movement using his right hand, he will use this pathway. Geschwind (1965) pointed out that in order to carry out a verbal command with the left hand, information must be processed by the right premotor cortex. Since it is extremely rare to find fibres that run obliquely in the corpus callosum, fibres either cross from Wernicke's area to the auditory association area on the other side or cross from the PMC on the left side to the PMC on the right side, and ultimately, the instruction is conveyed to the motor areas on the right side. Geschwind (1965) regarded the PMC as an intermediate stage between the sensory areas and the primary motor cortex, because—with the exception of the primary somatosensory cortex (SI)—the sensory areas project to the premotor and prefrontal areas rather than directly to the precentral region (Jones and Powell 1970; Chavis and Pandya 1976). According to Geschwind's schema, lesions of the arcuate fascicularis should disconnect the posterior language areas, which are important in comprehension, from the premotor areas, which are crucially involved in encoding motor programs. Therefore, the disconnection model of apraxia predicts that apraxic patients should have difficulties performing tasks to verbal command, but should correctly imitate gestures or manipulate objects and tools, since these tasks do not require language.

Geschwind's model cannot explain why apraxic patients with parietal lesions present with difficulties in imitating movements, or why they are sometimes clumsy when they use objects or tools (Heilman 1979; Heilman *et al.* 1982; Freund 1992; Goldenberg 1995; Halsband *et al.* 1995). Also, it is difficult for the model to explain why patients with sections of the corpus callosum sometimes show a substantial recovery of their apraxic symptoms despite a disconnection of the hemispheres.

Heilman (1979) put forward an alternative model which suggests that apraxia results from destruction of spatiotemporal representations of learned movements. In order to perform a skilled learned act, one must place particular body parts in particular positions in a particular temporal order. It is known that, even in the absence of specific cues, normal subjects are able to pantomime familiar skilled behaviours, which implies that the nervous system stores knowledge of motor skills. When this knowledge is called into use, it is retrieved from motor memory rather than being constructed *de novo* (Heilman and Rothi 1993). Heilman (1979) put forward a hypothesis to explain why patients with parietal lesions may not be able to pantomime, imitate, or use an object correctly. According to this model spatiotemporal representations of skilled movements are stored in the dominant parietal cortex, which is thought to instruct the premotor cortex for the necessary movements. Spatiotemporal movement representations direct the motor system to adopt the appropriate spatial positions of the relevant body parts over time, whereby the primary motor cortex innervates the specific motor neurones needed to carry out the skilled motor act (Asanuma 1989).

In agreement with Heilman's model it has been shown that the movement production impairment of patients with ideomotor apraxia is characterized predominantly by spatiotemporal errors (Poizner *et al.* 1990; Clark *et al.* 1994;

Hermsdörfer *et al.* 1996). Clark *et al.* (1994) reported errors in spatial accuracy and a spatiotemporal disintegration in apraxic patients in their execution of well-learned movements (slicing bread). These disturbances were also demonstrable when movements were not carried out under verbal commands. Apraxic patients showed deficits in the plane of motion, the shape of the trajectory, and in the coupling of hand speed and trajectory shape under various contextual cue conditions. These results provide strong evidence for Heilman's hypothesis (1979) that apraxia results from a fractionation of spatiotemporal representations of learned movements, rather than from a disconnection between the receptive language areas in the left hemisphere and the contralateral motor cortices (Geschwind 1965, 1975).

11.3 Apraxia and language

George Ettlinger (1969) highlighted the important issue of the relationship between the neural systems controlling language and action within the left hemisphere, and this has continued to be a matter of debate up to the present. He used evidence from cases of brain bisection, and came to the conclusion that apraxias may consist of two separate components:

(1) true apraxia, which he thought to be language-dependent and caused by left hemispheric lesions; and

(2) a disorder of dexterity as reflected by difficulties in imitating movements made by the examiner, which he thought to be the consequence of bilateral hemispheric lesions.

Nowadays it is well established that apraxia occurs in the overwhelming majority of cases following a lesion in the language-dominant hemisphere (see Poeck 1989, for a critical overview). The dominance of the left hemisphere in right-handers for both language and motor programming raises the question whether aphasic and apraxic disorders are the expression of a common underlying deficit of communication, or whether the two disorders are independent and only accidentally associated. Taken together, recent evidence supports the latter view, that the association between aphasia and apraxia may be due to the anatomical proximity of underlying structural correlates rather than to a common disorder. The human brain may be unique in the degree to which the vocal production system has become coupled with the neural mechanisms underlying praxic abilities.

In man there is evidence for a left hemisphere superiority on tasks involving complex sequential movements of the limb, and it has been shown that the majority of left hemispere apraxics are also aphasic (De Renzi *et al.* 1980; Kimura 1982). Kimura and Archibald (1974) reported that patients with left hemisphere damage were clearly impaired relative to a group with right hemisphere damage on a task requiring the copying of a sequence of hand movements. They argued that apraxia is due to a disruption of motor programming centres, which lie in the dominant hemisphere for both speech and non-speech behaviour. De Renzi *et al.* (1980) assessed the incidence of impairment in copying movements in right hemisphere and in left hemisphere damaged patients, all of whom were right handed. The limb ipsilateral to the lesion was used in all tests. In concordance with the investigation by Kimura and Archibald (1974), the impairments were found to be more frequent and severe in left-brain damaged patients than in right-brain damaged patients.

The relationship of aphasia and apraxia could be interpreted as a consequence of the fact that motor control of the limbs and of speech production both represent aspects of the control of integrated muscular sequences, the programming of which may be attributable to related neural mechanisms. Both language and skilful movements have the common characteristic that they require a highly complex sequencing ability and precise temporal adjustments. Sternberg *et al.* (1983) studied the relationship between the temporal control mechanisms for speech and hand movements performed by a skilled typist. They found a similar type of organization of the mean element and segment durations of two-syllable spoken words and typing sequences.

There are striking similarities in the temporal organization of speech and limb movements. Ostry and Cooke (1987) obtained kinematic measurements of tongue dorsum movements during the production of alternately stressed consonant–vowel sequences that were rhythmical in form. The authors found that the kinematic patterns for movements of the tongue dorsum were similar to those of voluntary flexion–extension movements about the elbow. This is consistent with the view that the nervous system produces kinematic patterns in different effector systems in comparable ways.

The underlying basis for a left hemisphere specialization in motor control is a highly controversial issue. Freeman (1984) suggested that the principal function of the left hemisphere may be to exercise a priority of control in situations appropriate to its action. In this way, the paradox of adequate right hemisphere control of the motor behaviour of the left hand in split-brain patients can be understood, since the normal priority of motor control by the left hemisphere in the control of motor behaviour in intact right-handed people would not be able to operate. This reasoning implies that motor control is largely attributable to the involvement of the dominant hemisphere in the control of highly overlearned motor behaviour. Corina *et al.* (1992) reported left hemisphere specialization of American sign and spoken language in deaf and hearing individuals. Their results suggest that left hemisphere specialization derives from the linguistic nature of the movement: no evidence of hemispheric asymmetry was found for production of either symbolic or arbitrary gestures. Other studies have emphasized the importance of both hemispheres in controlling a variety of motor tasks. For instance, tracking on a pursuit rotor (Heap and Wyke 1972), maze co-ordination (Haaland and Delaney 1981), screw rotation (Kimura 1979), and the control of single hand postures (Kimura and Archibald 1974; Jason 1986) have been shown to be impaired ipsilaterally after damage to the left or right hemisphere. Here a major problem seems to be the lack of homogeneity due to the diversity of behavioural tests and recording methods applied to different clinical populations. A thorough and analytical comparison of the contributions made by the various brain structures in both hemispheres that exert a direct influence on primary motor cortex in a given set of motor learning paradigms is needed.

11.4 Non-primary cortical motor areas: changing views

Apraxic disturbances are seen after lesions to the parietal or frontal lobes, or to their connecting fibres. Crucial areas are the sensory association cortex of the posterior parietal lobe and the non-primary cortical motor areas (see below). Also crucial is the rostral periventricular white matter, where anterior–posterior, callosal and cortico-subcortical connections can be damaged by relatively small lesions. Damage restricted to the prefrontal cortex or the pre- or postcentral gyrus does not result in apraxic disturbances. Furthermore, lesions restricted to subcortical structures do not produce apraxic deficits (Della Sala *et al.* 1992).

11.4.1 Premotor cortex, supplementary and pre-supplementary motor areas, and cingulate cortex

The premotor cortex (PMC) is part of the agranular frontal cortex rostral to the primary motor cortex and lateral to the supplementary motor cortex (SMA) (Humphrey 1979; Wiesendanger 1981; Weinrich and Wise 1982). There is disagreement in the literature as to the areal organization of the PMC (e.g. Passingham 1996). Recent evidence from anatomical and physiological studies suggest that it can be subdivided into at least two subsets of areas, one lying dorsally (PMCd) and another lying ventrally (PMCv) (Barbas and Pandya 1987; Humphrey and Tanji 1991; Kurata 1991; Wise *et al.* 1991). Figure 11.1 shows these subdivisions of area 6 in a surface view of the monkey brain as compared to the human brain. If the human inferior precentral sulcus is considered to be the homologue of the arcuate sulcus in monkeys, then the human PMCv may be regarded as including the banks of the precentral sulcus and the anterior part of the precentral gyrus (Freund 1991; Humphrey and Tanji 1991).

Recently, evidence has accumulated to indicate the existence of at least three additional non-primary motor areas on the medial surface, as well as the classical supplementary motor area (SMA) (Fig. 11.1b). There is a motor area lying immediately anterior to the SMA (Rizzolatti *et al.* 1990; Matelli *et al.* 1991) that has been termed pre-SMA (Tanji *et al.* 1991), and also two movement-related foci in the primate cingulate cortex, termed the rostral (CMr) and caudal (CMc) cingulate motor areas (Shima *et al.* 1991).

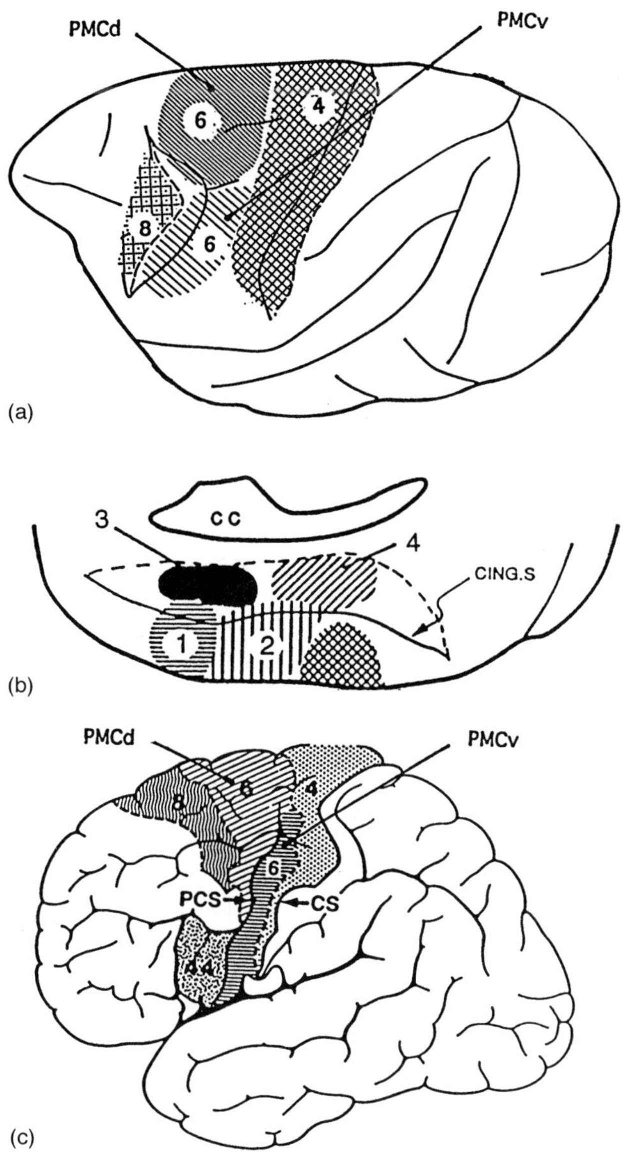

Fig. 11.1 Cortical motor areas in monkeys and man. (a) Dorsal (PMCd) and ventral premotor cortex (PMCv) within Brodmann's area 6 in the monkey. Areas 4 (primary motor cortex) and 8 (frontal eye-fields) are also indicated. (b) Subdivisions of non-primary motor cortex lying in the medial aspect of the monkey's cerebral cortex: 1, pre-supplementary motor area (pre-SMA); 2, supplementary motor area (SMA); 3, rostral cingulate motor area; 4, caudal cingulate motor area. (c) Surface view of a human brain, showing the distribution of Brodmann's cytoarchitectonic areas 4, 6, 8, and 44 on the precentral and frontal gyri: CS, central sulcus; PCS, precentral sulcus; PMCd, dorsal premotor cortex; PMCv, ventral premotor cortex.

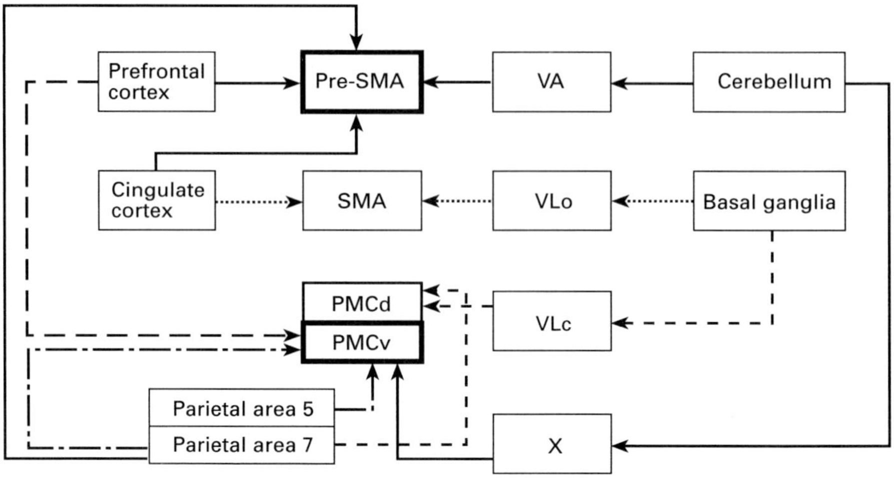

Fig. 11.2 Summary diagram indicating differences in the access to sensory information in the various non-primary motor areas: Pre-SMA, pre-supplementary motor area; SMA, supplementary motor area; PMCd, dorsal premotor cortex; PMCv, ventral premotor cortex; VA, VLo, VLc, X, subnuclei in the thalamus.

Striking differences in the access to sensory information are observed in these non-primary motor areas (Fig. 11.2). In contrast to the SMA, the PMC is known to have several sources of sensory information (Kubota and Hamada 1978). There are various routes by which the PMC receives visual and somatic information directly from the parietal cortex (Petrides and Pandya 1984; Matelli *et al.* 1986), and via cerebellar–thalamic projections (Glickstein *et al.* 1985; Matelli *et al.* 1989). It has been shown that the ventrolateral part of the cerebellar dentate nucleus projects to the PMC (Strick *et al.* 1993). Abundant projections from areas 5, 7, and SII form the major inputs to PMCv. In contrast, area 5 appears to be the sole source of projection to the PMCd from the parietal cortex (Kurata 1991). On the medial surface, the pre-SMA has more access to visual information than the SMA proper. It receives direct projections from the inferior parietal lobe, areas PG and PFG (Tanji *et al.* 1991; Luppino *et al.* 1993) and also afferents from the prefrontal cortex (Luppino *et al.* 1990, 1993; Matelli and Luppino 1992; Lu *et al.* 1994).

In agreement with these anatomical differences, it has been found that the non-primary motor areas play differential roles in sequential motor learning (Tanji and Shima 1994, 1996; Tanji *et al.* 1995; Passingham 1996). A current theme in research on this topic is the distinction between activities that are sensory-guided versus memory-guided, or internally versus externally driven (Tanji and Shima 1994, 1996; Tanji *et al.* 1995; Passingham 1996). Deiber *et al.* (1991) reported a greater activation in the SMA for tasks that were based on internal cues rather than on external cues, as measured by regional changes in cerebral blood flow (using positron emission tomography, PET). This is in accordance with brain-lesion studies in monkeys which have shown that damage to the SMA and to the pre-SMA leads to a significant impairment in the ability to generate a fixed sequence of three different movements to the same manipulandum (Halsband 1987), whereas animals with PMC lesions were unimpaired on this task (Halsband and Passingham 1982, 1985). In contrast, the behavioural effects of premotor lesions in monkeys (Halsband and Passingham 1982, 1985; Passingham 1985; Petrides 1985) and man (Halsband and Freund 1990; Halsband 1996) have demonstrated severe impairments of tasks in which subjects had to recall a movement on the basis of a sensory cue.

Furthermore, it has been shown that the non-primary motor areas on the medial surface are functionally distinct from the premotor cortex and the primary motor area by comparing single cell activity in visually instructed versus internally determined conditional motor tasks (Kurata and Wise 1988; Mushiake *et al.* 1991; Halsband *et al.* 1994; Tanji and Shima 1994), and in sensory-instructed versus self-initiated reaching movements (Romo and Schulz 1992). Mushiake *et al.* (1991) reported that SMA neurones were more active than PMC neurones when a monkey had to press a given sequence of buttons on the basis of internalized information stored in memory. In contrast, PMC neurones were more active than SMA neurones when the animal had to decide which button to press in accordance with current visual information. But in this task the animal had to perform the same movement to different locations in space, so that it remains unclear whether the crucial factor was performing sequences of movements, or memorizing spatial positions, or both. In order to clarify this question, Halsband and Tanji (1993) and Halsband *et al.* (1994) trained the animal on a conditional sequential motor task that ensured sequencing of multiple movements to the same manipulandum, rather than sequencing of continuous movements to different positions in space. A similar paradigm had already been applied successfully to study the effects of selective damage to the SMA, pre-SMA, and PMC in monkeys (Halsband 1987; Halsband and Passingham 1982).

In this study (Halsband and Tanji 1993; Halsband *et al.* 1994), single cell activity in four motor areas was analysed in a task which required the monkey to make three different movements (turn, push, pull), with intervening waiting periods, to the same manipulandum. The task was performed under two different conditions:

(1) the monkey had to generate the sequence from memory (internally determined); and

(2) the correct sequence of movements was performed by following lights illuminated one after each other (visually instructed).

The manipulandum returned to its original position after each movement. This paradigm was chosen in order to prevent the use of spatial cues in making the correct motor sequence. The same task was later applied and extended by Tanji and Shima (1994).

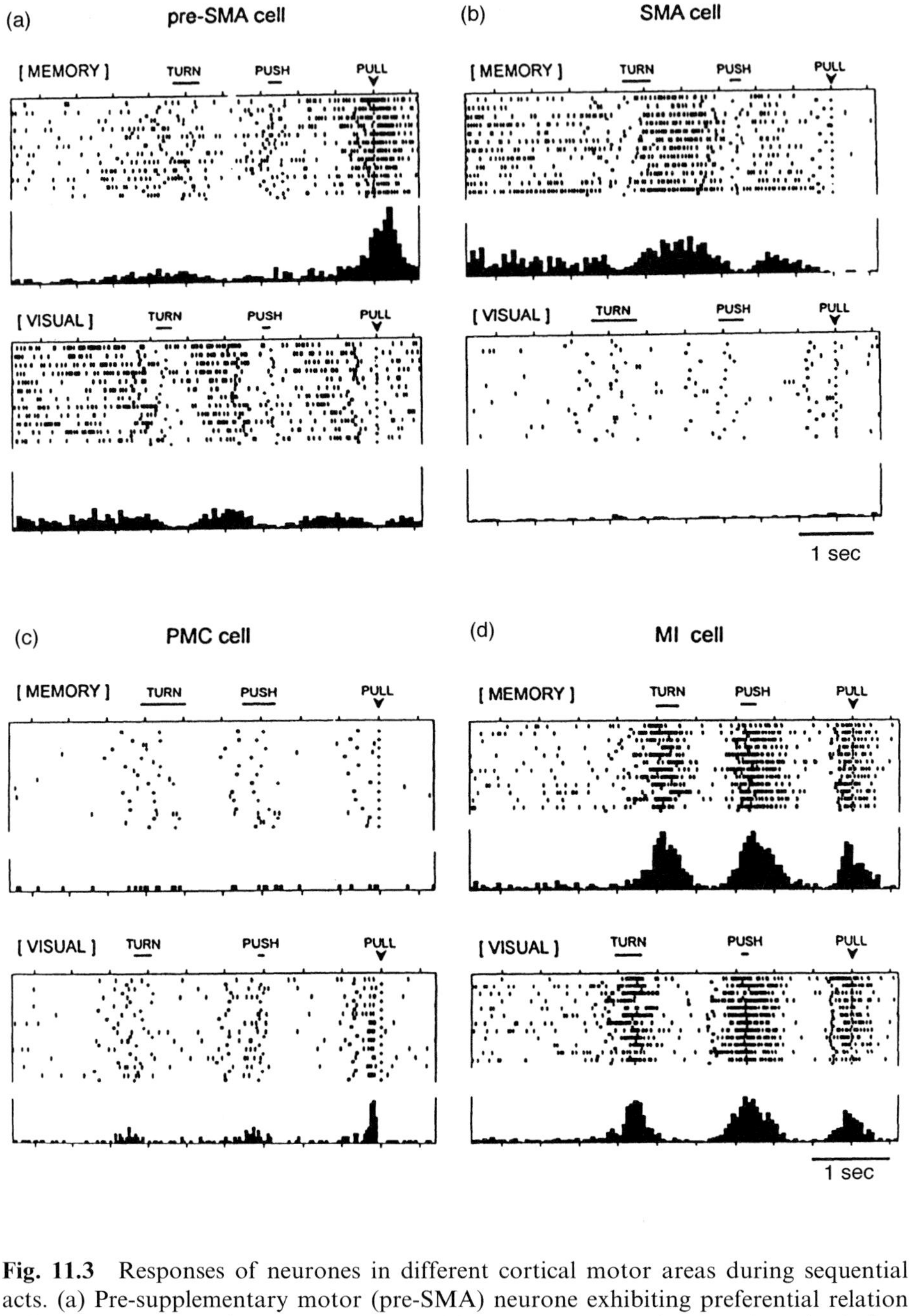

Fig. 11.3 Responses of neurones in different cortical motor areas during sequential acts. (a) Pre-supplementary motor (pre-SMA) neurone exhibiting preferential relation to internally generated motor sequences. This neurone was predominantly active before and during the third internally generated sequential movement (pull). It also exhibited preparatory activity in relation to the visually guided sequence task. In this mode, the neurone was predominantly active during the instruction and delay periods, but less

Among the 425 task-related neurones recorded in the study by Halsband *et al.* (1994), striking differences in neuronal activity were observed in the pre-SMA, SMA, PMC, and primary motor cortex (Fig. 11.3). More than half of the PMC neurones were preferentially or exclusively active in relation to visually instructed movements during both the pre-movement and movement periods. In accordance with the neuroanatomical findings of a greater sensory input to PMCv as compared to PMCd (Kurata 1991), a higher proportion of neurones recorded in the ventral part of the premotor cortex were active in relation to visually instructed movements (Fig. 11.4).

In contrast, SMA neurones were preferentially active when the correct motor sequence was determined on the basis of internalized information. The pre-SMA was found to contain a significantly higher proportion of neurones that were active during the delay and pre-movement period as compared to the movement period. This suggests a greater proportion of preparatory activity and cue responses in pre-SMA neurones as compared to the SMA proper (Matsuzaka *et al.* 1992; Stephan *et al.* 1995). Activity in the pre-SMA was more related to visually guided movements during the pre-movement period, but exhibited a preferential relationship to internally generated movements during the movement period. MI neurones exhibited comparable activity during the instruction, delay, pre-movement, and movement periods, regardless of whether the sequential motor task was visually or internally instructed. These findings are in agreement with a clear distinction between set-related cells in primary and non-primary cortex as reported by Germain and Lamarre (1993) and by Tanji and Shima (1994).

There is recent evidence for an observation/execution matching system in monkeys (Gallese *et al.* 1996; Rizzolatti *et al.* 1996) and humans (Fadiga *et al.* 1995; Rizzolatti *et al.* 1997). Rizzolatti *et al.* (1996) and Gallese *et al.* (1996) recorded neural responses in the ventral PMC (area F5) when the experimental animal observed movements without executing them, as well as when it produced the movements itself. In around 20 per cent of the recorded neurones a discharge was seen both when movements were observed and when they were

---

active during the pre-movement and movement periods. (b) Supplementary motor neurone (SMA) exhibiting a selective relationship to a remembered sequential movement. The SMA neurone was exclusively active when the animal performed the internally guided sequence task, but inactive when the sequence was prompted by visual cues. (c) Typical example of premotor cortex neurone (PMC) having an exclusive relation to the visually instructed sequential motor task. (d) Primary motor cortex neurone (MI) that is active equally during both visually guided and memory guided motor tasks. Times of occurrence of action potentials are displayed as dots, with each row representing a trial. Raster displays are aligned with the onset of the pull movement. Each histogram is made by summation of the neuronal data in each raster with a binwidth of 50 ms. (From Halsband *et al.* 1994.)

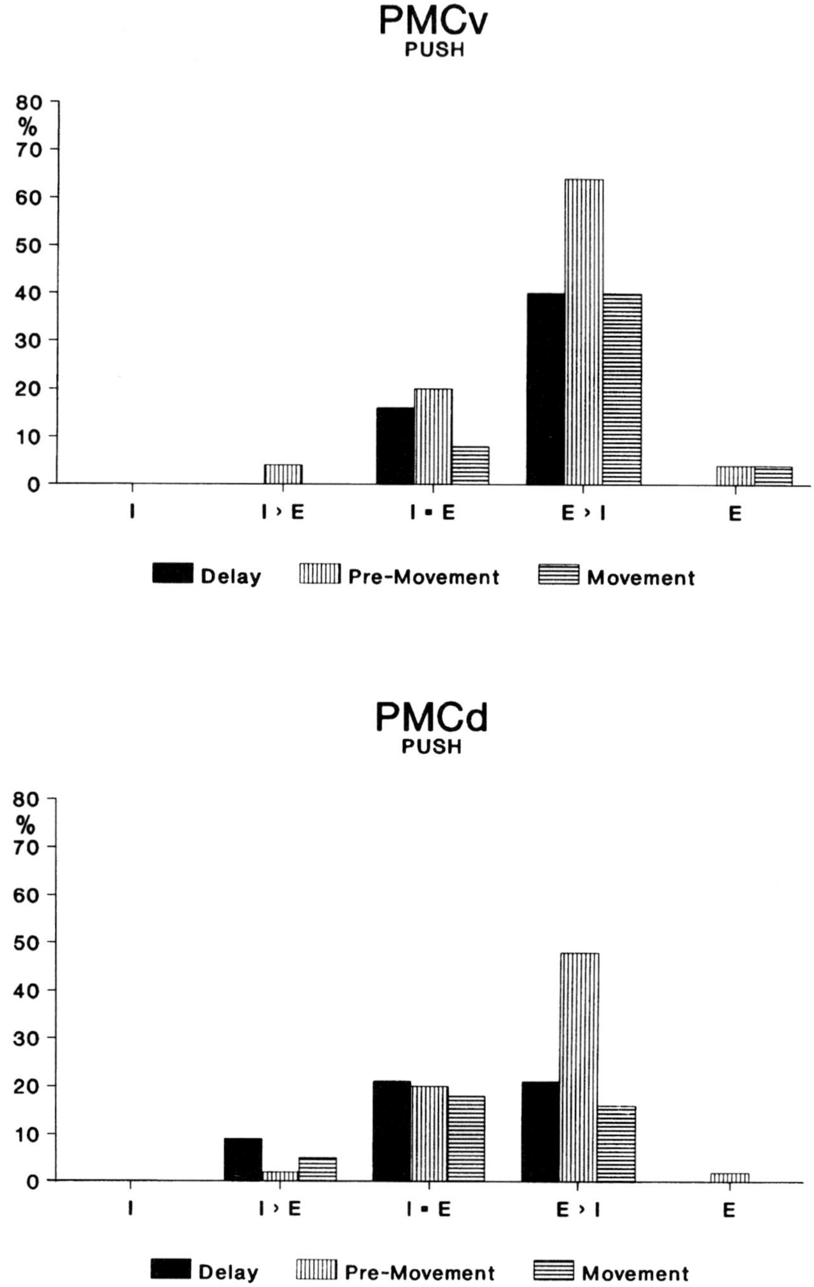

Fig. 11.4 Distribution of ventral premotor neurones (PMCv, top) and dorsal premotor neurones (PMCd, bottom), classified according to their association with the externally guided (E) versus the internally instructed (I) motor task. Neuronal distributions are

produced by the animal; these neurones were called 'mirror neurones'. The authors argued that mirror neurones reflect an abstract representation of the action.

One interpretation is that mirror neurones are related to motor preparation. When the monkey observes an action, it may start to prepare the same action. Brain activity mapping during the observation of actions and during motor imagery may thus show similar activation patterns. According to Jeannerod (1995) and Jeannerod and Decety (1995) the neurones responsible for the motor image formation are the same as those the subject will later activate during planning and preparation of the action. According to this view, these are neurones that represent actions internally. In contrast, Rizzolatti *et al.* (1996) and Gallese *et al.* (1996) favour the view that these neurones play a crucial role in the understanding of motor events.

The results of brain activation studies of motor imagery have emphasized the activity of several brain areas, including prefrontal areas, supplementary motor area, cerebellum, and basal ganglia. Interestingly, within the supplementary motor area the more anterior zone was more related to representational stages of action and to motor imagery as compared to the posterior zone of the SMA proper (Tyszka *et al.* 1994; Stephan *et al.* 1995). It remains an interesting question for future research whether a selective enhancement of neuronal activity can be found in the anterior SMA and pre-SMA in primates when the animal observes an action without performing it.

Deficits of simultaneous but independent movements of both hands have been observed after mesial frontal lesions in monkeys (Brinkman 1981; Wiesendanger 1986) and in patients (Laplane *et al.* 1977; Chan and Ross 1988; Halsband *et al.* 1995). There are functional similarities and differences of SMA and cingulate structures. Shima *et al.* (1991) reported that neurones in the rostral cingulate motor area exhibit neuronal activity akin to that in the SMA. Brinkman (1984) observed in SMA-lesioned monkeys that the two hands started to behave in a similar manner instead of sharing the task between them. Laplane *et al.* (1977) reported difficulties with bimanual movements in three patients with unilateral damage to the anterior part of SMA and anterior cingulate. These patients were not able to open one fist while simultaneously clenching the other and vice versa. Similarly, we have shown (Halsband *et al.* 1993) that patients with supplementary motor lesions have serious difficulties in generating movements with both hands in an alternating manner. Our most recent evidence also shows that patients with unilateral lesions to the anterior cingulate cortex sparing the SMA exhibit pronounced deficits in bimanual

---

displayed for the 'push' movement only. Classification criteria: I, exclusive relation to I (at $p < 0.001$); I > E, more related to I ($p < 0.05$); I = E, equally related (if the activity was not significantly different in the two modes at $p < 0.05$); E < I, more related to I ($p < 0.05$); E, exclusive relation to E ($p < 0.001$).

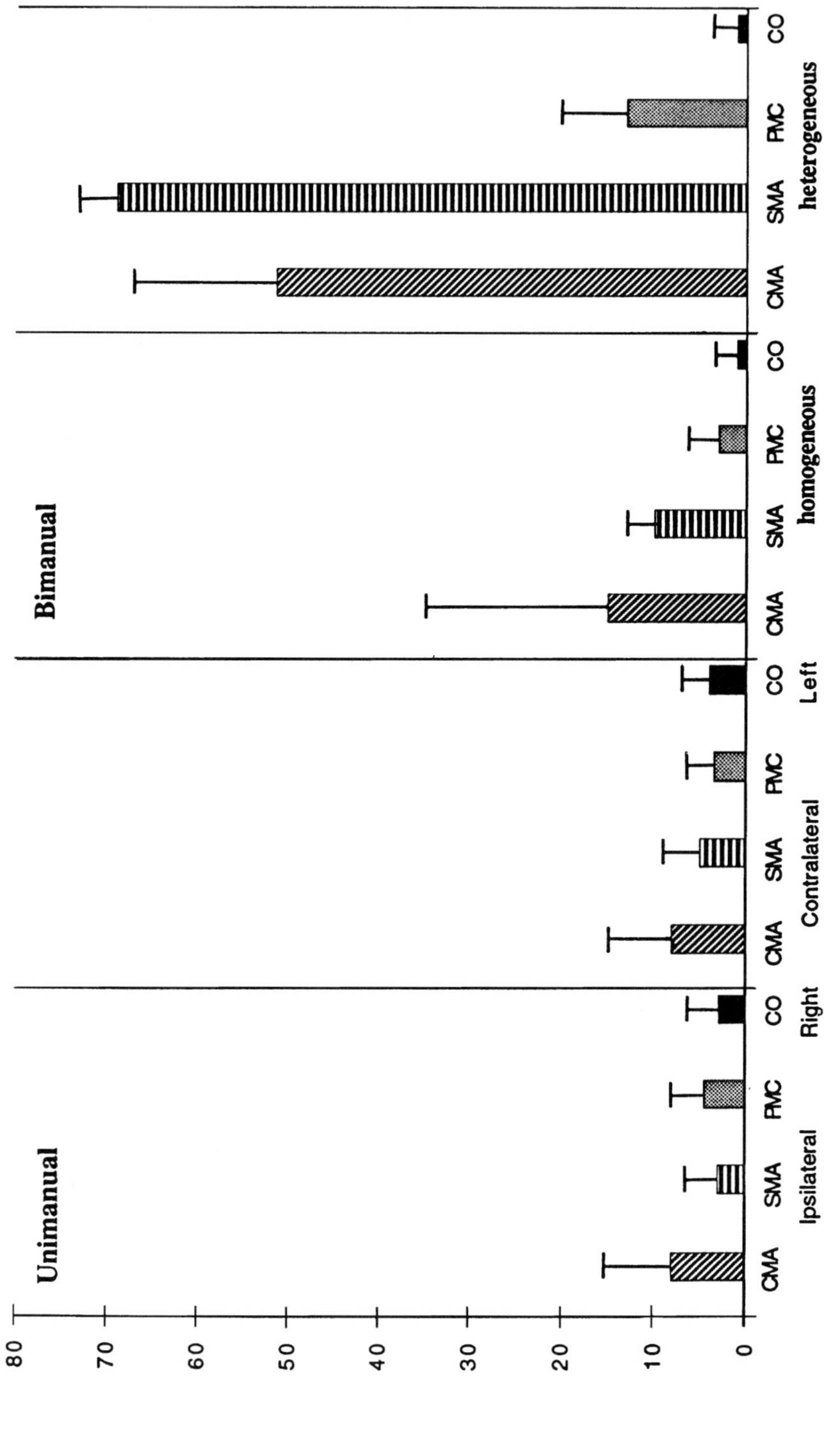
Unimanual
Bimanual
CMA
SMA
PMC
CO
Ipsilateral
Right
Contralateral
Left
homogeneous
heterogeneous
0
10
20
30
40
50
60
70
80

motor control (Stephan *et al.* 1997). In one of the tasks, subjects were requested to imitate 20 meaningful movements using both hands simultaneously. Half of the actions presented consisted of two homogeneous components whereby both hands performed an identical movement to an imagined object, such as wringing, or piano-playing with symmetrical finger movements. The other 10 actions consisted of heterogeneous movement patterns. In these, subjects were requested to use their left and right hand simultaneously and to perform two different pantomimed motor acts to an imagined object. For instance, when subjects imagined cooking a pudding they were instructed to pantomime pouring pudding powder into the boiling milk with their left hand while simultaneously stirring it with the other (right) hand. Bimanual performance was compared with the ability to pantomime 30 meaningful unimanual movements. The results revealed the most pronounced deficits in the bimanual heterogeneous condition, particularly in patients with cingulate lesions and in patients with damage to the SMA. Patients with lesions to the premotor cortex were less severely impaired in performing bimanual heterogeneous movements, although the difference from the performance of healthy control subjects was still statistically significant (Fig. 11.5).

At a first glance it appears that the severe deficit of bimanual motor control in patients with cingulate lesions is similar to that described in patients with unilateral SMA lesions. But our recent findings suggest that the two areas may be associated preferentially with different aspects of bimanual motor control: SMA with planning and preparation of movements, including bimanual motor acts, and anterior cingulate with co-ordination of bihemispheric movement execution (Stephan *et al.* 1997). Furthermore, we were able to establish on neuropsychological grounds a clear functional difference in visuomotor association learning in patients with cingulate and SMA lesions. Patients had to learn to associate six coloured stimuli with six different arm movements which were previously rehearsed. A control task involved an association between the same set of sensory stimuli and six spatial locations. It was found that patients with cingulate lesions were not impaired on either of these conditional learning tasks; in contrast, patients with SMA lesions were severely impaired when they had to recall a movement on the basis of a visual cue, but not for an association involving spatial location (Fig. 11.6).

Fig. 11.5 Percentage errors in pantomiming unimanual and bimanual movements in patients with unilateral lesions in non-primary cortical motor areas and in healthy controls. Bimanual movements were classified as homogeneous movement patterns, whereby both hands performed an identical movement, and heterogeneous movement patterns, whereby the left and right hand performed simultaneously two different motor acts to an imagined object. CMA, cingulate motor area; SMA, supplementary motor area; PMC, premotor cortex; CO, control subjects; vertical lines give the standard deviation.

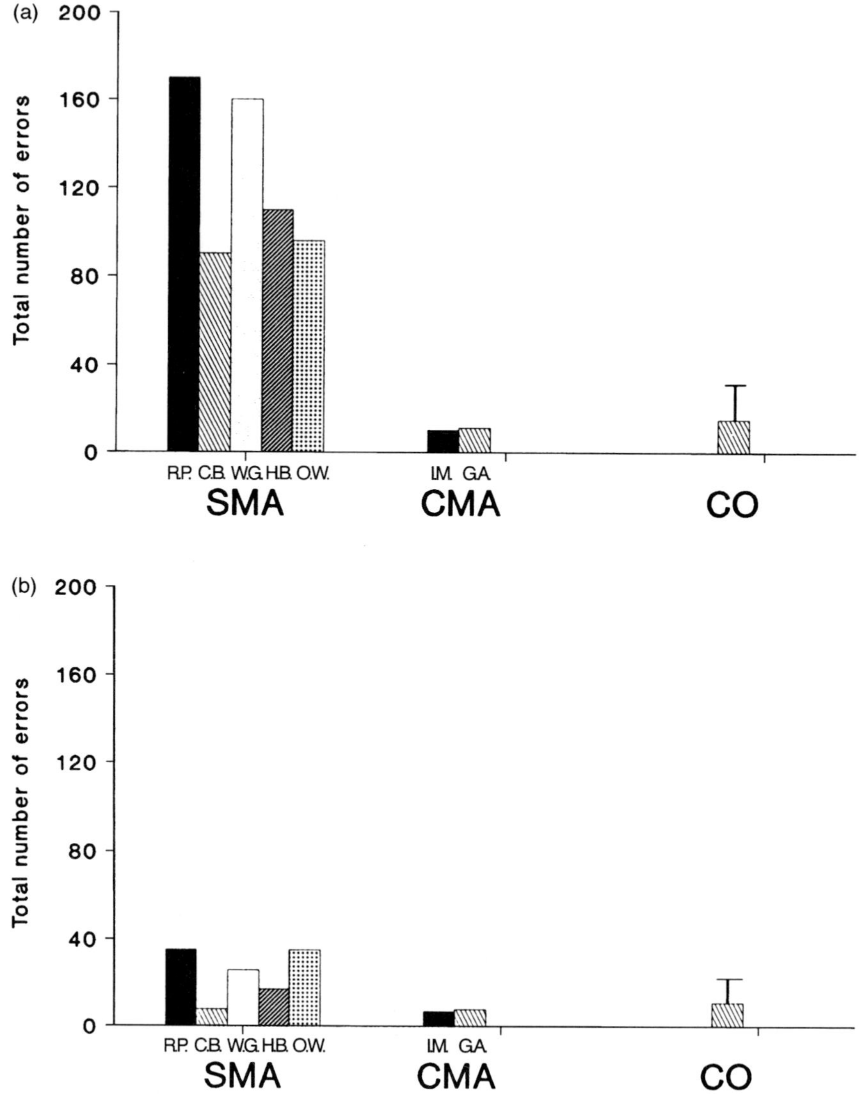

Fig. 11.6 Mean number of errors made by patients with damage to the supplementary motor area (SMA) and cingulate motor area (CMA) as compared with healthy control subjects (CO), on (a) a visual conditional motor task and (b) a spatial conditional task. The results are based on the total number of errors made by the subjects to criterion level (18/18 correct) in up to a maximum of 250 trials. Results are given for individual patients and for a group of control subjects.

11.4.2 Parietal cortex

There are reasons for supposing that the parietal cortex belongs to those regions that differ to a relatively large degree between monkey and man, so that special caution is warranted before generalizing across species when dealing with parietal functions (Passingham and Ettlinger 1974; Passingham, Chapter 15 this volume). There is evidence from neurophysiological and lesion studies in primates of functional differences and similarities of the upper parietal area (Brodmann's area 5, von Economo's PE) and the lower parietal cortex (Brodmann's area 7, von Economo's PG and PF) (Mountcastle *et al.* 1975; Hyvärinen 1982; Nixon *et al.* 1992). However, the application of these studies to the human brain is controversial since there are uncertainties as to the equivalence of the corresponding areas even at the cytoarchitectonic level.

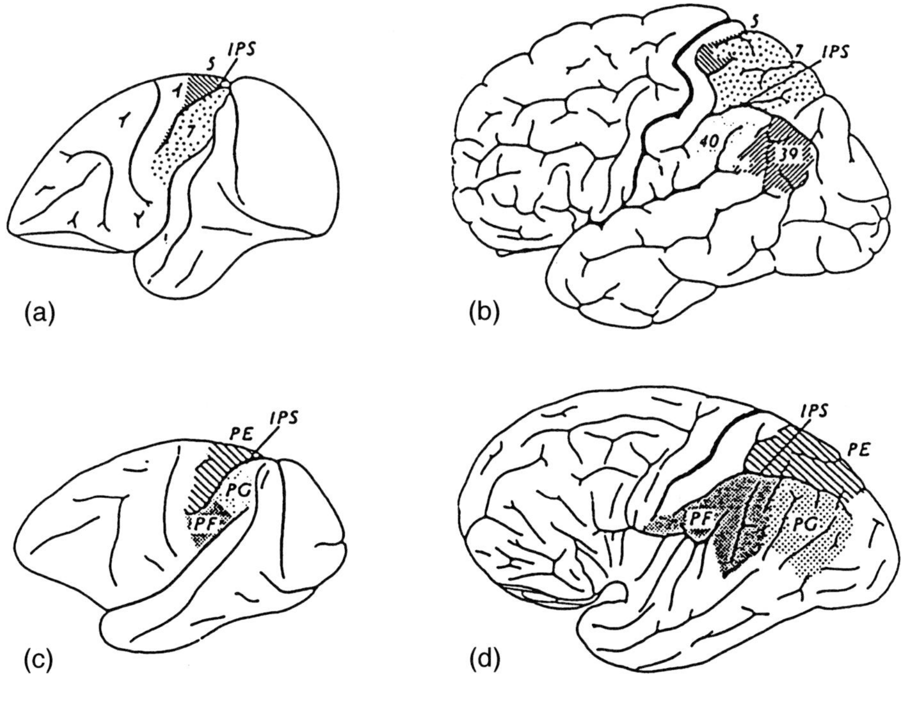

Fig. 11.7 Parietal regions in monkey (left) and human (right). (a) Brodmann's delineation of areas 5 and 7 in *Cercopithecus*; (b) Brodmann's classification of the parietal areas in the human brain; (c) subdivisions of the parietal regions in *Macaca mulatta* (after von Bonin and Bailey 1947); (d) subdivisions of the parietal cortex in the human brain (after von Economo 1929). IPS, Intraparietal sulcus.

Figure 11.7 shows the difference of the cytoarchitectonic divisions of the parietal cortex in the primate (left) and the human brain (right). According to Brodmann's classification, in the human brain the areas localized above the intraparietal sulcus are defined as areas 5 and 7, and in the lower parietal cortex as areas 39 and 40. However, the area 7 in monkeys is not equivalent to areas 39 and 40 in humans, but developed evolutionarily from a primordial region of the total parietal cortex (Brodmann 1909). Zilles (1990) reviewed the available neuroanatomical evidence thoroughly and came to the conclusion that areas 39 and 40 were to be interpreted as cortical convolutions of the higher polymodal association areas. In contrast, Bailey and von Bonin (1951) argued that the areas defined by von Economo (1929) and von Economo and Koskinas (1925) as PG and PF in the lower parietal cortex are identical in apes and humans. This lettering system has been the basis for experimental analysis on non-human primate brains (e.g. Pandya and Seltzer 1982) and for cytoarchitectonical observations on the human parietal cortex (Eidelberg and Galaburda 1984).

In monkeys, parietal lesions have not been followed by a motor condition similar to apraxia in humans. Despite the controversies about the delineation of the different forms of apraxia, there is agreement that lesions in the human supramarginal gyrus and the junctional areas between the parietal and the occipital and temporal lobe of the language-dominant hemisphere interfere with the conception and synthesis of voluntary movements (Freund 1987). It is to be assumed that the basis of apraxia is a disturbance of the choice and sequencing of movements which follow one another. Voluntary movements are affected regardless of whether they are mediated through the language-based motor system or the skeletal–muscular motor system. Apraxia is not a unitary process, but must be broken down according to the stages of defective comprehension and/or production and to the different sets of conditions to which it applies. The conceptualization and first-stage processing of motor behaviour seems to occur in neuronal repertoires that are similar or close to those circuitries engaged in the comprehension of language, gestures, or other purposive motor behaviour.

Accordingly, one of the basic questions in human apraxia research is whether the concept of a movement is stored in a neuronal structure that itself plays a decisive role in the execution of that movement, or whether representation and production are differentially organized. Recently, we have addressed the following: whether apraxic impairments are associated with a specific alteration in the recognition and understanding of motor acts, and whether the occurrence of deficits depends on the types of movements examined and the location of the lesion (Halsband *et al.* 1995, 1997). The study was based on 11 patients with unilateral lesions in the parietal cortex, 14 patients with lesions in the premotor cortex or the supplementary motor area, 3 patients with lesions in the primary motor cortex, and 16 healthy control subjects. Patients with neglect were excluded. Subjects were asked to imitate pantomimed motor acts as shown on a video screen, to describe the meaning of the actions, and to indicate the context in which they appear (e.g. to put one's hand up at school). Motor tasks included symbolic and meaningful gestures without object use (such as waving or saluting), pantomimed actions aimed at producing explicitly defined movements towards one's own body parts (e.g. combing one's hair or tooth-brushing), and motor acts with respect to an imagined object in extrapersonal space, such as hammering a nail into the wall.

Patients with parietal lobe lesions were significantly impaired on unimanual action production (imitating pantomimed motor acts); in contrast, no deficits occurred after damage to the PMC or MI. Interestingly, the most pronounced impairment was observed after left parietal lobe lesions when patients were asked to imitate gestures on their own bodies rather than imitating movements with reference to an external object. It seems likely that the basic deficit in these subjects concerns the ability to code and comprehend movements in relation to one's own body. According to Goldenberg (1995), faulty apprehension of spatial relationships between body parts manifests itself not only in imitation on oneself but also on a wooden manikin. His findings can be adduced as evidence for an overall disturbance of representation of the human body-schema independent of whether actions relate to the own body or to an external model. It is unclear as yet whether the disturbances relate selectively to the human body itself or whether such deficits would also appear in the use of animal models or arbitrary multi-part mechanical objects.

Recognition of pantomimed motor acts was unimpaired in patients with PMC or MI damage. In patients with parietal lobe damage there was a heterogeneous picture of disturbances of representation and production; some of the apraxic patients showed no deficits at all in the discrimination of actions perceptually, although their production was severely disturbed; in contrast, others showed deficits in both areas (Halsband *et al.* 1995, 1997). Since it was found that some patients showed great disturbances in the production of movements while having an intact comprehension of the meaningfulness of the action, the hypothesis that apraxic disturbances can be traced back to a basic disturbance of representation of the form or meaning of actions cannot be supported.

Roy and Square (1985) postulated a dissociation between conceptual and production components which is supported by the recent findings by Rapcsak *et al.* (1995). A patient with bilateral damage to the posterior parietal lobe was unable to pantomime simple movements with either the left or the right hand and showed great deficits in the use of real tools, albeit with some small improvement over her performance on imitation. However, the patient had no problems in interpreting and discriminating actions pantomimed by others.

The interaction between cognitive representation and production has recently been the focus of critical discussion in a review by Jeannerod and Decety (1995), where especially the meaning of context-specific components was questioned. The authors came to the conclusion that 'the motor impairments observed in apraxic patients result from a specific alteration in their ability to mentally evoke actions, or to use stored motor representations for forming mental images of actions. Thus, the deficit arises when the patient shifts from a strategy where object-orientated actions are processed automatically, to when the content of these actions has to be explicitly represented' (p. 730).

11.4.3 Conclusion

In conclusion, there is a dearth of understanding of the neuroanatomical correlates of apraxia. A major problem is that most previous studies have selected patients on the basis of the diagnosis of apraxia and then attempted to identify a single site of neuroanatomical pathology. More studies are needed that pursue the complementary strategy of identifying patients with specific lesions and then assessing their recognition of motor acts and their praxic abilities.

References

Asanuma, H. (1989). *The motor cortex*. Raven Press, New York.

Bailey, P. A. and von Bonin, G. (1951). *The isocortex of man*. University of Illinois Press, Urbana, IL.

Barbas, H. and Pandya, D. N. (1987). Architecture and frontal cortical connections of the premotor cortex (area 6) in the rhesus monkey. *Journal of Comparative Neurology*, **256**, 211–28.

Bay, E. (1965). The concepts of agnosia, apraxia and aphasia after a history of a hundred years. *Journal of the Mount Sinai Hospital*, **32**, 637–50.

Benton, A. L. (1969). Disorders of spatial orientation. In *Handbook of Clinical Neurology*, vol. 3, (ed. P. J. Vinken and G. W. Bruyn), pp. 664–87. North-Holland, Amsterdam.

Brinkman, J. (1981). Lesions in supplementary motor area interfere with a monkey's performance of a bimanual coordination task. *Neuroscience Letters*, **27**, 276–70.

Brinkman, C. (1984). Supplementary motor area of the monkey's cerebral cortex: short- and long-term deficits after unilateral ablation and the effects of subsequent callosal section. *Journal of Neuroscience*, **4**, 918–29.

Brodmann, K. (1909). *Vergleichende Lokalisationslehre der Grosshirnrinde*. Barth, Leipzig.

Carlesimo, G. A., Fadda, L., and Caltagirone, C. (1993). Basic mechanisms of constructional apraxia in unilateral brain-damaged patients: role of visuo-perceptual and executive disorders. *Journal of Clinical and Experimental Neuropsychology*, **15**, 342–58.

Chan, J.-L. and Ross, E. D. (1988). Left-handed mirror writing following right anterior cerebral artery infarction: evidence for non-mirror transformation of motor programs by right supplementary motor area. *Neurology*, **38**, 59–63.

Chavis, D. A. and Pandya, D. N. (1976). Further observations on corticofrontal connections in the rhesus monkey. *Brain Research*, **117**, 369–86.

Clark, M. A., Merians, A. S., Kothari, A., Poizner, H., Macauley, B., and Rothi, L. J. G. (1994). Spatial planning deficits in limb apraxia. *Brain*, **117**, 1093–106.

Cohen, N. J. (1984). Preserved learning capacity in amnesia: evidence for multiple memory systems. In *Neuropsychology of memory*, (ed. L. Squire and N. Butters), pp. 83–103. Gulford, New York.
Corina D. P., Vaid, J., and Bellugi, U. (1992). The linguistic basis of left hemisphere specialization. *Science*, **255**, 1258–60.
Critchley, M. (1953). *The parietal lobes*. Arnold, London.
Darley, F. L. (1982). *Aphasia*. Saunders, Philadelphia.
De Ajuriaguerra, J., Hécaen, H., and Angelergues, R. (1960). Les apraxies. Variétes cliniques et lateralisation lesionelle. *Revue Neurologique*, **102**, 566–91.
Deiber, M. P., Passingham, R. E., Colebatch, J. G., Friston, K. J., Nixon, P. D. *et al.* (1991). Cortical areas and the selection of movement: a study with positron emission tomography. *Experimental Brain Research*, **84**, 393–402.
Della Sala, S., Basso, A., Laiacona, M. *et al.* (1992). Subcortical localization of ideomotor apraxia: a review and an experimental study. In *Neuropsychological disorders associated with subcortical lesions*, (ed. G. Vallar, S. F. Cappa, and C. W. Wallesch), pp. 357–80. Oxford University Press, Oxford.
De Renzi, E. and Lucchelli, F. (1988). Ideational apraxia. *Brain*, **113**, 1173–88.
De Renzi, E., Motti, F., and Nichelli, P. (1980). Imitating gestures: a quantitative approach to ideomotor apraxia. *Archives of Neurology*, **37**, 6–10.
De Renzi, E., Pieczuro, A., and Vignolo, L. A. (1968). Ideational apraxia: a quantitative study. *Neuropsychologia*, **6**, 41–52.
Eidelberg, D. and Galaburda, A. M. (1984). Inferior parietal lobule. Divergent architectonic asymmetries in the human brain. *Archives of Neurology*, **41**, 843–52.
Ettlinger, G. (1969). Apraxia considered as a disorder of movements that are language-dependent: evidence from cases of brain bi-section. *Cortex*, **5**, 285–9.
Ettlinger, G., Warrington, E., and Zangwill, O. L. (1957). A further study of visual-spatial agnosia. *Brain*, **80**, 335–70.
Fadiga, L., Fogassi, L., Pavesi, G., and Rizzolatti, G. (1995). Motor facilitation during action observation: a magnetic stimulation study. *Journal of Neurophysiology*, **73**, 2608–11.
Faglioni, P. and Basso, A. (1985). Historical perspectives on neuroanatomical correlates of limb apraxia. In *Neuropsychological studies of apraxia and related disorders*, (ed. E. A. Roy), pp. 3–44. Elsevier, Amsterdam.
Freeman, R. B. (1984). The apraxias, purposeful motor behavior left-hemisphere function. In *Cognition and motor processes*, (ed. W. Prinz and A. F. Sanders), pp. 29–50. Springer, Berlin.
Freund, H.-J. (1987). Abnormalities of motor behavior after cortical lesions in humans. In *Handbook of physiology, nervous system*, Vol. 5, (ed. V. B. Mountcastle, F. Plum, and S. R. Geiger), pp. 763–810. American Physiological Society, Bethesda, MD.
Freund, H.-J. (1991). What is the evidence for multiple motor areas in the human brain? In *Motor control: concepts and issues*, (ed. D. R. Humphrey and H.-J. Freund), pp. 399–413. Wiley, Chichester.
Freund, H.-J. (1992). The apraxias. In *Diseases of the nervous system. Clinical neurobiology*, IIA, (ed. K. Asbury, G. M. McKhann, and W. I. McDonald), pp. 751–67. Wiley, Chichester.
Freund, H.-J. and Hummelsheim, H. (1985). Lesions of premotor cortex in man. *Brain*, **108**, 697–733.
Gallese, V., Fadiga, L., Fogassi, L., and Rizzolatti, G. (1996). Action recognition in the premotor cortex. *Brain*, **119**, 593–609.

Germain, L. and Lamarre, Y. (1993). Neuronal activity in the motor and premotor cotrices before and after learning the associations between auditory stimuli and motor responses. *Brain Research*, **611**, 175–9.

Geschwind, N. (1965). Disconnexion syndromes in animals and man. *Brain*, **88**, 237–94, 585–644.

Geschwind, N. (1975). The apraxias: neural mechanisms of disorders of learned movements. *American Scientist*, **63**, 188–95.

Glickstein, M., May, J. G., and Mercier, B. E. (1985). Corticopontine projection in the macaque: the distribution of labelled cortical cells after large injections of horseradish peroxidase in the pontine nuclei. *Journal of Comparative Neurology*, **235**, 343–59.

Godschalk, M., Lemon, R. N., Kuypers, H. G. J. M., and Ronday, H. K. (1984). Cortical afferents and efferents of monkey postarcuate area: an anatomical and electrophysiological study. *Experimental Brain Research*, **56**, 410–24.

Goldenberg, G. (1995). Imitating gestures and manipulating a mannikin—the representation of the human body in ideomotor apraxia. *Neuropsychologia*, **33**, 63–72.

Haaland, K. Y. and Delaney, H. D. (1981). Motor deficits after left or right hemisphere damage due to stroke or tumor. *Neuropsychologia*, **19**, 17–27.

Halsband, U. (1987). Higher disturbances of movement in monkeys. In *Motor control*, (ed. G. N. Gantchev, B. Dimitrov, and P. Gatev), pp. 79–85. Plenum Press, New York.

Halsband, U. (1996). Neuropsychologische und neurophysiologische Studien zum Motorischen Lernen. Habilitationsschrift aus der Neurologischen Klinik der Hohen Medizinischen Fakultät der Heinrich-Heine-Universität Düsseldorf.

Halsband, U. and Freund, H.-J. (1990). Premotor cortex and conditional motor learning in man. *Brain*, **113**, 207–22.

Halsband, U. and Freund, H.-J. (1993). Motor learning. *Current Opinion in Neurobiology*, **3**, 940–9.

Halsband, U. and Passingham, R. E. (1982). The role of premotor and parietal cortex in the direction of action. *Brain Research*, **240**, 368–72.

Halsband, U. and Passingham, R. E. (1985). Premotor cortex and the conditions for movement in monkeys (*Macaca fascicularis*). *Behavioural Brain Research*, **18**, 269–77.

Halsband, U. and Tanji, J. (1993). Cross-cultural comparison of trajectorial learning in German and Japanese subjects. *Canadian Journal of Neural Sciences*, **20**, 152.

Halsband, U., Ito, N., Tanji, J., and Freund, H.-J. (1993). The role of premotor cortex and the supplementary motor area in the temporal control of movement in man. *Brain*, **116**, 243–66.

Halsband, U., Matsuzaka, Y., and Tanji, J. (1994). Neuronal activity in the primate supplementary, pre-supplementary and premotor cortex during externally- and internally instructed sequential movements. *Neuroscience Research*, **20**, 149–55.

Halsband, U., Weyers, H. M., Schmitt, J., and Freund, H.-J. (1995). Gestik, transitive und intransitive Handlungsabläufe nach Läsionen der parietalen oder prämotorischen Areale. Vortrag auf der 26. *Jahrestagung der Deutschen Gesellschaft für Traumatologie und klinische Neuropsychologie*, p. 50.

Halsband, U., Weyers, H. M., Schmitt, J., Binkofski, F., Grützner, G., and Freund, H.-J. (1997). Recognition and imitation of pantomimed motor acts after unilatera parietal and premotor lesions: a perspective on apraxia. *Neuropsychologia*, in press.

Heap, M. and Wyke, M. (1972). Learning of a unimanual motor skill by patients with brain lesions: an experimental study. *Cortex*, **8**, 1–18.

Hécaen, H. and Albert, M. L. (1978). *Human neuropsychology*. Wiley, New York.

Heilman, K. M. (1973). Ideational apraxia—a re-definition. *Brain*, **96**, 861–4.
Heilman, K. M. (1979). Apraxia. In *Clinical neuropsychology*, (ed. K. M. Heilman and E. Valenstein), pp. 159–82. Oxford University Press, New York.
Heilman, K. M. and Rothi, L. J. G. (1985). Apraxia. In *Clinical neuropsychology*, (ed. K. M. Heilman and E. Valenstein), (2nd edn), pp. 131–50. Oxford University Press, New York.
Heilman, K. M. and Rothi, L. J. G. (1993). Apraxia. In *Clinical neuropsychology*, (ed. K. M. Heilman and E. Valenstein), (3rd edn), pp. 141–60. Oxford University Press, New York.
Heilman, K. M., Rothi, L. J., and Valenstein, E. (1982). Two forms of ideo-motor apraxia. *Neurology*, **32**, 342–6.
Hermsdörfer, J., Mai, N., Spatt, J., Marquardt, C., Veltkamp, R., and Goldenberg, G. (1996). Kinematic analysis of movement imitation in apraxia. *Brain*, **119**, 1575–86.
Humphrey, D. R. (1979). On the cortical control of visually directed reaching: contributions by non-precentral motor areas. In *Posture and movement*, (ed. R. E. Talbot and D. R. Humphrey), pp. 51–112. Raven, New York.
Humphrey, D. R. and Tanji, J. (1991). What features of voluntary motor control are encoded in the neuronal discharge of different cortical motor areas? In *Motor control: concepts and issues*, (ed. D. R. Humphrey and H.-J. Freund), pp. 413–43. Wiley, Chichester.
Hyvärinen, J. (1982). *The parietal cortex of monkey and man*. Springer, Berlin.
Jeannerod, M. (1995). Mental imagery in the motor context. *Neuropsychologia*, **33**, 1419–32.
Jeannerod, M. and Decety, J. (1995). Mental motor imagery: a window into the representational stages of action. *Current Opinion in Neurobiology*, **5**, 727–32.
Jones, E. G. and Powell, T. P. S. (1970). An anatomical study of converging sensory pathways within the cerebral cortex of the monkey. *Brain*, **93**, 793–820.
Jason, G. W. (1986). Performance of manual copying tasks after focal cortical lesions. *Neuropsychologia*, **24**, 181–91.
Kimura, D. (1979). Neuromotor mechanisms in the evolution of human communication. In *Neurobiology of social communication in primates: an evolutionary perspective*, (ed. H. D. Steklis and M. J. Raleigh), pp. 197–219. Academic Press, New York.
Kimura, D. (1982). Left-hemisphere control of oral and brachial movements and their relation to communication. *Philosophical Transactions of the Royal Society of London (Biological Sciences)*, **298**, 135–49.
Kimura, D. and Archibald, Y. (1974). Motor functions of the left hemisphere. *Brain*, **97**, 337–50.
Kleist, K. (1934). *Gehirnpathologie*. Barth, Leibzig.
Kubota, K. and Hamada, U. (1978). Visual tracking and neuron activity in the post-arcuate area in monkeys. *Journal of Physiology*, **74**, 294–312.
Kurata, K. (1991). Corticocortical inputs to the dorsal and ventral aspects of the premotor cortex of macaque monkeys. *Neuroscience Research*, **12**, 263–80.
Kurata, K. and Wise, S. P. (1988). Premotor and supplementary motor cortex in rhesus monkeys: neuronal activity during externally- and internally-instructed motor tasks. *Experimental Brain Research*, **72**, 237–48.
Laplane, D., Talairach, J., Meininger, V., Bancaud, J., and Orgogozo, J. M. (1977). Clinical consequences of corticectomies involving the supplementary motor area in man. *Journal of Neurological Sciences*, **34**, 301–14.
Lehmkuhl, G. and Poeck, K. (1981). A disturbance in the conceptual organization of actions in patients with ideational apraxia. *Cortex*, **17**, 153–8.

Liepmann, H. (1900). Das Krankheitsbild der Apraxie (motorischen Asymbolie). *Mitschriften der Psychiatry*, **8**, 15–44, 102–32, 182–97.
Liepmann, H. (1908). *Drei Aufsätze aus dem Apraxiegebiet*. Karger, Berlin.
Lu, M. T., Preston, J. B., and Strick, P. L. (1994). Interconnections between the prefrontal cortex and the premotor areas in the frontal lobe. *Journal of Comparative Neurology*, **341**, 375–92.
Luppino, G., Matelli, M., and Rizzolatti, G. (1990). Cortico-cortical connections of two electrophysiologically identified arm representations in the mesial agranular frontal cortex. *Experimental Brain Research*, **82**, 214–18.
Luppino, G., Matelli, M., Camarda, R. M., and Rizzolatti, G. (1993). Cortico-cortical connections of area F3 (SMA-proper) and area F6 (pre-SMA) in the macaque monkey. *Journal of Comparative Neurology*, **338**, 114–40.
Luria, A. R. (1966). *Higher cortical functions in man*. Tavistock, London.
Matelli, W. and Luppino, G. (1992). Anatomo-functional parcellation of the agranular frontal cortex. *Experimental Brain Research*, **22**, 85–102.
Matelli, W., Camarda, R., Glickstein, M., and Rizzolatti, G. (1986). Afferent and efferent projections of the inferior area 6 in the macaque monkey. *Journal of Comparative Neurology*, **251**, 281–98.
Matelli, W., Luppino, G., Fogassi, L., and Rizzolatti, G. (1989). Thalamic input to inferior area 6 and area 4 in the macaque monkey. *Journal of Comparative Neurology*, **280**, 468–88.
Matelli, W., Luppino, G., and Rizzolatti, G. (1991). Architecture of superior and mesial area 6 and the adjacent cingulate cortex in the macaque monkey. *Journal of Comparative Neurology*, **311**, 445–62.
Matsuzaka, Y., Aizawa, H., and Tanji, J. (1992) A motor area rostral to the supplementary motor area (presupplementary motor area) in the monkey: neuronal activity during a learned motor task. *Journal of Neurophysiology*, **68**, 653–62.
Mountcastle, V. B., Lynch, J. C., Georgopolous, A. P., Sakata, H., and Acuña, C. (1975). Posterior parietal association cortex of the monkey: command functions for operations within extrapersonal space. *Journal of Neurophysiology*, **38**, 871–908.
Mushiake, H., Inase, M., and Tanji, J. (1991). Neuronal activity in the primate premotor supplementary and precentral motor cortex during visually guided and internally determined sequential movements. *Journal of Neurophysiology*, **66**, 705–18.
Nixon, P. D., Burbaud, P., and Passingham, R. E. (1992). Control of arm movement after bilateral lesions of area 5 in the monkey (Macaca mulatta). *Experimental Brain Research*, **90**, 229–32.
Ostry, D. J. and Cooke, J. D. (1987). Kinematic patterns in speech and limb movements. In *Motor and sensory processes of language*, (ed. E. Keller and M. Gopnik), pp. 223–36. Erlbaum, Hillsdale, NJ.
Pandya, D. N. and Seltzer, B. (1982). Association areas of the cerebral cortex. *Trends in Neurosciences*, **5**, 386–90.
Passingham, R. E. (1985). Premotor cortex: sensory cues and movement. *Behavioural Brain Research*, **18**, 175–86.
Passingham, R. E. (1996). Functional specialization of the supplementary motor area in monkeys and humans. In *Advances in neurology*, Vol. 70, (ed. H. O. Lüders), pp. 105–16. Lippincott-Raven, New York.
Passingham, R. E. and Ettlinger, G. (1974). A comparison of cortical function in man and other primates. *International Reviews in Neurobiology*, **16**, 233–99.
Petrides, M. (1985). Deficits in non spatial conditional associative learning after periarcuate lesions in the monkey. *Behavioural Brain Research*, **16**, 95–101.

Petrides, M. and Pandya, D. N. (1984). Projections to the frontal cortex from the posterior parietal region in the rhesus monkey. *Journal of Comparative Neurology*, **228**, 105–16.

Platz, T. and Mauritz, K.-H. (1995). Human motor planning, motor programming, and use of new task-relevant information with different apraxic syndromes. *European Journal of Neuroscience*, **7**, 1536–47.

Poeck, K. (1989). Apraxie. In *Klinische Neuropsychologie*, (ed. K. Poeck), pp. 188–207. Thième, Stuttgart.

Poizner, H., Mack, L., Verfaellie, M., Rothi, L. J. G, and Heilman, K. M. (1990). Three-dimensional computer-graphic analysis of apraxia. *Brain*, **113**, 85–101.

Rapcsak, S. Z., Ochipa, C., Anderson, K. C., and Poizner, H. (1995). Progressive ideomotor apraxia: evidence for a selective impairment of the action production sytem. *Brain and Cognition*, **27**, 213–36.

Rizzolatti, G., Gentilucci, M., Camarda, R. M., Gallese, V., Luppino, G., and Matelli, M. (1990). Neurons related to reaching-grasping arm movements in the rostral part of area 6 (area 6ab). *Experimental Brain Research*, **82**, 337–50.

Rizzolatti, G., Fadiga, L., Gallese, V., and Fogassi, L. (1996). Premotor cortex and the recognition of motor actions. *Cognitive Brain Research*, **3**, 131–41.

Rizzolatti, G., Fadiga, L., Matelli, M., Bettinardi, V., Paulesu, E., Perani, D., and Fazio, F. (1997). Localization of grasp representation in humans by PET: 1. Observation versus execution. *Experimental Brain Research*, **111**, 246–52.

Romo, R. and Schulz, W. (1992). Role of primate basal ganglia and frontal cortex in the internal generation of movements. III. Neuronal activity in the supplementary motor area. *Experimental Brain Research*, **91**, 396–407.

Roy, E. A. and Square, P. A. (1985). Common considerations in the study of limb, verbal and oral apraxia. In *Neuropsychological studies of apraxia and related disorders*, (ed. E. A. Roy), pp. 111–59. North Holland, Amsterdam.

Roy, E. A., Square-Storer, P. A., Hogg, S., and Adams, S. (1991). Analysis of task demands in apraxia. *International Journal of Neuroscience*, **56**, 177–86.

Roy, E., Brown, L., and Hardie, M. (1993). Movement variability in limb gesturing: implications for understanding apraxia. In *Variability of motor control*, (ed. K. Newell and D. Corcos), pp. 261–82. Human Kinetics Publishers, Champaign, IL.

Shima, K., Aya, K., Mushiake, H., Inase, M., Aizawa, H., and Tanji, J. (1991). Two movement-related foci in the primate cingulate cortex observed in signal-triggered and self-paced forelimb movements. *Journal of Neurophysiology*, **65**, 188–202.

Squire, L. R. (1986). Mechanisms of memory. *Science*, **232**, 1612–19.

Steinthal, H. (1871). Cited by Thiele, R. (1928). *Aphasie, Apraxie, Agnosie*. Bunke Handbuch der Geisteskrankheiten. Springer, Berlin.

Stephan, K. M., Fink, G. R., Passingham, R. E., Silbersweig, D., Ceballos-Baumann, A. O., Frith, C. D. *et al.* (1995). Functional anatomy of the mental representation of upper extremity movements in healthy subjects. *Journal of Neurophysiology*, **73**, 373–86.

Stephan, K. M., Binkofski, F., Halsband, U., Schnitzler, A., Wunderlich, G., Tass, P. *et al.* (1997). Cingulate gyrus subserves bimanual synchrony: kinematic and functional imaging data, submitted.

Sternberg, S., Knoll, R. L., Monsell, S., and Wright, C. E. (1983). *Control of rapid action sequences in speech and typewriting*. AT & T Bell Laboratories Technical Communication, pp. 1–20. Murray Hill, NJ.

Strauss, H. (1924). Über konstruktive Apraxie. *Monatsschrift für Psychiatrie und Neurologie*, **63**, 739–48.

Strick, P. L., Hoover, J. E., and Mushiake, H. (1993). Evidence for 'output channels' in the basal ganglia and cerebellum. In *Role of the cerebellum and basal ganglia in voluntary movement*, (ed. N. Mano, I. Hamada, and M. R. DeLong), pp. 171–80. Elsevier, Amsterdam.

Stuss, D. T. and Benson, D. F. (1986). *The frontal lobes*. Raven Press, New York.

Tanji, J. and Shima, K. (1994). Role for supplementary motor area cells in planning several movements ahead. *Nature*, **371**, 413–16.

Tanji, J. and Shima, K. (1996). Contrast of neuronal activity between the supplementary motor area and other cortical motor areas. In *Advances in neurology*, Vol. 70, (ed. H. O. Lüders), pp. 95–105. Lippincott-Raven, New York.

Tanji J., Aizawa H., Shima, K., and Matsuzaka, Y. (1991). A forelimb motor task-related area rostral to the supplementary motor area. *Japanese Journal of Physiology*, **41**, 252.

Tanji, J., Shima, K., Matsuzaka, Y., and Halsband, U. (1995). Neuronal activity in the supplementary, presupplementary and premotor cortex of monkey. In *Functions of the cortico-basal ganglia loop*, (ed. M. Kimura and A. M. Graybiel), pp. 154–65. Springer, Berlin.

Taylor, J. (ed.) (1932). *Selected writings of John Hughlings Jackson*. Hodder and Stoughton, London.

Tyszka, J. M., Grafton, S. T., Chew, W., Woods, R. P., and Colletti, P. M. (1994). Parceling of mesial frontal motor areas during ideation and movement using functional magnetic resonance imaging at 1.5 tesla. *Annals of Neurology*, **35**, 746–9.

Von Bonin, G. and Bailey, P. (1947) *The neocortex of* Macaca mulatta. University of Illinois Press, Urbana, IL.

Von Economo, C. and Koskinas, G. N. (1925). *Die Cytoarchitektonik der Hirnrinde des erwachsenen Menschen*. Springer, Wien.

Von Economo, C. (1929). *The cytoarchitectonics of the human cerebral cortex*. Oxford University Press, London.

Warrington, E., James, M., and Kinsbourne, M. (1966). Drawing disability in relation to laterality of cerebral lesion. *Brain*, **89**, 53–82.

Weinrich, M. and Wise, S. P. (1982). The premotor cortex of the monkey. *Journal of Neuroscience*, **2**, 1329–45.

Wernicke, C. (1874). *Der aphasische Symptomenkomplex*. Cohn, Breslau.

Wiesendanger, M. (1981). Organization of secondary motor areas of cerebral cortex. In *Handbook of physiology*, Vol. 2, (ed. V. C. B. Brooks), pp. 1121–247. American Physiological Society, Bethesda, MD.

Wiesendanger, M. (1986). Recent development in studies of the supplementary area of primates. *Reviews in Physiology, Biochemistry and Pharmacology*, **103**, 1–59.

Wise, S. P., Alexander, G. E., Altman, I. S., Brooks, V. B., Freund, H.-J. *et al.* (1991). Group report: What are the specific functions of the different motor areas? In *Motor control: concepts and issues*, (ed. D. R. Humphrey and H.-J. Freund), pp. 463–85. Wiley, Chichester.

Zangwill, O. L. (1960). Le problème de l'apraxie idéatoire. *Revue Neurologique*, **102**, 595–603.

Zilles, K. (1990). Cortex. In *The human nervous system*, (ed. G. T. Paxinos), pp. 757–802. Academic Press, San Diego.

12

Perspectives on visuospatial neglect

MONIKA HARVEY

Among the behavioural disorders found in patients with hemispheric dysfunction, unilateral visual neglect is one of the most striking. The symptoms, although many and various, always include a tendency to ignore objects and parts of objects on the left (i.e. contralesional) side of the patient's egocentric space. In its most extreme forms, a patient may deny that the involved limbs are his own and object to their presence in his hospital bed. Other patients may fail to shave or dress the neglected side.

12.1 Historical background

12.1.1 The visual efficiency debate

Although visuospatial neglect has been described widely since the early twentieth century, the relevance and implications of the syndrome in terms of 'higher' functions have been debated ever since. Initially observed by Oppenheimer (1885), Bálint (1909), Holmes (1918), and Riddoch (1935), it was first discussed as a separate syndrome by Brain (1941, 1945). In 1941, he reported three patients with large right parietal lesions and a disorder of route-finding which he attributed to 'an inattention to, or neglect of the left half of visual space'. He suggested that this 'agnosia for the opposite half of space' was largely restricted to patients with minor (usually right) hemisphere lesions (Brain 1945), although he also pointed out that the apparent absence of the same symptoms in patients with lesions to the dominant (usually left) hemisphere might be due to masking from other effects, such as severe aphasia, disorientation, or different types of agnosia. Brain also firmly believed that the disorientation could not be attributed to a 'hemianopia in the left half-fields' nor be 'due to a loss of topographical memory' (Brain 1941). This view differed markedly from that of the influential German neurologist Bay (1950), who claimed that all so-called 'higher' perceptual disorders were secondary to sensory impairment, general intellectual loss, or language disturbance. In his very well and convincingly written treatise *Agnosie und Funktionswandel* (Bay 1950) he systematically analysed most of the agnosia cases reported in the German literature, including patient Schnei of Gelb and Goldstein (1920), and reduced them to mere sensory and intellectual impairments. Included in his critique was the syndrome of visual neglect (*optisch-räumliche Agnosie*) with a description of Schneller and Seidemann's patient (1932) whose neglect he explained as resulting from restricted visual fields and generally slow and clumsy behaviour, stating explicitly that 'the idea of an isolated neglect syndrome as a specific disorder of space perception is dispensable and by no means proven'(translated from Bay 1950, p. 140).

However, this view of agnosia, and within this the syndrome of neglect, as simply a sensory disorder was strongly argued against by George Ettlinger. In his 1956 paper, he took on board Bay's strong call for careful examination of more elementary visual processes but elegantly proved that these deficits *per se* could not explain agnosia (here used in a wider sense including neglect and topographical loss). Amongst other agnosic patients, he tested the incidence and magnitude of sensory deficits in three patients with neglect (grouped under visual–spatial agnosia) and concluded that, although their visual efficiency indices were low, they were well above another patient group who had such defects unaccompanied by spatial loss. He substantiated this view in a further joint paper with Elizabeth Warrington and Oliver Zangwill (Ettlinger *et al.* 1957) in which they described 10 cases of right-sided posterior lesions with visual–spatial agnosia: none of these patients gave any suggestion that their defects of visual discrimination bore any systematic relation to the visual–spatial disorder. They argued that the essential defect in these patients did not lie in a failure of sensory input but in *a failure to make effective use of this input at a central level.*

For neglect, this argument was nicely consolidated 20 years later in the ingenious study by Bisiach and Luzzatti (1978), which is now a classic. (On a personal note, I can attest that the study was greatly admired by George Ettlinger, and that none of his German students would pass an examination without understanding the implications of this study!) Patients with unilateral spatial neglect from right hemisphere damage were asked to describe from memory a highly familiar scene. In one condition they were to take the perspective of facing the cathedral located at the end of the major piazza in Milan. In a second condition they were to take the perspective of facing away from the cathedral. In the patients' descriptions of the piazza, left sided details were omitted *depending on the perspective taken.* The authors thus demonstrated unilateral spatial neglect on purely conceptual tasks, i.e. tasks that are soluble without sensory inflow and which contain an in-built control condition indicating the availability in memory of all necessary information. Neglect therefore had to be categorized as a 'higher' disorder independent of primary visual, or indeed intellectual, deficits.

12.1.2 The laterality debate

Apart from this issue, another debate surrounding neglect at that time was the issue of laterality: does neglect for one side of space occur more frequently with right- than with left-sided lesions, and if so, what significance can be attributed to such a bias? (Halsband *et al.* 1985). Brain's view of visuospatial neglect as a manifestation of predominantly right hemisphere damage was strongly supported by Zangwill's group (McFie and Zangwill 1960), who compared cases of constructional disability due to left hemisphere damage with a group of previously reported right hemisphere lesions, among them Ettlinger's 10 cases of agnosia (Paterson and Zangwill 1944, 1945; McFie *et al.* 1950; Ettlinger *et al.* 1957). They found that left-sided visuospatial neglect had been present in 14 of the 21 right hemisphere lesioned patients but right-sided neglect only in one of the eight left hemisphere lesioned patients. However, in contrast to these studies, Battersby *et al.* (1956), who specifically looked for evidence of visuospatial neglect in 85 patients with space-occupying lesions, found no significant difference as to the side of the lesion. Although they found the syndrome in 29 per cent of patients with non-dominant lesions and only in 9 per cent of patients with dominant lesions, they concluded that this difference was due to the fact that severe aphasia had precluded adequate testing in a further 29 per cent of the patients with dominant hemisphere lesions. So looking at it the opposite way round, they judged 62 per cent of the left hemisphere cases and 59 per cent of the right hemisphere cases to be without neglect (in the remaining 12 per cent of right hemisphere cases the diagnosis of neglect was uncertain). Gainotti (1968) then attempted to study the same problem by means of a battery of tests simple enough to be administered to all patients, including severe aphasics. He found that unilateral spatial neglect was not only significantly more frequent, but also definitely more severe in patients suffering from lesions of the right hemisphere. This was only partly confirmed by Costa *et al.* (1969), who also found a higher incidence of neglect in right hemisphere lesioned patients but, contrary to Gainotti, they reported that severity and patterns of deficit were alike in both left- and right-lesioned groups.

Various factors may underlie these divergent findings. Especially in the older studies, authors failed to specify their criterion for the diagnosis of unilateral visual neglect, so some differences must have been due to case selection. Also, Oxbury *et al.* (1974) pointed out that the two hemisphere groups of McFie and Zangwill differed in the incidence of both visual field defect and papilloedema, suggesting that the right hemisphere lesions may have been bigger than those of the left. Both Battersby *et al.* (1956) and Hécaen (1962) claimed that unilateral spatial neglect was associated with widespread cerebral dysfunction, and in both series neglect was associated with a high incidence of hemianopia.

Task was also discovered to be an important component regarding the differences between right and left hemisphere damage on neglect. Data obtained by Gainotti *et al.* (1972) and Colombo *et al.* (1976) showed that when the task required attention to be focused on small portions of space, then neglect for one half of the stimulus was almost only observed in right hemisphere damaged patients. On the contrary, when the task required exploration of large displays, no difference was observed between patients with right or left hemisphere damage, i.e. contralateral neglect was shown in both groups. Similarly Gainotti *et al.* (1986) reported that while both patients with left hemisphere damage and those with right hemisphere damage showed an asymmetric exploration of space in a 'searching for animals test', only those with right hemisphere damage showed a clear tendency to omit figures lying on the left side of the composite pattern in an 'overlapping figures test'.

A final critical factor, ignored at the time, involved the locus of the responsible lesion. Halsband *et al.* (1985) noted that during the period 1941–57 a consensus emerged that 'parietal damage was sufficient to give rise to the manifestations of neglect, although the advantages of modern computer-based radiological methods were not then available to exclude additional damage elsewhere'. Later research showed that neglect can also arise after temporo-occipital lesions (Battersby *et al.* 1956), frontal lesions (Chédru *et al.* 1973; Van der Linden *et al.* 1980), and subcortical lesions in structures such as the striatum (Healton *et al.* 1982; Stein and Volpe 1983), the thalamus (Henderson *et al.* 1982), and the claustrum (Ettlinger 1984*a*). More recently, extensive CT scan studies have linked neglect to a range of cortical and subcortical circuits (Vallar and Perani 1986; Vallar *et al.* 1994).

None the less, a general consensus emerged from all these studies that neglect is generally more frequent and severe after lesions of the right hemisphere (Critchley 1953; Gainotti 1968; Oxbury *et al.* 1974; De Renzi 1982; Heilman 1983; Gainotti *et al.* 1986;), an observation which was again nicely demonstrated in the work carried out by Ettlinger and his colleagues in Bielefeld (Halsband *et al.* 1985) in which the performance of 80 unselected patients with unilateral cerebral lesions was assessed on a systematically designed range of neglect tests. Thirty patients were identified as showing neglect, and in 27 of these cases the lesion was found to be right sided.

12.2 The neglect syndrome: confusion or reality?

12.2.1 Is neglect a unitary disorder?

In retrospect, it seems surprising now that despite the diversity of neglect phenomena, the disorder was still very much regarded as a unitary phenomenon throughout the seventies and eighties. Heilman *et al.* (1985*a*) defined a 'neglect syndrome', identifying a group of symptoms which were clinically recognizable and logically distinct (hemispatial neglect, hemi-inattention, hemiakinesia, extinction, and allaesthesia), and proposed a standardized terminology. Although they went further by pointing out that there were double dissociations among some of these neglect symptoms, in other words that there really was no such thing as a 'syndrome' of neglect, all major neglect theories prevalent at that time were based on a unitary neglect syndrome:

1. Bisiach's representational map hypothesis (Bisiach and Luzzatti 1978; Bisiach *et al.* 1981), alluded to above, attributed visuospatial neglect to a defective mental representation of space. Bisiach suggested that the mental representation of the environment is structured topographically and mapped

across the brain, arguing that the processes by which the visual image is built up may be split between the two hemispheres and that right hemisphere damage results in a representational failure for the left half of this image.

2. Kinsbourne's attentional hypothesis (Kinsbourne 1977, 1987) postulated that each hemisphere is responsible for shifting attention in a contraversive direction, either in the ipsilateral or contralateral half of space, and that damage to one hemisphere consequently unbalances the attentional system in favour of shifts contraversive to the intact side. He assumed that the leftward bias caused by the right hemisphere is weaker, with two consequences: first, the right hemisphere exerts a more balanced control over both sides of space and, secondly, a right hemisphere lesion releases a stronger contraversive bias from the left hemisphere, thus causing neglect.

3. Also within the attentional domain, Posner and his colleagues (Posner 1980; Posner *et al.* 1980) adopted a 'covert orienting' paradigm in which spatial attention is manipulated by presenting subjects with visual cues that specify to-be-attended locations, followed by targets that appear either at the cued (primed) location, or targets that appear at unattended locations. When using this paradigm in a clinical context, Posner *et al.* (1982, 1984) found that patients with right parietal damage showed little impairment in the detection of a left visual field stimulus when the spatial cue was also directed towards the left visual field. There was also no impairment (beyond the 'normal cost') when detecting right visual field stimuli when their attention had been directed to the left visual field. However, when a cue directed attention to the right visual field, patients often failed to detect a subsequent left visual field stimulus or, if they did, showed abnormally long response latencies. In a further experiment, it was found that patients with parietal lobe damage are worse in redirecting their attention in a contralesional than in a ipsilesional direction in *either* visual field (Posner *et al.* 1987). So it seemed to be the case that parietal patients had difficulty in reorienting to targets contralateral to the current focus of attention, a difficulty conceptualized by Posner and his colleagues as one of attentional 'disengagement'.

4. The 'directional hypokinesia' hypothesis of Heilman and colleagues (Heilman and Valenstein 1979; Heilman *et al.* 1985*a*,*b*, 1987) stated that each side of the brain possesses its own activating system and that, when one of these two systems is disrupted, the corresponding hemisphere cannot properly process sensory information and organize motor responses. To explain why unilateral spatial neglect occurs more frequently following right than left hemisphere lesions, they postulated that the left hemisphere controls orienting to stimuli on the right side of space only, whereas the right hemisphere controls orienting towards both sides.

Almost all of these models have their problems since they assume a unitary underlying disorder, thus reducing neglect either to an attentional failure assuming a single attentional executive (for a critique of this approach see Rizzolatti *et al.* 1994), or a movement execution deficit. In their 1985 paper,

Ettlinger and his colleagues did briefly address the issue of the unitary nature of the neglect syndrome, concluding that 'at this time it is uncertain whether neglect can still be regarded as a unitary defect, or whether different processes are disturbed in association with different forms of neglect' (Halsband *et al.* 1985). They assessed and categorized 80 unselected patients with unilateral lesions, identifying 30 of these as having contralateral neglect either of a visual (n = 5), auditory (n = 6), tactile (n = 5), motor (n = 4), or mixed (n = 10) kind. This extensive study, including a total of 114 patients, clearly has the stamp of Ettlinger's careful and rigorous experimental technique: few studies nowadays would meet his standards of patient and control subject selection, his care in designing the screening tasks, and his extra analyses and tests ensuring that there were no differences in either sex, age, or intellectual ability between the groups.

None the less, although the diversity of the neglect syndrome was clearly demonstrated in the study of Halsband *et al.* (1985), it was not until the numerous studies of Halligan and Marshall in the late eighties and early nineties that it became obvious that *even within the visual domain* the clinical and theoretical picture of spatial neglect had to be far more complex than previously assumed. These authors found neglect for near (personal) but not far (extrapersonal) space (Halligan and Marshall 1991), for line bisection but not cancellation (Halligan and Marshall 1992), and for bisection of long but not short lines (Halligan and Marshall 1988). This work was complemented by that of other researchers showing neglect for faces but not other equally complex stimuli (Young *et al.* 1990) or neglect for imagery but not real-life objects (Guariglia *et al.* 1993). So here the implication was not merely that neglect may operate differently across varying sensory domains or tasks, but that it may even apply differentially within a given task, across different spatial scales or different stimulus patterns (Milner and Harvey 1994). This is, of course, a daunting prospect and the frustration engendered by it led Halligan and Marshall to the provocative title of their 1992 paper 'Left visuospatial neglect: a meaningless entity?'.

Although one might be tempted to abandon in despair all hope of understanding neglect, it seems more constructive to accept that there are different types of neglect and thus, in the absence of a theory-driven taxonomy, hope to become able to compare one patient with another by devising satisfactory ways of teasing apart the different factors contributing to their neglect symptoms. Some attempts have now been made in this direction.

12.2.2 Current distinctions

Several studies have shown that there are patients with a broadly defined *perceptual*-type neglect who demonstrate an attentional/representational failure resulting in a misperception of space, whereas other patients with neglect of a mainly *directional* nature fail to direct their actions properly (Bisiach *et al.*, 1990, Tegnér and Levander, 1991, Liu *et al.*, 1992, Milner *et al.*

1993, Harvey *et al.* 1995*a*). In the initial study (Bisiach *et al.* 1990) a pulley device was employed which allowed line bisection in a 'congruent' and an 'incongruent' condition. In the congruent condition, moving a manipulandum rightwards would bisect a presented line rightwards as well. Bisecting a line to the right of its true midpoint is behaviour typically shown by neglect patients. However, the directions of motion differed from each other in the incongruent condition; in this case movement of the manipulandum to the right would result in a leftward bisection. Bisiach *et al.* (1990) showed that a number of neglect patients exhibit some form of *perceptual* neglect, so that when asked to bisect the line they would actually move the manipulandum leftwards in order to set the transection pointer rightwards from the midpoint of a line. Conversely, patients with the *directional* form of neglect performed movements into their right hemispace only, thus transecting lines to the *left* of the centre in the incongruent condition (presumably in order to avoid making a leftward movement).

A slightly different procedure was introduced by Tegnér and Levander (1991). Their patients performed a line cancellation task either with normal viewing or through a 90° angled mirror. When the patient looked at the display through the mirror, the lines on the left of the display were seen in the right half of the mirror, whereas the lines on the right side of the display were seen in the left half. In normal viewing, all patients showed the typical neglect behaviour with omissions of lines on the left side of the display. They differed, however, in the way they behaved in the mirror condition: some patients now cancelled only in the left hemispace (thus showing perceptual neglect, since the lines *appeared* to be in their right hemispace), whereas others still cancelled lines in the right hemispace (despite these lines appearing to lie on the left), thus indicating directional neglect. Additionally, Milner *et al.* (1993) and Harvey *et al.* (1995*a*) have shown that patients with perceptual-type neglect experience a distortion of their subjective space so that a bisection mark (the so-called 'landmark') placed centrally on a line appears to be offset to the left. Harvey *et al.* (1995*a*) presented this landmark task to eight neglect patients, asking them to point to the end the bisection mark appeared closer to. In contrast to control patients whose responses were randomly distributed, seven of the eight neglect patients consistently indicated the mark as being closer to the left side, whereas the eighth patient pointed mainly to the right throughout the experiment. Presumably any perceptual bias in this patient was outweighed by a rightward response bias.

Unfortunately, there have been no systematic studies to investigate whether these different tasks partition, in their different ways, the set of neglect patients into essentially the same taxonomic subsets. However, other dissociations have been found, and so far the most accepted ones are personal versus extrapersonal neglect, perceptual versus directional, and spatial versus object-based neglect (reviewed by Walker 1995). So in conjunction with Marshall *et al.* (1993) and Walker (1995) I would argue that there is no such entity as visuospatial neglect, just as there is no such entity as aphasia.

The term aphasia is used as a clinical shorthand for language disorders, without any expectation of reference to a specific language problem. Similarly, there is no reason why neglect should not be defined in the same general way, i.e. as a problem affecting the spatial distribution of awareness and behaviour, with each instance necessitating a specific assessment as to its precise nature. As Marshall and colleagues argue 'Why should we assume that spatial competence is any less complex than language competence, and hence less liable to show qualitatively distinct forms?' With this in mind, future research into the nature of the disorder should be addressing these different types separately, thus allowing a deeper understanding and more specific rehabilitation.

12.3 Neglect and theories of visual processing

12.3.1 Extinction and neglect

Although the striking clinical features and problems of rehabilitation of visuospatial neglect justify the study of the syndrome as such, this is only half the picture. Assuming there are different types of neglect, what does that tell us about theories of visual processing, about the neural circuits of attention, the modularity of the visual system, or indeed the meaningful analogies to be drawn across species for certain classes of behaviour?

There is no straightforward answer to any of these questions but early attempts were made by George Ettlinger when he started to address questions of the differences and commonalities among human and non-human primates during the 1970s. As early as 1962 he noted that no evidence of visual neglect in monkeys with unilateral posterior parietal lesions could be found (Ettlinger and Kalsbeck 1962), although they did show reaching defects in both half-fields with the contralesional hand. Given evidence that in humans, unlike monkeys, visual reaching impairment could often be restricted to the contralesional half-field only (e.g. Brain 1941), he argued in 1970 that 'there appear to be genuine differences between man and monkey in respect to the neural system which, when damaged, gives rise in man to visual neglect and inaccurate reaching for visual targets' (Drewe *et al.* 1970). In a later article (Ettlinger 1984*b*), he conceded that reaching impairments in men and monkeys might be similar in nature, but stuck to the idea of visual neglect as a possible discontinuity, since it occurred frequently in humans in association with parietal lesions but, he argued, in the monkey only in association with frontal lesions. Ettlinger also correctly pointed out that the study of Heilman *et al.* (1970), frequently cited as evidence of visual neglect in monkeys after parietal lesions, really only documented *extinction* (extinction being generally defined as the report of the presence of only one of two stimuli presented simultaneously).

In his later reappraisal of the Ungerleider and Mishkin concept of spatial versus object vision (the former putatively mediated by the dorsal, the latter by the ventral stream of visual processing), Ettlinger (1990) stressed again that unilateral posterior lesions in monkeys gave rise to extinction but not neglect, a point that has received renewed interest since the reported double dissociations between neglect and extinction in humans. Patients have been described who show neglect but not extinction, and other patients who show extinction but not neglect (De Renzi *et al.* 1984; Barbieri and De Renzi 1989; Liu *et al.* 1992). Secondly, there is an approximately equal incidence of extinction after left and right brain lesions, which is not the case for neglect. There seem to be anatomical differences in addition to these symptomatic dissociations: Vallar *et al.* (1994) noted that although extinction and neglect *together* are typically associated with damage to the right temporo-parieto-occipital junction, extinction alone is specifically *not* associated with damage to this area. All these data seem to indicate that extinction might not just be a mild form of neglect but a different disorder altogether.

Taking this argument further, Milner (1997) argues that extinction *but not* neglect may be regarded as a *dorsal stream* phenomenon. It has long been known that the visual responses of many of the neurones in the primate posterior parietal cortex are enhanced when the receptive-field stimulus is concurrently the target for a saccadic or manual movement (Bushnell *et al.* 1981). This neuronal enhancement is associated with spatially selective attention to the visual target stimulus. However, there is also good evidence (reviewed by Milner and Goodale 1995) that the posterior parietal cortex processes information about spatial location and even geometric object features in order to provide egocentric visual guidance for a range of motor acts. In *humans*, lesions which cause optic ataxia—a disordered visual control of the arm, fingers, and hand—are centred in the intraparietal sulcus and adjacent superior parietal lobule (Bálint 1909, translated by Harvey 1995; Perenin and Vighetto 1988). Similarly, lesions causing the slowing of saccadic eye movements to visual targets are centred in posterior parts of the intraparietal sulcus (Pierrot-Deseilligny *et al.* 1987, 1991). So brain lesions in this superior part of the parietal lobe have been found to be associated with both visual extinction and optic ataxia (Perenin and Vighetto 1988) but not neglect (Vallar and Perani 1986). If it is thus assumed that extinction is associated with a system guiding egocentric movements, damage to this system should be expected to be more apparent in the patient's motor output than in perceptual reports. Exactly this has been found by Bisiach *et al.* (1989): right brain damaged patients reported the occurrence of a contralesional stimulus less often when they used a manual rather than a verbal response mode. Of course, many patients with neglect also show extinction; but this might be due to the fact that most of the lesions causing neglect are large (Bisiach *et al.* 1981) and are therefore likely to disrupt more than one functional system.

12.3.2 Perceptual and object-based neglect

Bearing in mind the currently accepted distinctions within the neglect syndrome, certain other predictions might be made. The lesion evidence suggests that perceptual neglect is mainly due to temporo-parietal lesions whereas the directional type seems to involve appreciable damage to frontal and/or basal ganglia areas (Bisiach *et al.* 1990, Tegnér *et al.* 1991, Liu *et al.* 1992, Harvey *et al.* 1995*b*). This anatomical distinction is interesting again in relation to the so-called neglect phenomena seen in primates. George Ettlinger noted in a 1990 critique that 'neglect that follows certain unilateral frontal lesions in the monkey . . . appears unlike the parietal neglect in man' (Ettlinger 1990). It seems to be transient, irrespective of laterality, multimodal, and predominated by limb hypokinesia. He argued that this form of neglect might be homologous to neglect after frontal lesions in humans. If one agrees with this view, it would seem unlikely that perceptual neglect would be demonstrable in primates (1) due to the nature of the lesion—parietal damage does not seem to produce neglect in monkeys; and (2) due to the nature of the impairment—perceptual neglect seems to be a disruption of a spatial–representation network rather than of a visuomotor system such as the frontal eye field. Milner and Harvey's demonstration of impaired size perception in patients with perceptual neglect (Milner and Harvey 1995) seems to suggest that neglect affects the processing of visual stimuli at a 'late' stage when certain object properties such as size have already been processed. Indeed, as Milner (1997) argues, some of the impairments in neglect patients can only be explained by assuming that their brain damage disrupts processing beyond the point where the perceptual system distinguishes between different classes of visual pattern (e.g. faces; Young *et al.* 1990). In line with this argument are the findings that perceptual neglect generally results from damage to the right inferior parietal lobule, a region which evidently receives highly processed information relating to object identity (Warrington and Taylor 1973).

The frequent co-occurrence of neglect symptomatology in more than one sensory modality (Halsband *et al.* 1985) suggests that the system damaged in perceptual neglect is a multimodal one. There is no prima-facie reason why such a system should not exist in the monkey cortex and, for example, multimodal networks have been identified in parieto-temporal cortex which could constitute a precursor (Jones and Powell 1970; Bruce *et al.* 1981). Current evidence suggests that the major source of visual information to these areas is to be found in the ventral rather than the dorsal stream of visual processing. None the less, to my knowledge no studies have been done that have demonstrated perceptual neglect (as opposed to extinction) in primates following a posterior lesion, although, for example, the landmark test (Milner *et al.* 1992) could easily be adapted to do so, and was in fact based on a task first devised for use with monkeys.

It is notable that patients with 'object-based' neglect usually have lesions in the temporo-parietal region (Driver and Halligan 1991; Driver *et al.* 1994; Walker *et al.* 1996). Neglect of an object-based representation occurs for one side of the object only, independent of the location of that object in space. It is highly probable that, as with patients with other varieties of perceptual neglect, the problems experienced by these patients are due to damage to a system that depends upon detailed information about object structure, thus allowing the system to represent spatial relationships intrinsic to those objects. Should this be the case I would argue that object-based neglect (and indeed perceptual types of neglect in general) should not be easily ameliorated by leftward eye movements and should indeed be independent of extinction and visuomotor behaviour. A number of studies have investigated eye movement behaviour of neglect patients and have invariably found it to be impaired (Ishiai *et al.* 1989; Hornak 1992; Karnath and Fetter 1995). However, to my knowledge only a couple of studies so far have addressed the crucial question of whether abnormal eye movements are caused by neglect or vice versa (Walker and Young 1996; Walker *et al.* 1996). The patient R.R. described by Walker *et al.* (1996), who showed object-based neglect, failed to report the left side of chimeric faces even when his first saccades landed on the left side of these stimuli. In a further experiment Walker and Young (1996) showed that R.R. made left saccades to scan the image and correctly named the object when a left half object was presented to the left of initial fixation. Hence his failure to identify and scan the left side of chimeric objects cannot simply be attributed to an inability to make contralesional saccades. Instead, it seems that his defective eye movements are a consequence of his object-based neglect and not vice versa, a finding which fits well with the present notion of perceptual and object-based neglect as disruptions of representational networks located in the right inferior parietal lobe. More research into the cause and effect of eye movements in patients with identified types of neglect will be necessary, but it is interesting that George Ettlinger and colleagues already proposed their independence in 1957. When describing a neglect patient, they state that 'a test was devised . . . to ascertain whether this patient's unilateral neglect was due to failure to turn his eyes towards objects lying on his left-hand side . . . This result suggests that unilateral neglect occurs even under conditions in which the patient is constrained by opto-kinetic nystagmus to fixate objects in the left half of extra-personal space' (p. 342). In characteristic fashion, George Ettlinger thus made pioneering observations, 40 years ago, to exclude not only sensory but also oculomotor disorders as primary causal factors in neglect.

References

Bálint, R. (1909). Seelenlähmung des 'Schauens', optische Ataxie, räumliche Störung der Aufmerksamkeit. *Monatsschrift für Psychiatrie und Neurologie*, **25**, 51–81.

Barbieri, C. and De Renzi, E. (1989). Patterns of neglect dissociation. *Behavioral Neurology*, **2**, 13–24.

Battersby, W. S., Bender, M. B., Pollack, M., and Kahn, R. L. (1956). Unilateral 'spatial agnosia' ('inattention') in patients with cerebral lesions. *Brain*, **79**, 68–93.

Bay, E. (1950). *Agnosie und Funktionswandel*. Springer, Berlin.

Bisiach, E. and Luzzatti, C. (1978). Unilateral neglect of representational space. *Cortex*, **14**, 129–33.

Bisiach, E., Capitani, E., Luzzatti, C., and Perani, D. (1981). Brain and conscious representation of outside reality. *Neuropsychologia*, **19**, 543–51.

Bisiach, E., Vallar, G., and Geminiani, G. (1989). Influence of response modality on perceptual awareness of contralesional visual stimuli. *Brain*, **112**, 1627–36.

Bisiach, E., Geminiani, G., Berti, A., and Rusconi, M. L. (1990). Perceptual and premotor factors in unilateral neglect. *Neurology*, **40**, 1278–81.

Brain, W. R. (1941). Visual disorientation with special reference to lesions of the right hemisphere. *Brain*, **64**, 113–30.

Brain, W. R. (1945). Speech and handedness. *Lancet*, **2**, 837–42.

Bruce, C., Desimone, R., and Gross, C. G. (1981). Visual properties of neurones in a polysensory area in superior temporal sulcus of the macaque. *Journal of Neurophysiology*, **55**, 1057–75.

Bushnell, M. C., Goldberg, M. E., and Robinson, D. L. (1981). Behavioral enhancement of visual responses in monkey cerebral cortex. I. Modulation in posterior parietal cortex related to selective visual attention. *Journal of Neurophysiology*, **46**, 755–72.

Chédru, F., Leblanc, M., and Lhermitte, F. (1973). Visual searching in normal and brain-damaged subjects (contribution to the study of unilateral inattention). *Cortex*, **9**, 94–111.

Colombo, A., De Renzi, E., and Faglioni, P. (1976). The occurrence of visual neglect in patients with unilateral cerebral disease. *Cortex*, **12**, 221–31.

Costa, L. D., Vaughan, H. C., Horwitz, M., and Ritter, W. (1969). Patterns of behavioral deficit associated with visual spatial neglect. *Cortex*, **5**, 242–62.

Critchley, M. (1953). *The parietal lobes*. Edward Arnold, London.

De Renzi, E. (1982). *Disorders of space exploration*. Wiley, New York.

De Renzi, E., Gentilini, P., and Pattacini, F. (1984). Auditory extinction following hemispheric damage. *Neuropsychologia*, **22**, 733–44.

Drewe, E. A., Ettlinger, G., Milner, A. D., and Passingham, R. E. (1970). A comparative review of the results of neuropsychological research on man and monkey. *Cortex*, **6**, 129–63.

Driver, J. and Halligan, P. W. (1991). Can visual neglect operate in object-centred coordinates? An affirmative single-case study. *Cognitive Neuropsychology*, **8**, 475–96.

Driver, J., Baylis, G. C., Goodrich, S. J., and Rafal, R. D. (1994). Axis based neglect of visual shapes. *Neuropsychologia*, **32**, 1353–65.

Ettlinger, G. (1956). Sensory deficits in visual agnosia. *Journal of Neurology, Neurosurgery and Psychiatry*, **19**, 297–307.

Ettlinger, G. (1984*a*). Subcortical neglect. *Neurology*, **34**, 261.

Ettlinger, G. (1984*b*). Humans, apes and monkeys: the changing neuropsychological viewpoint. *Neuropsychologia*, **22**, 685–96.

Ettlinger, G. (1990). 'Object vision' and 'spatial vision': the neuropsychological evidence for the distinction. *Cortex*, **26**, 319–41.

Ettlinger, G. and Kalsbeck, J. E. (1962). Changes in tactile discrimination and in visual reaching after successive and simultaneous bilateral posterior parietal ablations in the monkey. *Journal of Neurology, Neurosurgery, and Psychiatry*, **25**, 256–68.

Ettlinger, G., Warrington, E., and Zangwill, O. L. (1957). A further study of visual-spatial agnosia. *Brain*, **80**, 335–61.

Gainotti, G. (1968). Les manifestations de négligence et d'inattention pour l'hémispace. *Cortex*, **4**, 64–91.

Gainotti, G., Messerli, P., and Tissot, R. (1972). Qualitative analysis of unilateral spatial neglect in relation of cerebral lesions. *Journal of Neurology, Neurosurgery and Psychiatry*, **35**, 545–50.

Gainotti, G., D'Erme, P., Monteleone, D., and Silveri, M. C. (1986). Mechanisms of unilateral spatial neglect in relation to laterality of cerebral lesions. *Brain*, **109**, 599–612.

Gelb. A. and Goldstein, K. (1920). *Psychologische Analysen hirnpathologischer Fälle*. J. A. Barth, Leipzig.

Guariglia, C., Padovani, A., Pantano, P., and Pizzamiglio, L. (1993). Unilateral neglect restricted to visual-imagery. *Nature*, **6434**, 235–7.

Halligan, P. W. and Marshall, J. C. (1988). How long is a piece of string? A study of line bisection in a case of visual neglect. *Cortex*, **24**, 321–8.

Halligan, P. W. and Marshall, J. C. (1991). Left neglect for near but nor far space in man. *Nature*, **350**, 498–500.

Halligan, P. W. and Marshall, J. C. (1992). Left visuo-spatial neglect: a meaningless entity? *Cortex*, **28**, 525–35.

Halsband, U., Gruhn, S., and Ettlinger, G. (1985). Unilateral spatial neglect and defective performance in one half of space. *International Journal of Neuroscience*, **28**, 174–95.

Harvey, M. (1995). 'Psychic paralysis of gaze, optic ataxia, spatial disorder of attention'. Translated from Bálint (1909) 'Seelenlähmung des 'Schauens', optische Ataxie, räumliche Störung der Aufmerksamkeit'. *Cognitive Neuropsychology*, **12**, 266–82.

Harvey, M., Milner, A. D., and Roberts, R. C. (1995*a*). An investigation of hemispatial neglect using the landmark task. *Brain and Cognition*, **27**, 59–78.

Harvey, M., Milner, A. D., and Roberts, R. C. (1995*b*). Differential effects of line length on bisection judgements in hemispatial neglect. *Cortex*, **31**, 711–22.

Healton, E. B., Navarro, C., Bressman, S., and Brust, J. C. M. (1982). Subcortical neglect. *Neurology*, **32**, 776–8.

Hécaen, H. (1962). Clinical symptomatology in right and left hemisphere lesions. In *Interhemispheric relations and cerebral dominance*, (ed. V. B. Mountcastle), pp. 215–43. The John Hopkins Press, Baltimore.

Heilman, K. M. (1983). Localization of lesions in neglect. In *Localization in Neuropsychology*, (ed. A. Kertesz), pp. 471–9. Academic Press, New York.

Heilman, K. M. and Valenstein, E. (1979). Mechanisms underlying hemispatial neglect. *Annals of Neurology*, **5**, 166–70.

Heilman, K. M., Pandya, D. N., and Geschwind, N. (1970). Trimodal inattention following parietal lobe ablations. *Transactions of the American Neurological Association*, **95**, 259–61.

Heilman, K. M., Valenstein, E., and Watson, R. T. (1985*a*). The neglect syndrome. In *Handbook of clinical neurology I (45): Clinical neuropsychology*, (ed. J. A. M. Frederiks), pp. 153–83. Elsevier, Amsterdam.

Heilman, K. M., Bowers, D., Coslett, H. D., Whelan, H., and Watson, R. T. (1985*b*). Directional hypokinesia: Prolonged reaction time for leftward movements in patients with right hemisphere lesions and neglect. *Neurology*, **35**, 855–9.

Heilman, K. M., Bowers, D., Valenstein, E., and Watson, R. T. (1987). Hemispace and hemispatial neglect. In *Neurophysiological and neuropsychological aspects of spatial neglect*, (ed. M. Jeannerod), pp. 115–50. Elsevier, Amsterdam.

Henderson, V. W., Alexander, M. P., and Naeser, M. (1982). Right thalamic injury, impaired visuospatial perception and alexia. *Neurology*, **32**, 235–40.

Holmes, G. (1918). Disturbances of visual orientation. *British Journal of Ophthalmology*, **2**, 449–68.

Hornak, J. (1992). Ocular exploration in the dark by patients with visual neglect. *Neuropsychologia*, **30**, 547–52.

Ishiai, S., Furukawa T., and Tsukagoshi, H. (1989). Visuospatial processes of line bisection and the mechanisms underlying unilateral spatial neglect. *Brain*, **112**, 1485–502.

Jones, E. G. and Powell, T. P. S. (1970). An anatomical study of converging sensory pathways within the cerebral cortex of the monkey. *Brain*, **93**, 793–820.

Karnath, H. O. and Fetter, M. (1995). Ocular space exploration in the dark and its relation to subjective and objective body orientation in neglect patients with parietal lesions. *Neuropsychologia*, **33**, 371–7.

Kinsbourne, M. (1977). Hemi-neglect and hemisphere rivalry. In *Advances in neurology*, (ed. E. A. Weinstein and R. P. Friedland), pp. 41–7. Raven Press, New York.

Kinsbourne, M. (1987). Mechanisms of unilateral neglect. In *Neurophysiological and neuropsychological aspects of spatial neglect*, (ed. M. Jeannerod), pp. 69–89, Elsevier, Amsterdam.

Liu, G. T., Bolton, A. K., Price, B. H., and Weintraub, S. (1992). Dissociated perceptual-sensory and exploratory-motor neglect. *Journal of Neurology, Neurosurgery, and Psychiatry*, **55**, 701–6.

McFie, J. and Zangwill, O. L. (1960). Visual-constructive disabilities associated with lesions of the left cerebral hemisphere. *Brain*, **83**, 243–60.

McFie, J., Piercy, M., and Zangwill, O. L. (1950). Visual-spatial agnosia associated with lesions of the right cerebral hemisphere. *Brain*, **73**, 167–90.

Marshall, J. C., Halligan, P. W., and Robertson, I. H. (1993). Contemporary theories of unilateral neglect: a critical review. In *Unilateral neglect: Clinical and experimental studies*, (ed. I. H. Robertson and J. C. Marshall), pp. 311–29. Lawrence Erlbaum Associates, Hove.

Milner, A. D. (1997). Neglect, extinction and the cortical streams of visual processing. In *Parietal lobe contributions to orientation in 3D space*, (ed. P. Thier and H. O. Karnath), pp. 3–22. Springer–Verlag, Heidelberg.

Milner, A. D. and Goodale, M. A. (1995). *The visual brain in action*. Oxford University Press, Oxford.

Milner, A. D. and Harvey, M. (1994). Toward a taxonomy of spatial neglect. *Neuropsychological Rehabilitation*, **4**, 177–81.

Milner, A. D. and Harvey, M. (1995). Distortion of size perception in visuospatial neglect. Current Biology, **4**, 85–9.

Milner, A. D., Brechmann, M., and Pagliarini, L. (1992). To halve or to halve not: an analysis of line bisection judgements in normal subjects. *Neuropsychologia*, **30**, 515–26.

Milner, A. D., Harvey, M., Roberts, R. C., and Forster, S. V. (1993). Line bisection errors in visual neglect: misguided action or size distortion? *Neuropsychologia*, **31**, 39–49.

Oppenheimer, H. (1885). Über eine, durch eine klinisch bisher nicht verwertete Untersuchungsmethode, ermittelte Form der Sensibilitätsstörung bei einseitigen Erkrankungen des Großhirns. *Neurologisches Zentralblatt*, **4**, 529–33.

Oxbury, J. M., Campbell, D. C., and Oxbury, S. M. (1974). Unilateral spatial neglect and impairments of spatial analysis and visual perception. *Brain*, **97**, 551–64.

Paterson, A. and Zangwill, O. L. (1944). Disorders of visual space perception associated with lesions of the right cerebral hemiphere. *Brain*, **67**, 331–58.

Paterson, A. and Zangwill, O. L. (1945). A case of topographical disorientation associated with a unilateral cerebral lesion. *Brain*, **68,** 188–212.

Perenin, M.-T. and Vighetto, A. (1988). Optic ataxia: a specific disruption in visuomotor mechanisms. I. Different aspects of the deficit in reaching for objects. *Brain*, **111**, 643–74.

Pierrot-Deseilligny, C., Rivaud, S., Penet, C., and Rigolet, M.-H. (1987). Latencies of visually guided saccades in unilateral hemispheric cerebral lesions. *Annals of Neurology*, **21**, 138–48.

Pierrot-Deseilligny, C., Rivaud, S., Gaymard, B., and Agid, Y. (1991). Cortical control of reflexive visually guided saccades. *Brain*, **114**, 1473–85.

Posner, M. I. (1980). Orienting of attention. *Quarterly Journal of Experimental Psychology*, **32**, 3–25.

Posner, M. I., Snyder, C. R. R., and Davidson, B. J. (1980). Attention and the detection of signals. *Journal of Experimental Psychology: General*, **109**, 160–74.

Posner, M. I., Cohen, Y., and Rafal, R. D. (1982). Neural systems control of spatial orienting. *Philosophical Transactions of the Royal Society of London, B*, **298**, 187–98.

Posner, M. I., Walker, J. A., Friedrich, F. J., and Rafal, R. D. (1984). Effects of parietal injury on covert orienting of attention. *Journal of Neuroscience*, **4,** 1863–74.

Posner, M. I., Walker, J. A., Friedrich, F. J., and Rafal, R. D. (1987). How do the parietal lobes direct covert attention? *Neuropsychologia*, **25**, 135–45.

Riddoch, G. (1935). Visual disorientation in homonymous half-fields. *Brain*, **58**, 376–82.

Rizzolatti, G., Riggio, L., and Sheliga, B. M. (1994). Space and selective attention. In *Attention and Performance XV. Conscious and nonconscious information processing*, (ed. C. Umilta and M. Moscovitch), pp. 231–65. MIT Press, Cambridge, MA.

Schneller, H. and Seidemann, H. (1932). Zur Frage der optisch-räumlichen Agnosie. *Monatsschrift für Psychiatrie*, **81**, 97.

Stein, S. and Volpe, B. T. (1983). Classical 'parietal' neglect syndrome after subcortical right frontal lobe infarction. *Neurology*, **33**, 797–9.

Tegnér, R. and Levander, M. (1991). Through a looking glass. A new technique to demonstrate directional hypokinesia in unilateral neglect. *Brain*, **114**, 1943–61.

Vallar, G. and Perani, D. (1986). The anatomy of unilateral neglect after right-hemisphere stroke lesions. A clinical/CT-scan correlation study in man. *Neuropsychologia*, **24**, 609–22.

Vallar, G., Rusconi, M. L., Bignamini, L., Geminiani, G., and Perani, D. (1994). Anatomical correlates of visual and tactile extinction in humans: a clinical CT scan study. *Journal of Neurology, Neurosurgery and Psychiatry*, **57**, 464–70.

Van der Linden, M., Seron, X., Gillet, J., and Bredart, S. (1980). Héminégligence par lésion frontale droite. A propos de trois observations. *Acta Neurologica Belgica*, **80**, 298–310.

Walker, R. (1995). Spatial and object-based neglect. *Neurocase*, **1**, 371–83.

Walker, R. and Young, A. W. (1996). Object-based neglect: an investigation of the contributions of eye movements and perceptual completion. *Cortex*, **32**, 279–95.

Walker, R., Findlay, J. M., Young, A. W., and Lincoln, N. B. (1996). Saccadic eye movements in object-based neglect. *Cognitive Neuropsychology*, **13**, 569–615.

Warrington, E. K. and Taylor, A. M. (1973). The contribution of the right parietal lobe to object recognition. *Cortex,* **9**, 152–64.

Young, A. W., De Haan, E. H. F., Newcombe, F., and Hay, D. C. (1990). Facial neglect. *Brain*, **28**, 391–415.

13

Cognition in great apes

RICHARD W. BYRNE

13.1 Preliminary: what are great apes?

Apes differ from other primates most obviously in a package of anatomical adaptations associated with locomotion (Aiello and Dean 1990). Whereas monkeys are quadrupeds with a horizontal body carriage, apes are brachiators, adapted to move from branch to branch suspended from the hands. In the small-bodied gibbons, or 'lesser apes', brachiation is refined into an elegant and rapid means of swinging propulsion, but in the well-named great apes, arm-swinging is measured and slower. In great apes, therefore, long-distance travel is done on the ground for preference, where the apes' long arms put most weight on their short back legs; the fists, or the knuckles in African species (but not the flat of the hands as in monkeys), play only a minor support role. Knuckle- or fist-walking is energetically inefficient, but the anatomy of the hand and shoulder that enables apes to feed suspended from branch tips prevents normal quadrupedalism.

In the Miocene there were many species of ape, but few are known today (Pilbeam 1984); now the great apes comprise only two species of chimpanzee, one or perhaps two species of gorilla (Ruvolo 1994), and the orang-utan. In addition, modern cladistic taxonomy using biomolecular similarity has firmly placed the human as a species of great ape, rather than in a sister taxon (Sarich and Wilson 1967; Bailey *et al.* 1992; Horai *et al.* 1992). The old terms, 'pongid' and 'hominid', have acquired quite different modern meanings as realization has grown that humans are more closely related to chimpanzees and gorillas than either of them are to Asian apes. The ancestors of all African great apes, including the human, separated from the orang-utan line at about 14–16 million years ago (Ma). Almost all evidence suggests that the gorilla line diverged next, at around 7–8 Ma, later splitting into very distinct eastern and western forms. The human and chimpanzee lineages finally separated only at about 5–6 Ma. Much more recently, a chimpanzee population south of the Congo river became so distinct that they are now classed as a separate species: the pygmy chimpanzee. In contrast, the orang-utan populations of Borneo and Sumatra, though just as distinct in biomolecular terms, remain very similar in behaviour and morphology. (The term pongid is retained for the orang-utan line, while hominid is now reserved for the past 5–6 Ma of separate human evolution—characterized by bipedality. No common term for the 'African great apes' clade has yet been agreed.)

13.2 Evolution revealed by the comparative method

The interest to psychologists in understanding the cognition of non-human primates lies in the potential for reconstructing the evolution of information-processing skills. Complex features, shared by a related group of living species, are most likely to have originated by common descent from a single ancestor population (Ridley 1986). By discovering the distribution of cognitive abilities of living monkeys and apes, we can trace back to the cognitive characteristics of remote human ancestors (Byrne 1995). The utility of this 'comparative method', always obvious to some psychologists, has been brought to the fore by our modern realization that humans are 'just another African great ape'. (On the other hand, the oft-repeated and quite correct assertion that we share 99 per cent of our DNA with chimpanzees is harder to interpret; we also share a surprisingly large fraction with a tomato plant.) Such a broad-based approach is in contrast to that favoured by some schools of experimental psychology, which compare 'the human' with 'the animal' (laboratory strains of rat, usually white or hooded). This almost guarantees that dramatic human uniqueness is found, and has often led to an assumption that human cognition is wholly unrelated to animal 'mind', if there is any such thing. However, the extreme improbability of a single 'macro-mutation' producing a radical reorganization of any complex adaptation, including cognition, must be realized (Dawkins 1986). Natural selection efficiently accumulates small beneficial changes; this produces great changes over long timescales, but the probability of a genetic mutation for a major change resulting in anything but death is infinitesimal. The likelihood of a single 'gene for language' or a 'gene for mind' arising suddenly is not great.

Using the comparative method implies 'continuity' of intellect between humans and other living primates. However, this is not based on the hope of finding a smooth, graded series of living forms, stretching from the lemur to the (obviously superior) human, like a *scala natura*. The only continuity that certainly exists can be seen in the thought experiment of tracing up a lineage, backward in time from a modern species to a point of divergence, then forward in time down the other branch to another modern species. Between every adjacent pair of generations along this imagined route, any difference in intellect will be small. By contrast, expecting continuity between modern forms is unrealistic. Evolution often proceeds by means of radiation into many novel niches, producing 'bushy' trees, followed by gradual extinction of lineages until the tree of many modern species is a sparse one (Foley 1994). This accentuates discontinuities, and the fewer the surviving close relatives a species has, the more we see it as 'unique'. Quite apart from this loss of information, there is no guarantee that mental prowess will even be monotonically related to evolutionary distance from humans. Large brains are very costly, in developmental and energetic terms; the brain of a human child consumes 50 per cent of basal metabolic rate (BMR) at one stage of development (Hofman 1983*a,b*). There is therefore every reason for brain size to decrease sometimes with evolutionary time: specifically, whenever its adaptive pay-off is reduced. For instance island species, exposed to less competition than their mainland counterparts, generally have smaller relative brain size (Eisenberg 1981). Some primate lineages might therefore have specialized in other capacities which allow them to dispense with advanced cognition.

Another false path to be avoided is an implicit search for living 'models' for human ancestors. True, species exist which are loosely called living fossils, differing little from their own remote ancestors. This is most common where the species is adapted to a highly stable environment, such as the deep ocean, or where it inhabits a surviving fragment of a once-common environment, such as hot mineral water pools around volcanic upwellings. However, these cases are unusual, and would not have been accepted without good evidence of both modern and extinct forms. When we build up such evidence for human ancestors, it *may* be shown that some modern primates are adequate models of human ancestors—or not. The important process is the use of comparative evidence to identify the evolutionary history of traits, avoiding premature identification with living species (Tooby and DeVore 1987). The discarded 'reconstructions' of human ancestors, littering old textbooks and museum displays, mainly testify to the errors that can be introduced by not resisting this very natural human search for analogy.

This chapter will first establish a 'baseline' of animal cognition, against which to compare the cognition of great apes. The proper group to use for this is the Old World monkeys,[1] diverging from the ape line at about 30 Ma. Then, evidence that great apes differ cognitively from monkeys will be reviewed. Unfortunately, as yet the picture of cognitive differences between the various great apes is sketchy; the pattern seen in recent years is for an ability, first detected with the much-studied common chimpanzee, to be later found in other, and perhaps all, ape species. Once the genuine differences among the apes are worked out, it will be possible to trace human cognitive evolution in some detail from 14 Ma to 5 Ma, but at present this would be premature speculation. Finally, a theory will be sketched of how great ape cognition could have arisen from that of primitive primates, providing a platform for the later evolution of the unique human capacities.

13.3 Cognition in monkeys

When compared to other mammal orders, primates are relatively large-brained (Martin 1990). However, there is variation within the order, and in particular

[1] The gibbons, diverging at 18–20 Ma, might seem a better choice, but there are two problems. First, all extant species are closely related—within the same genus—so if the group is highly derived, as their specialization for arboreal agility has led many to suggest, they may be a poor source of evidence about the primitive population from which they and great apes derive. Secondly, the gibbons are simply poorly known, apart from ecological studies.

the strepsirhines[2] (prosimians, with tarsier excluded) do not differ from typical mammals, whereas haplorhines (simian primates and tarsiers) have brains that average twice as large as typical mammals of their size (Passingham 1981).This suggests that even at 40 Ma the haplorhine lineage had begun to specialize in intelligence of some sort, and there is now converging evidence on the nature of the abilities that their larger brains enabled. Most research, laboratory and field, has concentrated on the Old World monkeys and apes[3] (the catarrhine primates), and evidence of rapid learning and social complexity is now well established for a range of species.

Although much laboratory testing of learning has been plagued by confounds with sensory and motor capacities and the difficulty of equating motivation (Warren 1973; Macphail 1982), it is now clear that large-brained primates learn with great rapidity. For instance, Passingham has shown that in learning the rule behind repeated similar visual discrimination tasks, Old World monkeys far out-perform a range of other mammals (Passingham 1982). Primates also show great curiosity: the simple experiment of placing novel objects in front of individuals of different species showed that primates directed more responses to the objects than rodents, marsupials, edentates, or insectivores, and their interest waned slower than that of carnivores (Glickman and Sroges 1966). (Note that carnivores are also a relatively large-brained order.) Curiosity and explorative behaviour may well be related to diet: haplorhine primates are unusual in needing to put together a balanced diet from plants, while lacking the specialized stomachs of most plant feeders (Chivers *et al.* 1984). Similarly, the dexterity of the primate hand is chiefly used in feeding. However, the rapid learning abilities of primates seem to be far in excess of anything needed for learning how to identify and locate foods (Humphrey 1976); indeed the impressive foraging memories of birds like jays, nutcrackers, and some tits are underwritten by relatively tiny brains (Krebs *et al.* 1989).

Primates may be unique in social complexity. Unlike most mammals, monkeys rely on the support of other individuals, far more than on individual power. This is so marked in Old World monkeys that the young effectively 'inherit' the rank of their mothers, thanks to the continual support of the mother in conflicts (Datta 1983). Support is not simply based on kinship: alliances can be built up using social grooming (Dunbar 1991). Even a single bout of grooming with a non-relative raises the attentiveness of the recipient to the groomer's calls of distress hours later (Seyfarth and Cheney 1984). However, strong and lasting relationships are based on many hours of mutual grooming (Dunbar 1988). For this reason, Old World monkeys groom far

[2] The strepsirhine primates retain a typical mammalian reliance on olfaction, aided by a wet rhinarium, whereas the haplorhine primates depend more on their excellent vision, which is typically binocular and trichromatic.

[3] The relative paucity of evidence on New World monkeys is not problematic for establishing our 'baseline' for ape cognition, since the New World line diverged earlier, but it limits deductions about the original utility of large brains.

more than is necessary for hygiene. Also, when allies come into conflict, they may deliberately ‘reconcile’ with approach and grooming soon afterwards, and pairs that reconcile are more likely to support each other in the future (de Waal and van Roosmalen 1979). The intervention of ‘third parties’ in conflicts over rewards or rank is not unknown in non-primates (e.g. dolphins, hyenas, zebras: Harcourt and de Waal 1992), but social support in catarrhines seems to be unique in that allies are chosen for the qualities of rank and power they can bring to the alliance (Harcourt 1992).

There is other evidence that monkeys are sensitive to characteristics of individuals. In conflicts, monkeys often ‘redirect’ aggression on to subordinates, and their choice of victim—kin of their persecutor—shows they are aware of the relationship (Cheney and Seyfarth 1986, 1989). When third parties are involved, this can progress a further step, when kin of one fighting monkey attack the kin of the other, almost like a vendetta. Knowledge of kinship in third parties has also been shown experimentally, by teaching crab-eating macaques a task that can only be solved by choosing the daughter (or sister, in another experiment) of a monkey shown in a cue photograph (Dasser 1988). And observationally, when the reaction of vervet monkey mothers to playback of infant lost calls was noted, it was found that non-mothers looked towards the mother of the infant whose call was broadcast, even before she reacted on some occasions (Cheney and Seyfarth 1980, 1990). Vervets even know the membership of neighbouring troops, which they have never entered: when a call was artificially broadcast from the ‘wrong’ troop’s range, females reacted with surprise, yet vervet females remain in the same troop throughout life (Cheney and Seyfarth 1982).

Living in long-lasting and often cohesive groups with individuals who are necessarily competitors for food and mating brings potential for conflict. The use of deception to manipulate the behaviour of companions is likely to be a consequence of this, and so far has chiefly been described in primates, for which many records of putative deception have been submitted by experienced researchers in response to survey requests (Byrne and Whiten 1990; but see Hauser, 1997). Data collected by unstructured observations must necessarily be treated with caution, and in analysing this corpus Andrew Whiten and I independently rated each record as ‘tactical deception’ only if it met the strict criteria of:

(1) deliberate use;
(2) intent to obtain a goal;
(3) involving social manipulation of another individual;
(4) resulting in the other individual necessarily being deceived.

Nevertheless, we agreed that 117 of the 253 records met the criteria, and these were spread over all taxa of monkeys and apes (Byrne and Whiten 1992). Furthermore, there is now evidence that neocortical enlargement (the main source of variance of overall brain size among non-human primates) is directly correlated with social skill. Correcting for the number of studies of a given taxon, the frequency with which tactical deception has been recorded is well predicted by the relative size of the neocortex in the brain (Byrne 1993*a*, 1996).

13.4 Do great apes differ from monkeys in cognition?

Monkeys therefore emerge, by comparison with most mammals, as socially complex and socially knowledgeable, able to manipulate their companions, intellectually curious, and dextrous with their hands. The social skills of monkeys are directly related to their neocortical enlargement, which seems to be the source of their very superior learning abilities. However, these differences from other mammals are most likely to be *quantitative* ones; comparable social complexity and rapid-learning ability can be expected in other taxa with large brains, such as carnivores and toothed whales.

Great apes, although larger brained than any monkey by virtue of their overall large sizes, show no greater enlargement of the neocortex than monkeys, and relative to body size their brains are also of similar size (Dunbar 1992). On this basis, we might predict they would show—at similar frequencies to some monkeys—support for kin, alliances among non-relatives, signs of knowing the kinship and habits of third parties, grooming targeted at particularly useful allies, reconciliation when conflict perturbs a lasting relationship, and the use of tactical deception to manipulate social companions. These expectations are entirely borne out (Cheney and Seyfarth 1990; Byrne 1995), although the detailed knowledge of social companions shown by vervet monkeys has not yet been demonstrated in apes. Is there, then, any reason to attribute a difference between monkey and great ape cognition?

Although I shall argue for a firm 'yes' to this question, several difficulties in assessment of evidence must be recognized. Where monkeys and apes have been deliberately posed the same problems with the same rewards, it is sometimes striking that monkeys fail and apes succeed. However, the challenge of 'some species can't do X' has often in the past been met by experimentalists who find a way of persuading them to do it, or by observationalists who finally record the rare circumstance in which they do it spontaneously. In any case, absence of evidence is never evidence of absence, and 'excuses' can be made for the failures of monkeys. The more distant relationship that monkeys have to humans gives them an inherent disadvantage in several ways. *Staring* at the face has a different communicative function for a monkey than for an ape or human, often conveying a threatening message, and many tasks depend on information available from faces. Monkeys' *behavioural style* is more impetuous and uncontrolled (especially in the capuchins and macaques popular in laboratory studies), compared with the more mannered and contemplative style of great apes. This may favour monkeys on some problems and apes on others; but human testers are surely more likely to devise problems amenable to their own, ape-like style of approach. And several of the clearest signs suggesting advanced mentality in great apes come from *enculturated* individuals (i.e. home-reared by humans), and can only be contrasted with data from wild or zoo-reared monkeys, because there is still a lack of data from home-reared monkeys (Tomasello *et al.* 1993; Tomasello 1994). It is not clear quite how and why human rearing affects great apes, but it certainly does, in ways that make their behaviour seem more human-like. In fact, sometimes cases where both monkeys and apes perform what is superficially the same action are more robust evidence of a *difference* than cases of outright 'failure' in monkeys: subtle details in the form or flexibility of the behaviour in the two cases can identify convincingly different mental mechanisms and ontogeny.

13.4.1 Dealing with the social world

When young monkeys visibly learn from their mothers, or adult monkeys deceive their companions, it is tempting for people to see the actions as 'intentional', in the special sense of adjusted to the mental states of other individuals: maternal actions intended to promote specific learning, or manipulative tactics used with an intent to create false beliefs. However, this is often not entailed by the evidence. Our analysis of a large corpus of records of tactical deception in primates concluded that most records, including all where the agent was a monkey, could be explained by postulating an individual history of coincidental reinforcements—one that was entirely possible for the species concerned (Byrne and Whiten 1991, 1992). Rapid learning can thus give rise to tactics that *function* by deception in a complex social environment. Moreover, in the only experimentally elicited case of tactical deception in a monkey (a mangabey developed over three trials the tactic of leading a competitor away from food), it was concluded that learning, not insight, was the means (Coussi-Korbel 1994). A functional analysis of 'teaching' similarly found little evidence of intentional pedagogy in monkeys (Caro and Hauser 1992).

However, for great apes, some evidence for intentional deception and teaching exists. Only 85 per cent of the records of tactical deception could be explained (away) as rapid learning: for the remaining 18 cases, only grossly implausible past circumstances might have conditioned the tactics (Byrne and Whiten 1991). For these 18, an intentional origin by anticipatory planning was considered a more parsimonious explanation. Interestingly, whereas tactical deception was spread over all taxa of haplorhine primates, intentional tactical deception was concentrated in great apes, of all four species (Byrne and Whiten 1992). Evidence for intentional teaching is even more fragmentary, and entirely derives from the common chimpanzee. In captivity, a 'language-trained' ape was noted to use demonstration and hand-moulding (techniques by which she had been trained) to teach her infant to sign, and the infant did learn 70 signs without input from humans (Fouts *et al.* 1989). In West Africa, where chimpanzees habitually crack nuts by pounding rounded hammer-stones on flat anvil-stones, mothers have been observed performing the actions unnaturally slowly and repetitively, after they had watched their juveniles fail at the task (Boesch 1991). Although mothers of chimpanzees and gorillas remove potentially dangerous items from infants (Hiraiwa-Hasegawa 1986; Byrne and Byrne 1991), no other cases of active teaching have been recorded. However, hammer-and-anvil use is the slowest of all tool-using traditions to be acquired in development (McGrew 1992), so is presumably at the limit of chimpanzee manual skill and most in need of scaffolding by maternal intervention.

These suggestions of mental-state attribution from observational data have been supported by experimental tests, although none is conclusive (Whiten 1994). Chimpanzees, but not rhesus monkeys, quickly discriminate the proffered pointing cues of humans who have reason to know which cup is baited, from pointing by humans 'presumed ignorant' who were absent during the baiting. Furthermore, they generalize this discrimination to other kinds of 'ignorance', resulting from being behind a screen, or from wearing a paper bag over the head (Povinelli *et al.* 1990, 1991). However, in all cases the discrimination is not *immediate*, so very fast instrumental learning is not excluded (Heyes 1993; Povinelli 1994). Chimpanzees also learn to discriminate between humans who share food with them, and those who do not, giving information about food preferentially to the former. Again, however, the discrimination takes time, and testing with capuchin monkeys gives identical results (Woodruff and Premack 1979; Mitchell and Anderson 1997). More persuasive is the behaviour of a chimpanzee when it is denied a reward by *accident* by one human, who 'falls' and spills the coveted orange drink, as opposed to *maliciously* by another, who pours it away deliberately. The result is clear: the chimpanzee avoids asking the 'mean' trainer in future, but continues to request from the 'clumsy' one (Povinelli 1991).

Other experimental data have been advanced in support of mental-state attribution, but may be explicable in other terms. For instance, both chimpanzees and rhesus monkeys readily learn the Mason two-player task, where one individual can see which cup is baited but only the other can reach a handle which brings the food to both parties. However, when their roles are reversed, monkeys begin learning more or less from scratch; chimpanzees immediately perform at a high level, suggesting that they understand the logic of the task (Povinelli *et al.* 1992*a,b*). Also, despite the common expression 'monkey see, monkey do' apparent demonstrations of imitation of actions by monkeys have all proved amenable to simpler explanation (Visalberghi and Fragaszy 1990). But in great apes, chimpanzees (experimentally) and orang-utans (observationally) have been shown able to copy novel actions by observation alone (Russon and Galdikas 1993, 1995; Custance *et al.* 1994). However, neither understanding another's role in a joint action, nor understanding another's behaviour sufficiently to copy it, seem to me to be compelling evidence of an understanding of mental states. Rather, I prefer to treat these cognitive capacities as part of an ape's ability to deal with the physical world of actions and objects (Byrne 1997).

13.4.2 Dealing with objects and actions

In several ways, comprehension of the physical world and comprehension of behavioural operations on physical objects seems more sophisticated in great apes than in monkeys.

Much of this evidence relates to tool use, which is shown spontaneously by all great apes in captivity and by chimpanzees and orang-utans in the wild, but by few species of monkey even in captivity. One monkey that does use tools readily is the capuchin, *Cebus* spp., and much careful experimentation has been devoted to this species. Given the right captive circumstances, capuchins use and will even make tools to solve each of the types of task for which chimpanzees use tools in the wild (Visalberghi 1987; Westergaard and Fragaszy 1987; Fragaszy and Visalberghi 1989; Westergaard and Suomi 1993). But when the behaviour of these monkeys is examined closely—their reinforcement history, the type of errors made, their abilities to generalize—a number of observations suggest that their success is based on insightless learning (Visalberghi and Trinca 1987; Visalberghi and Limongelli 1994). For instance, capuchins that have learnt to push a peanut out of a horizontal transparent tube with a particular stick will, when that stick is removed, attempt to probe with objects absurdly too thick to go in the hole, or too short to be effective, or not even rigid. They appear to have no outline idea, or *representation*, of what an adequate tool should be. In contrast, young chimpanzees in the wild have ample opportunity to make such silly errors, but they do not (Goodall 1986). That chimpanzees select only more-or-less appropriate objects to use as tools, instead of all the sorts of absurd ones they *could* choose, shows that they have a mental specification of what is needed. And indeed, captive chimpanzees tested in just the same way as the capuchin seldom made its distinctively 'absurd' errors (Visalberghi *et al.* 1995). To oversimplify the comparison somewhat, monkeys show fast learning of tool tasks, but apes show *representational understanding* of tools.

Wild chimpanzees sometimes make appropriate probe tools *before* moving, often over 100 m away and out of sight, to a termite mound where the probes are used (Goodall 1986). Appropriately selected hammer-stones are sometimes carried even further, to the site of nuts needing cracking (Boesch and Boesch 1984). These observations show that mental representations of objects, specified for the purpose, can be activated *in advance* of the stimulus configuration of the task. It is not clear whether the representations can also be activated when the individual has no intention of tackling the task, as is the case for mental representations in humans; but nor is it obvious how we could know.

The difference between monkey and ape tool use is even greater than these issues of representation suggest. True, laboratory capuchins and wild chimpanzees both probe for food, hammer things open, and so forth. However, the capuchin is typically presented with a highly simplified world: an obvious hole, food visible within it, and a choice of only a few moveable items, one of which is usually an adequate probe. The wild chimpanzee is 'presented' with a termite mound, initially without holes in it, in the African bush (McGrew 1977, 1992). (To be precise, there may be a few dozen, rather inconspicuous, termite nests in the home range of 40–50 km^2 of forest and bush. A random day's walk would miss all of them.) The range of objects with which a mound might be probed (or prodded, or struck) is huge; yet very few of these natural objects are tried. Even the hole has to be *made*, and this can only be done in certain parts of the mound in which termites are readying to emerge, at a certain time of year (the emergence tubes are then capped with softer mud). The edible termites are not visible at all. Probing must be done delicately: hasty poking destroys the tool; hasty pulling out dislodges any attached termites. There is, in short, a lot more to learn: termite fishing is an *elaborated* skill. Nor is termite fishing the only elaborated skill that wild chimpanzees show; ant-dipping for safari ants involves deft bimanual co-ordination and precise timing in addition to making a different type of tool, and nut-cracking involves using two tools in conjunction, as hammer and anvil, which may have to be brought together to the nut source.

Other ape populations do not use tools in food gathering and preparation, but nevertheless demonstrate comparably advanced cognition. Mountain gorillas, for instance, in order to deal with the *physical* defences of plants —stings, spines, hard cases, clinging hooks—in the preparation of their leaf and stem foods, develop complex programs of skilled manual action (Byrne and Byrne 1991, 1993). As with chimpanzee tool use, deft use of precision grips, delicate co-ordination of the two hands in different roles, and strong laterality within individuals are found. The programs comprise several discrete *stages*, as is shown by gorillas' ability to iterate subroutines to build up a larger handful of part-processed material, and by their ability to insert optional processes at some points—usually cleaning the part-processed handful. Iteration and optional stages enable us to see some of the structural organization in the behaviour, which is *hierarchical* (Byrne and Russon 1997). At physiological levels, no doubt most behaviour is hierarchical in structure; but these are *learned* programs. The ability to build up hierarchically structured routines, using one program as an embedded subroutine in another, is commonplace in human problem solving, but I know of no evidence that any monkey or non-primate shows this ability (current work on orang-utans suggests similarly elaborate routines: Russon submitted).

The complex feeding techniques of mountain gorillas are acquired quickly by infants. Significantly, although there is great idiosyncratic variation in all the details of grip type and laterality, each gorilla acquires a similar overall organization. Since there are many other possible ways of processing the plants, this standardization suggests that the outline of the procedure is imitated. Although the developmental trajectory is not yet known, it appears that gorillas have the ability to imitate the overall form of actions but acquire the details individually. This skill, which I have called 'program-level imitation' (Byrne 1993*b*, 1994), plausibly underlies the various reports of imitation of complex novel actions in orang-utans and chimpanzees noted above.

Thus, in various great apes, there is some evidence for mental representation of objects and structures (remembering *that*, not just remembering *how*), anticipatory use of representations to guide future behaviour, the ability to build up novel hierarchical organizations of behaviour, and the copying of the overall organization of another's behaviour. My suspicion is that all four capabilities are general in the great apes, and related to each other (Byrne 1995). Together, they provide apes with a quite different approach to the physical world: an approach that in humans we would call *problem–solving*: the ability to abstract the relevant structure from fluid action and from constellations of objects, thereby to duplicate observed structures of behaviour or select appropriately matching objects, and perhaps in a simple way to reason (compute) with mental representations. If this account is correct, then it would be appropriate to speak of apes *thinking*; this would point to an earlier origin for human non-verbal thought than for the verbal thought, unique to humans, that dominates our conscious reflection.

13.5 The evolutionary origin of ape cognition

A case has been made for the presence in all extant great apes of a representational understanding of the physical world, of hierarchically organized actions, and of the cause-and-effect relations among objects, along with some (perhaps rudimentary) ability to represent the mental worlds of other individuals. How might such a special adaptation as mental representation have evolved? Social and ecological pressures are often seen as *alternative* selective pressures that might have resulted in enhanced intelligence in primates, but what I would like to suggest here is that perhaps both are needed in a full story of how pre-human intelligence evolved.

As haplorhine primates, the ancestral apes of 14–16 Ma in which representational understanding first evolved were already relatively larger-brained than most competing mammals. The origins of this specialization of brain tissue—and, in particular, of neocortex—are strongly indicated by recent studies of brain allometry. In Old World monkeys, the relative enlargement of the neocortex is closely correlated with the typical size of the social group, a rough-and-ready index of the social complexity the species can deal with (Dunbar 1992, 1995). But a similar index of environmental complexity (the residual of range size for a species, after the major effect of body size is removed) has no relation to neocortical or brain enlargement. This favours the 'Machiavellian intelligence' hypothesis (Byrne and Whiten 1988), which attributes the intelligence of monkeys and apes to the selection pressure posed by living in long-lasting social groups, the problem of dealing with competition from conspecific companions. Rather than aggression, which acts to disrupt groups, more subtle tactics of manipulation such as deception and co-operation would be favoured, requiring intelligence. Since the competitors are also part of the breeding population, each increase in intelligence contributes to an arms-race of escalating social complexity, limited only by the high cost of brain tissue. In the pioneering early statements of this hypothesis, the exact nature of the resulting 'social intelligence' was unspecified (Jolly 1966), or implied to involve mental state attribution (Humphrey 1976). Modern evidence, however, suggests an interpretation merely in terms of greatly enhanced learning abilities, underwritten by an enlarged neocortex (Byrne 1995; Byrne and Whiten 1997).

Yet this hypothesis goes nowhere in explaining the apparent difference between monkeys and apes in the nature of their intelligence, since apes and monkeys do not differ systematically in typical group size, nor in neocortical enlargement. Instead, representational understanding may have an origin in the complex feeding niche of apes (Byrne 1997). In the great ape common ancestor, the challenge to feed efficiently was much greater than for any monkey, because of the larger body size of apes, and their inefficient locomotion by brachiation. When competition from monkeys later emerged, this would be exacerbated by their more specialized digestions, allowing unripe fruit and a wider range of plants to be consumed. All apes are excellent at remembering where and when sources of sporadically available food are to be found, but so are monkeys: having a good 'cognitive map' does not distinguish monkeys from apes. In contrast, all great apes today show food processing techniques that are technically demanding in some way, whereas monkeys do not. I propose, therefore, that this is where the cognitive 'edge' came in, increasing feeding efficiency in those great apes that evolved a representational understanding of objects and actions. (Those that did not, left no descendants, for the same reasons.) This enabled the development of complex and elaborated feeding techniques, and (where it was functional) representational use of tools. Secondarily, and incompletely, this ability generalized to social problems, allowing some representation of the unobservable mental states of other individuals.

Unlike some alternatives, this hypothesis does *not* require postulation of tool-using in the common ancestor of modern great apes, and the implausible subsequent loss of the behaviour in most of its descendants (Parker and Gibson 1979). Nor does it rely on a particular task, such as extractive foraging or cognitive mapping (Milton 1988), presenting a special challenge to apes—but strangely not to other species of mammal that show such skills. And it is capable of accounting for an ape/monkey difference in cognition, whereas the Machiavellian intelligence hypothesis cannot.

In the subsequent 5–6 Ma of (specifically) hominid evolution to the present, there is scope for many further cognitive adaptations. Which actually occurred is currently a matter of controversy. On the one hand, some evolutionary psychologists argue for intricate, domain-specific cognitive structures (Barkow *et al.* 1992), adapted to particular problem circumstances with survival value in a Pleistocene hunter–gatherer culture: mate selection, exchange, detection of non-reciprocations, and so forth. On the other, studies of 'ape language' in individuals treated like human children have now shown receptive understanding of such syntactical niceties as assignment of reference by relative clauses (Savage-Rumbaugh *et al.* 1993), raising the serious possibility that even aspects of language can be instantiated in 'general purpose' brain tissue. Now that these big questions are finally being asked within psychology, we can expect great progress on this most shadowy of topics.

References

Aiello, L. and Dean, C. (1990). *An introduction to human evolutionary anatomy*. Academic Press, London.

Bailey, W. J., Hayasaka, K., Skinner, C. G., Kehoe, S., Sieu, L. C., Slightom, J. L., and Goodman, M. (1992). Re-examination of the African hominoid trichotomy with additional sequences from the primate ß-globin gene cluster. *Molecular Phylogenetics and Evolution*, **1**, 97–135.

Barkow, J. H., Cosmides, L., and Tooby, J. (ed.) (1992). *The adapted mind: evolutionary psychology and the generation of culture*. Oxford University Press, Oxford.

Boesch, C. (1991). Teaching among wild chimpanzees. Animal Behaviour, **41**, 530–2.

Boesch, C. and Boesch, H. (1984). Mental map in wild chimpanzees: an analysis of hammer transports for nut cracking. *Primates*, **25**, 160–70.

Byrne, R. W. (1993*a*). Do larger brains mean greater intelligence? *Behavioural and Brain Sciences*, **16**, 696–7.

Byrne, R. W. (1993*b*). Hierarchical levels of imitation. Commentary on M. Tomasello, A. C. Kruger and H. H. Ratner 'Cultural learning'. *Behavioural and Brain Sciences*, **16**, 516–17.

Byrne, R. W. (1994). The evolution of intelligence. In *Behaviour and evolution*, (ed. P. J. B. Slater and T. R. Halliday), pp. 223–65. Cambridge University Press, Cambridge.

Byrne, R. W. (1995). *The thinking ape: evolutionary origins of intelligence*. Oxford University Press, Oxford.

Byrne, R. W. (1996). Relating brain size to intelligence in primates. In *Modelling the early human mind*, (ed. P. A. Mellars and K. R. Gibson), pp. 49–56. Macdonald Institute for Archaeological Research, Cambridge.

Byrne, R. W. (1997). The technical intelligence hypothesis. An additional evolutionary stimulus to intelligence. In *Machiavellian intelligence II: extensions and evaluations*, (ed. A. Whiten and R. W. Byrne), pp. 289–311. Cambridge University Press, Cambridge.

Byrne, R. W. and Byrne, J. M. E. (1991). Hand preferences in the skilled gathering tasks of mountain gorillas (*Gorilla g. beringei*). *Cortex*, **27**, 521–46.

Byrne, R. W. and Byrne, J. M. E. (1993). Complex leaf-gathering skills of mountain gorillas (*Gorilla g. beringei*): Variability and standardization. *American Journal of Primatology*, **31**, 241–61.

Byrne, R. W. and Russon, A. (1998). Learning by imitation: a hierarchical approach. *Behavioral and Brain Sciences*, in press.

Byrne, R. W. and Whiten, A. (1988). *Machiavellian intelligence: social expertise and the evolution of intellect in monkeys, apes and humans*. Clarendon Press, Oxford.

Byrne, R. W. and Whiten, A. (1990). Tactical deception in primates: the 1990 data-base. *Primate Report*, **27**, 1–101.

Byrne, R. W. and Whiten, A. (1991). Computation and mindreading in primate tactical deception. In *Natural theories of mind*, (ed. A. Whiten), pp. 127–41. Basil Blackwell, Oxford.

Byrne, R. W. and Whiten, A. (1992). Cognitive evolution in primates: evidence from tactical deception. *Man*, **27**, 609–27.

Byrne, R. W. and Whiten, A. (1997). Machiavellian intelligence. In *Machiavellian intelligence II: extensions and evaluations*, (ed. A. Whiten and R. W. Byrne), pp. 1–23. Cambridge University Press, Cambridge.

Caro, T. M. and Hauser, M. D. (1992). Is there teaching in non–human animals? *Quarterly Review of Biology*, **67**, 151–74.

Cheney, D. L. and Seyfarth, R. M. (1980). Vocal recognition in free-ranging vervet monkeys. *Animal Behaviour*, **28**, 362–76.

Cheney, D. L. and Seyfarth, R. M. (1982). Recognition of individuals within and between groups of free-ranging vervet monkeys. *American Zoologist*, **22**, 519–29.

Cheney, D. L. and Seyfarth, R. M. (1986). The recognition of social alliances among vervet monkeys. *Animal Behaviour*, **34**, 1722–31.

Cheney, D. L. and Seyfarth, R. M. (1989). Reconciliation and redirected aggression in vervet monkeys. *Behaviour*, **110**, 258–75.

Cheney, D. L. and Seyfarth, R. M. (1990). *How monkeys see the world: inside the mind of another species*. University of Chicago Press, Chicago.

Chivers, D. J., Wood, B. A., and Bilsborough, A. (1984). *Food acquisition and processing in primates*. Plenum Press, New York.

Coussi–Korbel, S. (1994). Learning to outwit a competitor in mangabeys (*Cercocebus t. torquatus*). *Journal of Comparative Psychology*, **108**, 164–71.

Custance, D. M., Whiten, A., and Bard, K. A. (1994). The development of gestural imitation and self-recognition in chimpanzees (*Pan troglodytes*) and children. In *Current primatology*: Vol. 2: *Social development, learning and behaviour*, (ed. J. J. Roeder, B. Thierry, J. R. Anderson, and N. Herrenschmidt), pp. 381–7. Université Louis Pasteur, Strasbourg.

Dasser, V. (1988). Mapping social concepts in monkeys. In *Machiavellian intelligence: social expertise and the evolution of intellect in monkeys, apes and humans*, (ed. R. W. Byrne and A. Whiten), pp. 85–93. Clarendon Press, Oxford.

Datta, S. B. (1983). Relative power and the acquisition of rank. In *Primate social relationships: An integrated approach*, (ed. R. A. Hinde), pp. 93–103. Blackwell, Oxford.

Dawkins, R. (1986). *The blind watchmaker*. Longman, London.

de Waal, F. and van Roosmalen, A. (1979). Reconciliation and consolation among chimpanzees. *Behavioral Ecology and Sociobiology*, **5**, 55–6.

Dunbar, R. I. M. (1988). *Primate social systems*. Croom Helm, London.

Dunbar, R. I. M. (1991). Functional significance of social grooming in primates. *Folia Primatology*, **57**, 121–31.

Dunbar, R. I. M. (1992). Neocortex size as a constraint on group size in primates. *Journal of Human Evolution*, **20**, 469–93.

Dunbar, R. I. M. (1995). Neocortex size and group size in primates: a test of the hypothesis. *Journal of Human Evolution*, **28**, 287–96.

Eisenberg, J. E. (1981). *The mammalian radiations: an analysis of trends in evolution, adaptation, and behavior*. Universtiy of Chicago Press, Chicago.

Foley, R. A. (1994). Speciation, extinction and climatic change in hominid evolution. *Journal of Human Evolution*, **26**, 275–90.

Fouts, R. S., Fouts, D. H., and Van Cantford, T. E. (1989). The infant Loulis learns signs from cross-fostered chimpanzees. In *Teaching sign language to chimpanzees*, (ed.

R. A. Gardner, B. T. Gardner, and T. E. Van Cantford), pp. 280–92. State University of New York Press, New York.

Fragaszy, D. M. and Visalberghi, E. (1989). Social influences on the aquisition and use of tools in tufted capuchin monkeys (*Cebus apella*). *Journal of Comparative Psychology*, **103**, 159–70.

Glickman, S. E. and Sroges, R. W. (1966). Curiosity in zoo animals. *Behaviour*, **26**, 151–8.

Goodall, J. (1986). *The chimpanzees of Gombe: patterns of behavior*. Harvard University Press, Cambridge, MA.

Harcourt, A. (1992). Coalitions and alliances: are primates more complex than non-primates? In *Coalitions and alliances in humans and other animals*, (ed. A. H. Harcourt and F. B. M. de Waal), pp. 445–71. Oxford University Press, Oxford.

Harcourt, A. H. and de Waal, F. B. (ed.) (1992). *Coalitions and alliances in humans and other animals*. Oxford University Press, Oxford.

Hauser, M. D. (1997). Minding the behaviour of deception. In *Machiavellian intelligence II: extensions and evaluations*, (ed. A. Whiten and R. W. Byrne), pp. 112–43. Cambridge University Press, Cambridge.

Heyes, C. M. (1993). Anecdotes, training, trapping and triangulating: do animals attribute mental states? *Animal Behaviour*, **46**, 177–88.

Hiraiwa–Hasegawa, M. (1986). A note on the ontogeny of feeding. In *The chimpanzees of the Mahale Mountains*, (ed. T. Nishida), pp. 277–83. University of Tokyo Press, Tokyo.

Hofman, M. A. (1983*a*). Encephalization in hominids: evidence for the model of punctuationalism. *Brain, Behavior and Evolution*, **22**, 102–17.

Hofman, M. A. (1983*b*). Energy metabolism, brain size and longevity in mammals. *Quarterly Review of Biology*, **58**, 495–512.

Horai, S., Satta, Y., Hayashi, S., and Takahata, N. (1992). Man's place in hominoidea revealed by mitochondrial DNA genealogy. *Journal of Molecular Evolution*, **35**, 32–43.

Humphrey, N. K. (1976). The social function of intellect. In *Growing points in ethology*, (ed. P. P. G. Bateson and R. A. Hinde), pp. 303–17. Cambridge University Press, Cambridge.

Jolly, A. (1966). Lemur social behaviour and primate intelligence. *Science*, **153**, 501–6.

Krebs, J. R., Sherry, D. F., Healy, S. D., Perry, V. H., and Vaccarino, A. L. (1989). Hippocampal specialization in food–storing birds. *Proceedings of the National Academy of Sciences USA*, **86**, 1388–90.

McGrew, W. C. (1977). Socialization and object manipulation by wild chimpanzees. In *Primate biosocial development*, (ed. S. Chevaklier-Slonikoff and F. E. Poirier), pp. 261–88. Garland Press, New York.

McGrew, W. C. (1992). *Chimpanzee material culture: implications for human evolution*. Cambridge University Press, Cambridge.

Macphail, E. (1982). *Brain and intelligence in vertebrates*. Clarendon Press, Oxford.

Martin, R. D. (1990). *Primate origins and evolution*. Chapman Hall, London.

Milton, K. (1988). Foraging behaviour and the evolution of intellect in monkeys, apes and humans. In *Machiavellian intelligence: social expertise and the evolution of intellect in monkeys, apes and humans,* (ed. R. W. Byrne and A. Whiten), pp. 285–305. Clarendon Press, Oxford.

Mitchell, R. W. and Anderson, J. R. (1997). Pointing, withholding information, and deception in capuchin monkeys (*Cebus apella*). *Journal of Comparative Psychology*, in press.

Parker, S. T. and Gibson, K. R. (1979). A developmental model for the evolution of language and intelligence in early hominids. *The Behavioural and Brain Sciences*, **2**, 367–408.

Passingham, R. E. (1981). Primate specializations in brain and intelligence. *Symposia of the Zoological Society of London*, **46**, 361–88.

Passingham, R. E. (1982). *The human primate*. W. H. Freeman, Oxford.

Pilbeam, D. A. (1984). The descent of hominoids and hominids. *American Science*, **250**, 84–96.

Povinelli, D. J. (1991). Social intelligence in monkeys and apes. Unpublished Ph.D. thesis, Yale University.

Povinelli, D. J. (1994). Comparative studies of mental state attribution: a reply to Heyes. *Animal Behaviour*, **48**, 239–41.

Povinelli, D. J., Nelson, K. E., and Boysen, S. T. (1990). Inferences about guessing and knowing by chimpanzees *(Pan troglodytes)*. *Journal of Comparative Psychology*, **104**, 203–10.

Povinelli, D. J., Nelson, K. E., and Boysen, S. T. (1992*a*). Comprehension of role reversal in chimpanzees: evidence of empathy? *Animal Behaviour*, **43**, 633–40.

Povinelli, D. J., Parks, K. A., and Novak, M. A. (1991). Do rhesus monkeys (*Macaca mulatta*) attribute knowledge and ignorance to others? *Journal of Comparative Psychology*, **105**, 318–25.

Povinelli, D. J., Parks, K. A., and Novak, M. A. (1992*b*). Role reversal by rhesus monkeys; but no evidence of empathy. *Animal Behaviour*, **44**, 269–81.

Ridley, M. (1986). *Evolution and classification: the reformation of cladism*. Longman, London.

Russon, A. E. (1997). The nature and evolution of intelligence in orangutans (*Pongo pygmaeus*). *Primates*, submitted.

Russon, A. E. and Galdikas, B. M. F. (1993). Imitation in free-ranging rehabilitant orangutans. *Journal of Comparative Psychology*, **107**, 147–61.

Russon, A. E. and Galdikas, B. M. F. (1995). Constraints on great ape imitation: model and action selectivity in rehabilitant orangutan *(Pongo pymaeus)* imitation. *Journal of Comparative Psychology*, **109**, 5–17.

Ruvolo, M. (1994). Molecular evolutionary processes and conflicting gene trees: The hominoid case. *American Journal of Physical Anthropology*, **94**, 93–113.

Sarich, V. and Wilson, A. (1967). Immunological time scale for hominid evolution. *Science*, **158**, 1200–3.

Savage–Rumbaugh, E. S., Murphy, J., Sevcik, R. A., Brakke, K. E., Williams, S. L., and Rumbaugh, D. M. (1993). Language comprehension in ape and child. *Monographs of the Society for Research in Child Development*, **58**, 1–252.

Seyfarth, R. and Cheney, D. (1984). Grooming alliances and reciprocal altruism in vervet monkeys. *Nature*, **308**, 541–2.

Tomasello, M. (1994). The question of chimpanzee culture. In *Chimpanzee cultures*, (ed. R. W. Wrangham, W. C. McGrew, F. B. M. de Waal, and P. G. Heltne), pp. 301–17. Harvard University Press, Cambridge, MA.

Tomasello, M., Savage–Rumbaugh, E. S., and Kruger, A. C. (1993). Imitative learning of actions on objects by children, chimpanzees, and enculturated chimpanzees. *Child Development*, **64**, 1688–705.

Tooby, J. and DeVore, I. (1987). The reconstruction of hominid behavioral evolution through strategic modeling. In *The evolution of human behavior: primate models*, (ed. W. G. Kinzey), pp. 183–238. State University of New York, Albany.

Visalberghi, E. (1987). Acquisition of nut-cracking behaviour by two capuchin monkeys (*Cebus apella*). *Folia Primatologica*, **49**, 168–81.

Visalberghi, E. and Fragaszy, D. M. (1990). Do monkeys ape? In *'Language' and intelligence in monkeys and apes*, (ed. S. T. Parker and K. R. Gibson), pp. 247–73. Cambridge University Press, Cambridge.

Visalberghi, E. and Limongelli, L. (1994). Lack of comprehension of cause-effect relationships in tool-using capuchin monkeys (*Cebus apella*). *Journal of Comparative Psychology*, **103**, 15–20.

Visalberghi, E. and Trinca, L. (1987). Tool use in capuchin monkeys: distinguishing between performing and understanding. *Primates*, **30**, 511–21.

Visalberghi, E., Fragaszy, D. M., and Savage-Rumbaugh, E. S. (1995). Performance in a tool-using task by common chimpanzees *(Pan troglodytes)*, bonobos *(Pan paniscus)*, an Orangutan *(Pongo pygmaeus)*, and capuchin monkeys *(Cebus apella)*. *Journal of Comparative Psychology*, **109**, 52–60.

Warren, J. M. (1973). Learning in vertebrates. In *Comparative Psychology: a modern survey*, (ed. D. A. Dewsbury and D. A. Rethlingshafer), pp. 471–509. McGraw Hill, New York.

Westergaard, C. G. and Fragaszy, D. (1987). The manufacture and use of tools by capuchin monkeys (*Cebus apella*). *Journal of Comparative Psychology*, **101**, 159–68.

Westergaard, G. C. and Suomi, S. J. (1993). Use of a tool-set by capuchin monkeys (*Cebus apella*). *Primates*, **34**, 459–62.

Whiten, A. (1994). Grades of mindreading. In *Origins of an understanding of mind*, (ed. C. Lewis and P. Mitchell), pp. 47–70. Lawrence Erlbaum, Hove, UK.

Woodruff, G. and Premack, G. (1979). Intentional communication in the chimpanzee: The development of deception. *Cognition*, **7**, 333–62.

14

Mental representation in human and monkey neuropsychology

ROSALIND M. RIDLEY and HARRY F. BAKER

14.1 Introduction

Analysis of mental representation in normal humans has become the cornerstone of cognitive psychology since the decline of Behaviorism. More recently the concept of mental representation has become important in understanding cognitive development in young children (Perner 1993) and in the mental disability of patients with certain developmental disorders (Frith 1989) or neurotrauma (Bisiach and Luzzatti 1978). In the study of localization of neuropsychological function, the correlation of symptoms with neuropathological findings in patients has been supplemented by studies in animals, particularly primates, on a variety of cognitive tests following experimental neurosurgery. It is therefore appropriate to apply the analysis of mental representation to comparative neuropsychology and, in particular, to consider the level of mental representation required by tasks that are used to test cognition in animals, in order to assess their relevance to human mental dysfunction.

14.2 Mental representation

14.2.1 What are mental representations?

External representations are man-made things 'in the real world' which represent or depict other things. Two important features of representations are: (1) they have to have a subject, i.e. they have to be *of* something, and (2) they have to represent that subject *as* something. For example, a photograph *of* a horse might represent it *as* standing up. The photograph represents the horse *by*, but not *as*, coloured patches on paper. Representations in the real world comprise those which 'mimic' and those which 'symbolize' something. Mimicry, or analogue models, include pictures, maps, diagrams, and onomatopoeia, while symbols are related to each other according to rules in order to produce propositional models which form the basis of language, symbolic logic, and mathematics.

Mental representations are things 'in the mind' that represent things 'in the real world'. Mental representations (like external representations) depict the subject *as* having certain characteristics. For example, a visual percept of a biscuit can represent it *as* brown and round. Mental representation occurs during cognitive activities such as 'knowing', 'thinking about', and 'remembering' things which either do, did, will, or could exist in the outside world. Mental representations are the products of mental processes and as such exist in consciousness, whereas the processes which gave rise to them do not (Nisbett and Wilson 1977; Prinz 1992). On being asked to think, for example, of an animal, a mental representation of one animal comes to mind, i.e. it is brought into consciousness, but the mental processes by which it got there remain opaque. The concepts of mental representation and consciousness are intimately related, such that the exercise of considering mental representation in animals raises issues of consciousness in animals and brings into focus the question of whether, in animal models of human ability, the animal mentation is occurring at an appropriate cognitive level to render the model valid.

14.2.2 What mental representations are not

The term 'mental representation' does not refer to 'information in the nervous system' or to 'the neural correlate of mental activity'. Activity in the nervous system is determined by, but does not represent, the outside event. In the same way that the photograph represents a horse *as* standing in a field *by* the pattern of patches on the page, so a percept represents a scene *as* a landscape *by* the pattern of neural activity in the posterior neocortex. The tendency to refer to any neural activity as a 'representation in the brain' should be avoided. This includes the topographical layout of sensory information in cortex, e.g. the 'homunculus' of the sensorimotor cortex, or the retinotopic layout of the visual cortex. Even though the neuroanatomist may detect this layout, the mind does not view the visual cortex in order to achieve perception.

The occurrence of behaviour cannot be taken as evidence of a mental representation. Lower animals perform extraordinary feats of instinctive behaviour, but it would be retrograde to posit the existence of mental representation to explain this behaviour—the wasp does not have a mental representation of the nest it is trying to build. Indeed the whole point of the discussion of mental representation is to escape from anthropomorphism on the one hand, and doctrinaire Behaviorism on the other, and to divide the explanation of human and animal behaviour into that which is dependent on conscious awareness and that which is not. A concept of 'unconscious representation' pervades some literature on such subjects as subliminal perception, blindsight, unilateral neglect, 'guessing without recollection', and the content of semantic stores. But since *mental* representations only exist experientially, i.e. in consciousness, an 'unconscious representation' is a contradiction in terms.

14.2.3 Levels of mental representation

Leslie (1987) argues that there are three levels of mental representation. *Primary* representations are about the world as it now is, i.e. the immediate and continuous present. Thus percepts of the outside world and statements of invariant relationships (facts about the way the world is) are primary representations. Primary representations are tied to the outside world in that they are, or were, generated by outside events. *Secondary* representations are 'decoupled' from the world as it now is, in that they are about things as they could be, as they once were, or as they will be. Secondary representations allow two important cognitive developments, hypothesis and recollection. Hypothesis means the ability to think of (i.e. mentally represent) alternatives to the present, to engage in pretence, and to anticipate the future. Recollection means the ability to reconstruct as memories, events, and scenes from the past (i.e. the common sense meaning of memories) as opposed to the wider definition of learning (i.e. the modification of behaviour as a result of experience). Primary and secondary representations are structurally similar. They differ, not in their content, but in how they relate to the outside world. Primary representations are generated from sensory input, either from the present (as in perception) or from a past perception (as in knowing a fact), whereas secondary representations, by virtue of being decoupled from the outside world, are created in working memory by means of an internally initiated mechanism.

The third level of representation is *meta-representation* and occurs only when it is necessary to represent a representation. But a meta-representation is not just a copy of a representation; the meta-representation must depict the subject *as* being a representation (Pylyshyn 1978). Macaques are able to perceive and remember photographs as stimuli (Gaffan 1992*b*) but their ability to relate the content of the picture to the 'real' equivalent has not been assessed. Chimpanzees can match pictures to real objects and objects to pictures (Hayes and Hayes 1952; Davenport and Rogers 1971) but it is not clear that this is done on the basis of appreciation of the representational relationship (Winner and Ettlinger 1979) rather than simple similarity (e.g. both photograph and object are the same colour). Chimpanzees recognize themselves in the mirror but monkeys behave as if the reflection is another monkey (Gallup 1975). Monkeys may fail, not because they do not have a concept of self (which they may or may not have) but because they are unable to represent the relationship between their real selves and themselves in the mirror. Indeed, it may be their 'sense of self' which prevents them from seeing the reflection as also 'themself'. Similarly, the mental states of oneself and others will usually be handled as a simple fact (primary representation), but a mental meta-representation is required to depict the fact that mental representations have a specific relation to the real world. Meta-representational analysis is necessary to understand that a misrepresentation, i.e. a mismatch between what someone believes and what is the case, has occurred and to modify people's beliefs independently of the real situation, i.e. to deceive. Thus meta-representation is an important aspect of some types of social interaction, but it is by no means necessary for all social interaction. It is important for understanding animal social behaviour to establish the phylogenetic stage at which these higher levels of mental representation appear. It is widely held that apes (especially chimpanzees) form meta-representations, as evidenced by their apparent ability to deceive and be deceived (Dawkins 1993) but the proof that monkeys (and other mammals) operate at this level is lacking (Cheney and Seyfarth 1990).

This description of meta-representation uses the prefix 'meta' in the recursive sense (e.g. meta-analysis is a combined analysis of several other analyses of some other subject). But the prefix 'meta' is also used in the non-recursive sense of modification (e.g. meta-morphosis is about a change of shape, not about the shape of shapes). Mental representations have cognitive 'labels' which have been called 'meta-representational comments' (Perner 1993) but, for the sake of distinction from its use in the recursive sense, we shall refer to this type of representation as epi-representation. The most important type of 'label' for cognition is one that labels a representation as being 'a perception', 'a known fact', 'a memory', and so on. The experiential quality that labels information as 'a memory' rather than 'just a known fact' has been referred to by Tulving (1985) as 'episodic trace information'. Since the loss of episodic memories with their associated trace information is the primary feature of amnesia, we need to consider, when attempting to produce a primate model of amnesia, whether monkeys benefit from epi-representational labelling, i.e. whether their memories have the experiential quality of recollection.

14.3 Mental representation and cognition

14.3.1 Cognitive uses of levels of representation

Perner (1993) has suggested that young infants can only form primary representations, and therefore function only in a 'single-updating' mode, but that by the age of 18 months they begin to form secondary representations and are then able to function in a 'multi-model' mode. For ease of reading we shall refer to these two modes as 'single' and 'multi'. The 'single' mode keeps track of reality through perception and long-term storage of usually invariant relationships. It can accommodate, in parallel, many independent facts about different subjects, but it is unable to entertain different possibilities about the same subject at the same time in the form of rules or propositions. This requires 'multi' processing. Ethologists can, potentially, describe all animal behaviour in terms of rules. The problem for the cognitive psychologist is to determine whether the animal is applying a rule *as* a rule (and therefore using 'multi' processing) or is merely behaving in a way that is predictable by an outsider. The ability of monkeys to perform tasks in which they make the correct response on the first presentation of a new stimulus implies, at first sight, that they are applying a rule. This occurs, for example, in the 'delayed non-matching to sample' (DNMS) task in which the monkey is rewarded for choosing, from a pair of stimuli, the stimulus that was not presented as the 'sample' on the preceding trial. Care is needed, however, in this analysis since even very primitive animals exhibit the capacity for generalization across stimuli (an animal may 'freeze' in response to all loud noises including novel loud noises). Monkeys may learn always to choose the larger of two objects but this may be achieved by feature extraction, i.e. the monkey may respond to 'bigness' as a feature applicable across many objects. Similarly 'novel' and 'familiar' are properties of objects to which the monkey may make the same response across many trials even though the objects are drawn from a large selection. More interesting is how the monkey comes to make this predictable choice: is it by a slow, incremental improvement, implying a 'single' system homing in on 'bigness' or 'familiarity'; or is it by a rapid switch to correct responding, implying the successful application of a rule?

14.3.2 The explicit versus implicit distinction

In clinical neuropsychology, the terms explicit and implicit are often used to describe different aspects of memory (Schacter 1987), but they actually refer to the way in which *any* information is *experienced* when it influences behaviour. Thus information experienced in the explicit domain appears in consciousness (it can be 'declared'; Squire 1992), whereas implicit information is not experienced independently of the behaviour that it modifies (it can only be 'demonstrated'). The implicit domain is therefore outside the realm of representation. In memory, the explicit domain refers to the conscious product of retrieval mechanisms but does not refer to a type of memory store. Episodic memories are constructed from an unconscious store, and the reconstructed representation changes with each repetition (Bartlett 1932). The semantic store is also unconscious and, by virtue of a dense network of interconnections between facts, contains information that may never have been directly acquired or expressed (i.e. represented) before, e.g. Aristotle had a liver. This creative, flexible relationship between what is recollected in consciousness and the data from which it is drawn indicates that these stores do not contain multiple 'representations' of potentially thinkable thoughts but rather contain information in some other form which is, none the less, capable of being expressed representationally. Squire (1992) has described some types of non-declarative memory as 'procedural'. These include habituation, classical conditioning, perceptual learning, motor skill learning, and possibly learnt emotional responses, and refer to changes in the probability of neural activation in specific neural pathways.

Much cognitive theory about normal humans appeals for its justification to experiential phenomenology (do you remember this from experience or just know it as a fact?). Attempting to study cognition in monkeys obliges the researcher to look outside this framework. Such an approach may also be of value in clinical neuropsychology where the experience of the patient is outside that of the clinician and is often paradoxical. Tulving (1989) refers to the 'doctrine of concordance' between experience, knowledge, and behaviour, i.e. that we experience what we know and know what we experience, and that our behaviour (especially in answering introspective questions) reflects that experience and knowledge. This may appear to be true in normal function but it is not clear that the same relationship will hold for people with brain damage, or for other species. In particular, the notion that awareness must be accompanied by self-awareness (Hirst 1995) would appear not necessarily to apply following certain neurotraumas, and need not apply to animals.

14.3.3 Mental representation in monkeys

Primates have been used for CNS studies in three main areas: visual perception, memory, and psychosis. According to people who doubt that animals have consciousness, even the study of perception in monkeys is not possible. But most psychologists credit mammals with the primary representations necessary for perception. Memory and psychosis present more subtle problems for representational analysis and are considered below.

Learning and memory is assessed in monkeys using the manual or automated Wisconsin General Test Apparatus (WGTA). The monkey is presented with a series of discrete trials on which it must choose one of, usually, two stimuli (objects or screen-displayed patterns) in order to obtain a reward. Most tasks given to monkeys can be classified into one of three types: trial-independent, trial-unique, and trial-dependent tasks (Ridley and Baker 1991). Trial-independent tasks are about invariant relationships and can therefore be acquired with only 'single' processing, while trial-unique and trial-dependent tasks require the knowledge of a rule and therefore require 'multi' processing.

In trial-independent tasks the monkey is presented with trials on which the relationship between stimulus and reward is the same on every trial (e.g. always choose A not B). Mishkin *et al.* (1984) have argued that the performance of simple trial-independent visual discriminations, even where many such pairs are presented in a random order across trials (concurrent learning), requires acquisition of a procedural skill or 'habit' and therefore occurs in the implicit domain. The definition of a skill, however, is that it is demonstrable only by the *quality* of an action (Squire 1986), whereas the monkey's state of knowledge in this task is measured by its ability to make correct *choices*, not by the facility (e.g. speed) with which it makes the response. Choosing the 'correct' stimulus may require different movements on different trials, and learning a new task with new stimuli requires the same basic movements to be made as for the old task. Motor skill is not crucial since clumsy or slow responses are just as acceptable as well-executed movements. It is unlikely that acquisition of a perceptual skill is required to perform these tasks, since—except where similar pattern stimuli are used—the ability of monkeys to perform trial-unique tasks indicates that they are capable of distinguishing immediately between most object stimuli. As Harlow (1949) pointed out 'by the time the monkey has run 344 discriminations, he does not possess 344 habits, bonds, connections or associations'. Learning this type of task does not seem to require episodic memory in the sense of remembering the events of the previous trial, since varying the intertrial intervals from a few seconds to 24 hours has little effect on learning rate (Malamut *et al.* 1984). Learning this type of task across many trials is best described as the acquisition of semantic knowledge about the meaning (reward association or value) of different stimuli rather than as habit formation. *Using* semantic knowledge (as opposed to the dormant long-term storage of semantic knowledge) is usually regarded as being in the explicit domain. We are arguing, therefore, that the behaviour of monkeys in the WGTA constitutes deliberate choices of objects based on acquired knowledge about the relationship between objects, rewards, and sometimes responses, and is in the explicit domain.

When a monkey has learnt a trial-independent visual discrimination and is then presented with the reversal of that task (the previously unrewarded stimulus is now rewarded and *vice versa*), it typically finds this reversal difficult but, with many subsequent serial reversals, each reversal becomes easier (see, for example, Ridley *et al.* 1989). This suggests that the first reversal is handled (poorly) with a 'single' processor but that, with practice, serial reversals are performed with a 'multi' processor that can acquire a 'reversal learning set', i.e. the animal approaches each task with the proposition that the discrimination might be either way round. Harlow (1949) suggested that learning sets (the application of a propositional rule to task solution) 'releases the animal from Thorndykian bondage'. This is a graphic description of the emancipation of the monkey from the restrictiveness of 'single' processing.

In trial-unique tasks the relationship between stimulus and reward only holds for one trial, e.g. choose only those stimuli that have not already been presented in this test session (Ridley and Baker 1991). In those trial-unique tasks in which wholly novel objects are used, the rule may be only to make an invariant 'novel' versus 'familiar' discrimination. But in those trial-unique tasks in which a relatively small set of recycled objects are used, so that all stimuli are familiar, successful performance may require recollection of the recent presentation of some of the objects, i.e. an episodic memory.

Trial-dependent tasks are those in which the relationship between stimulus and reward varies across trials, e.g. choose A and then B on alternate trials. Some trial-dependent tasks, e.g. spatial and object alternation and delayed matching using only two repeatedly presented objects, would also seem to require episodic memory of the outcome of the previous trial. Other trial-dependent tasks, such as conditional learning (if A go Y, if B go Z), do not require episodic memory of the previous trial to perform the task, but they may require episodic memory for the monkey to compare both types of trial and form the *a priori* hypothesis of the relationship between A, B, Y and Z. Thus while not strictly a test of episodic memory, such memories may be helpful during acquisition.

Discrimination learning sets where, in a large number of two-choice object discriminations, performance exceeds 90 per cent correct on the second and subsequent presentation of each pair of objects, also require memory of the outcome of the first trial of each sequence. Lesions within the frontal lobes impair the formation of learning sets where the monkey has to learn to choose the non-preferred object of each pair (Mishkin 1964), as well as spatial alternation (Stamm 1964), and object alternation (Pribram and Mishkin 1956). This suggests that the frontal lobes may be specialized for 'multi' processing, particularly the use of propositions or rules.

Conditional tasks ('choose object A (not B) in context X, but choose object B (not A) in context Y') are trial-dependent in the sense that the correct response to A or B is dependent on whether this is an X trial or a Y trial. A 'single' processor will regard 'A' as either rewarded or not rewarded, but will not be able to entertain the proposition that 'A' may or may not be rewarded in different circumstances. It is, however, possible to solve this conditional task by creating four separate compound stimuli 'A in context X', 'A in context Y', etc. These four compound stimuli can then be handled by a 'single' processor. Monkeys may be encouraged to approach a conditional task via compound stimuli by presenting the different types of trial in consecutive runs of trials so that each component is learnt separately, even though final performance has to be achieved with the trials presented in a random sequence. This procedure serves to overcome the impairment on this conditional task which is produced by lesions of the septohippocampal system (Ridley and Baker 1997; Ridley *et al.* 1996), indicating that this part of the brain may participate in 'multi' processing. Monkeys with fornix transection may also be helped to perform conditional tasks if the components are separated by providing different secondary reinforcers (Gaffan *et al.* 1984*b*) or by requiring different motor responses for each component (Gaffan and Harrison 1988). Whether monkeys approach a conditional problem by attending separately to the specific combinations which they then laboriously analyse by 'single' processing, or whether they attend to wider aspects (in space and time) of the task and then need a 'multi' model processor to produce a propositional solution to the task, seems to depend on prior training and the precise method of task presentation. These subtle differences may help explain the curious list of tasks which monkeys with septohippocampal lesions, particularly fornix transections, can and cannot perform (Ridley and Baker 1997).

14.4 Specific areas of cognition

14.4.1 Recognition

Recognition adds a particular experiential quality to a perception and is usually regarded as occurring in the explicit domain. Memory for the previous encounters which lead to an object now being recognized is, however, often unavailable at the time that recognition takes place. In this respect, recognition draws on prior knowledge implicitly, since it is not necessary to produce a secondary representation of that prior knowledge in working memory in order to recognize an object as 'familiar' or, conversely, as 'novel'. An important distinction should be drawn, however, between perceptual recognition (*this thing is vaguely familiar*), semantic recognition (*I know what type of thing this is*), and episodic recognition (*this is the same one as I saw earlier*). The first two do not require secondary representation of the previous events upon which the decision is based, whereas the last type of recognition does. This difference is embodied in the 'dual process' model of recognition, which suggests that parallel systems operate, one to evoke recollection of previous encounters and another to attach a sense of familiarity to the perception of a previously encountered object (Mandler 1980; Jacoby and Dallas 1981). Amnesic patients presented with examples of famous and non-famous faces and subsequently re-presented with these, together with a new set of faces, tended to judge many of the previously presented non-famous faces as famous (Squire and McKee 1993). This implies that, in these patients, implicit recognition of the previously presented items was intact but, because explicit recollection of these items was absent, they were judged as 'presumably famous' rather than 'recently encountered'. This suggests that perceptual recognition may be spared in amnesia if it is assessed by an indirect strategy. In many recognition tests, many patients may choose to interpret the task as asking 'do you recollect the occurrence of this item in the first presentations?' rather than 'does this item have a quality of familiarity?'. Unless bizarre test items are used, all the stimuli may be recognized in the sense of being familiar. Under these circumstances it is not surprising that test scores of 'recognition' and 'recall' are well correlated, and poor, in amnesic patients (Haist *et al.* 1992) even when priming (another measure of the implicit domain) is completely intact (Squire *et al.* 1985). There is some evidence to suggest, however, that recognition, especially if measured by familiarity, can be spared in amnesic patients, particularly those with focal neurotrauma limited to the hippocampus, fornix, or mamillary bodies (Volpe *et al.* 1986; Aggleton and Shaw 1996).

It is claimed that recognition can be assessed in monkeys (Gaffan 1974). Various versions of trial-unique testing are used but the most common consists of presenting the monkey with a 'sample' trial on which one object is shown and chosen by the monkey and then, after a predetermined delay, that object together with another are presented on the choice trial and the monkey is rewarded for choosing the new object. This is called 'delayed non-matching to sample' or DNMS. But some of these recognition tasks require discrimination between 'very familiar' versus 'wholly novel' objects (Gaffan *et al.* 1984*a*) while others require recognition of the most recently presented objects in comparison to others, all of which have been presented before (Gaffan 1974; Gaffan and Weiskrantz 1980). The latter requires explicit recollection of the items in the list, but it may only be necessary for the monkey to experience 'indifference' or 'surprise' (an implicit influence on perception) in order to perform the familiar/novel discrimination. Even where the recognition tasks require the most recently presented object to be identified, it is not clear that this requires matching the choice objects to a conscious recollection of the *event* of presentation of the sample object. It could be argued that the monkey needs only to *know* which objects have already been presented in order to do this task. The difficulty which monkeys with temporal lobe lesions exhibit on this task with delays of some minutes (Mishkin 1978), in comparison to their ability to learn concurrent discriminations with delays of 24 hours (Malamut *et al.* 1984), is at first sight surprising. But in the concurrent task the animal only has to learn about certain fixed characteristics about the objects (e.g. which of these are rewarded), which requires 'single' processing whereas DNMS requires one object to be seen as a current choice object and as a previous sample object. This requires 'multi' processing. The difference between trial-independent tasks, which monkeys with medial temporal lesions can learn, and those trial-unique tasks which they cannot perform, may not lie in the distinction between unconscious procedural habit and declarative episodic memory. Rather, it may be that although both types of task are performed in the explicit declarative domain, the former relies on 'single' processing leading to the acquisition of semantic knowledge, and the latter relies on 'multi' processing which is a prerequisite for recollection of an episodic memory.

14.4.2 Working memory

Baddeley has argued that many cognitive activities require the use of a working memory system which has at least three components: a central executive system, together with two subservient systems—a visuospatial sketch pad and a phonological loop (Baddeley and Hitch 1974). The content of the two subservient systems is conscious in the sense that the sketch pad comprises 'visual imagery' and the loop is sustained by rehearsal of 'inner speech', both of which are conscious events.

As a concept, working memory is more complex than short-term memory. Both describe temporary memory effects occurring over periods of less than a few minutes. One crucial difference, however, is that short-term memory and related concepts, such as echoic, iconic, or primary memory, refer to the ability to keep active a simple piece of perceptually acquired information, and therefore employ only primary representations, whereas one of the functions of working memory is to hold, in temporary store, information which is either a recollection of the past, a constructed possible alternative to the present, or a proposition about the future, and therefore requires secondary representation. Working memory would not be able to function without 'multi' processing.

The frontal lobes are crucially involved in working memory, although right and left posterior cortical areas may also be involved, respectively, in spatial and object-based components of working memory (Smith and Jonides 1995). Funahashi *et al.* (1989) have shown that neurones in the frontal cortex hold 'representations' of stimuli during the short delay time of a delayed response task after the offset of the sample stimulus and before the choice stimuli have been presented. These authors are using the term 'representation' in the sense of 'neural correlate' but their use of the term 'on line' seems to imply that they also mean 'in mind', i.e. that this neural activity is the neural correlate of information consciously held in working memory. Further work (Wilson *et al.* 1993) has shown that the dorsolateral frontal cortex receives information about the whereabouts of visual stimuli from occipital cortex via a dorsal, parietal route, while inferior frontal cortex receives information about the identity of visual stimuli from occipital cortex via a ventral, temporal route. Since monkeys with frontal lesions are neither spatially disorientated (unlike monkeys with parietal lesions; Sugishita *et al.* 1978) nor agnosic (unlike monkeys with prestriate or temporal cortex lesions; Cowey and Gross 1970; Mishkin 1972), it may be supposed that these posterior areas are required for the 'single' processing of perceptual analysis, whereas an interaction between these areas and frontal areas is necessary for 'multi' processing, including the maintenance of spatial and object information in working memory after the stimulus has been removed.

14.4.3 Primate models of amnesia

Since amnesia is the inability to recall information explicitly into consciousness, i.e. from a long-term store into a usable working memory, an animal model of the disorder must concentrate on this mental activity. Since only humans have a natural propositional language, which uses the phonological loop, a model of amnesia might best be sought in animals by examining the evidence for a visuospatial memory. Gaffan and Harrison (1989) have argued that monkeys with fornix transection have a specific loss of 'scenic memory', i.e. the ability to recall the layout of objects in space, and are therefore 'amnesic'. Fornix-transected monkeys are, however, able to learn to discriminate between large numbers of objects when the spatial layout is not relevant (see, for example, task 3 in Gaffan 1994) or to choose between objects on the basis of the bodily spatial orientation which they have just made (Expt 2, tasks 1 and 2, in Murray *et al.* 1989). This pattern of performance suggests that these monkeys are unable to produce allocentric visuospatial imagery from long-term memory but can use egocentrically defined spatial information. Gaffan (1992*a*) has also argued that the reason why fornix-transected animals are impaired on some versions of DNMS, while they are able to learn some versions of the more difficult delayed stimulus–reward association task (see, for example, Expt 2 of Gaffan *et al.* 1984*b*), is that in the former task they need to decide whether the stimulus is in the middle of the display (and that this is therefore a sample trial) or whether each stimulus is in a lateral position (and that this is therefore a choice trial). In the latter task, however, the monkey only has to remember the reward association, and does not need to differentiate between sample and choice trials. One problem with this interpretation is that it presupposes that the monkey does not see the difference between the presence of one or two stimuli. Although this explanation is linked to a spatial impairment, the explanation is actually similar to the broader argument put forward in this chapter. We would suggest that a monkey operating with only a 'single' processor would be unable to cope with the conditional aspect of the task (if 'A' is a sample stimulus, choose 'A', if 'A' is a choice stimulus choose 'B').

The most frequently used measure of amnesia in monkeys is performance on the DNMS task, which it is claimed measures a pure mnemonic loss (Mishkin 1978). While the impairment on this task shown by monkeys with medial temporal lobe lesions (Mishkin 1978) or dorsomedial thalamic lesions (Aggleton and Mishkin 1983) is used to support the claim that this task measures amnesia, performance on the task is more severely impaired by lesions of the rhinal cortex (Meunier *et al.* 1993) or medial frontal lobes (Bachevalier and Mishkin 1986), damage to which is not usually associated with amnesia in humans. Impairment by fornix-transected monkeys on these delay tasks depends critically on details of trial presentation (see next paragraph), which are not compatible with the animals' difficulty being simply one of the general decay of memory traces across time.

Gaffan *et al.* (1984*b*) have applied the distinction between 'congruent' and 'incongruent' learning (Capaldi 1971) to an analysis of primate learning tasks. Capaldi points out that tasks such as spatial or object alternation, in which the memory for reward has to be used as information indicating non-reward at a later time (the incongruent concept 'reward means no reward'), cannot be explained by simple learning theory. Gaffan argues that monkeys with fornix transection (which he regards as amnesic) cannot learn incongruent tasks but they can learn similar congruent tasks. His distinction is essentially the same as that which we have been making between 'single' and 'multi' processing since 'reward means non-reward' clearly cannot be handled by a 'single' processor. Monkeys with fornix transection can learn to choose, on re-presentation, the rewarded object from a previously presented pair but not the previously unrewarded object (Gaffan *et al.* 1984*b*). They also find it easier to learn to choose the familiar object if the sample stimulus was not rewarded (delayed matching to non-baited sample) than if it was rewarded (delayed matching to baited sample: Gaffan *et al.* 1984*c*). The latter task is 'incongruent' because 'novelty' (as a property of the sample object) means reward on sample trials, but 'novelty' (as a property of the alternative object on choice trials) means non-reward on choice trials. If this source of confusion is removed by presenting the sample with and then without reward, fornix-transected animals are not impaired (Expt 2 in Gaffan *et al.* 1984*a*). Monkeys with hippocampal ablations can learn to choose the place where they have seen reward (spatial delayed response; Mishkin 1954) but cannot learn to choose the place where they have not seen reward (spatial alternation; Mahut 1971). These differences have a great deal to do with differences in cognitive processing but little to do with the decay of memory traces across time.

If it is supposed that clinical amnesia is one, very conspicuous, consequence of the loss of one form of cognitive processing, rather than a specific loss of dedicated memory-serving systems, then amnesic patients should exhibit impairments on broad aspects of cognitive testing in addition to memory loss. As in the primate experiments, these impairments may be sought in tests of acquisition rather than of remembering. We were able to test one Korsakoff amnesic patient's learning ability on a visuospatial task, which monkeys with septohippocampal lesions have difficulty learning, and on a concurrent discrimination task, which monkeys with these lesions can learn (Frith *et al.* 1992). Both tasks were given to the patient in a semi-formal setting using large numbers of postcards. Each correct response was rewarded with a penny which the patient accumulated and exchanged for cigarettes. Superficially the patient approached both tasks with the same degree of conscious awareness in that he made comments about the postcards and chatted about his strategy for finding the pennies. The patient was unable to learn the visuospatial task in 350 trials, although a neurotic control patient learnt the task in 14 trials and a group of normal controls learnt in a mean of 20 trials. The Korsakoff patient was, however, able to learn 10 concurrent discriminations (where the intertrial interval in real time, and in the number of intervening trials, was more extended than in the visuospatial task) in 165 trials, while the neurotic control patient learnt the task in 112 trials. This suggests that the amnesic patient, like the lesioned monkeys, had difficulty with a specific type of cognitive processing.

14.4.4 Frontal lobe function

In addition to its function in recollecting the past, secondary representation is required for considering alternatives to the current situation and for imagining the future, while remaining oriented to the present. Keeping the real and the hypothetical situation 'on line' at the same time is required for planning, creativity, and pretence. These abilities are usually regarded as being within the province of the frontal lobes. Patients with frontal lobe damage frequently exhibit 'stimulus-bound' behaviour (where they have difficulty in not responding in the most direct way to encountered objects; Lhermitte 1983), distractibility (where their attention is captured by any passing salient event; Rylander 1939), and perseveration (where they continue to respond in the same way to a stimulus after a change in circumstances has rendered that behaviour inappropriate; Milner 1963). An organism functioning at the level of a 'single' processor will respond only to the primary representations of current perceptual input, and, because there will be no other modulatory influences, the organism will respond in the most direct way. Particularly salient percepts will intrude into behavioural control, even if they are not relevant to the ongoing behaviour, and behaviour which is already under stimulus control will continue to occur even if other information (including successful completion of the behavioural act) indicates that the behaviour should now stop. Thus the superficially contradictory effects of stimulus-bound perseveration and distractibility following frontal lobe damage are both predicted by the supposition that the organism is operating with a 'single' processor only.

Other features of frontal lobe damage in humans include inconsequentiality (in which the patient is undeterred by the prospect of a long-term deleterious outcome of their actions), poor problem solving (where this involves setting up a strategy with interim goals; Shallice 1982), and a lack of creativity in thought and action (which results from a difficulty in the effortful generation of data from long-term memory; Janowsky *et al.* 1989*a*). Normal function requires the person to generate ideas or take account of situations which are not present in the environment at the time the behaviour occurs, and therefore it needs 'multi' processing.

Patients with frontal lobe damage also perform badly in a wide variety of social situations (see, for example, Eslinger and Damasio 1985). In some cases this can be attributed simply to the patient's inability to use information from the past, or about the future or the background context, which needs to be taken into account in even simple social interactions. But in other cases the difficulty may arise from an inability to form secondary representations of other people's thoughts and, more specifically, from a failure to form a meta-representation of the relationship between another person's beliefs and either the outside world or one's own beliefs.

Damage to the frontal lobes produces subtle but important effects on memory, many of which are concerned with epi-representational information rather than with representational data *per se*. Thus patients with frontal damage are particularly likely to lose the 'feeling of knowing' even when they respond accurately on memory tests (Janowsky *et al.* 1989*b*). Frontal damage may impair source memory, i.e. produce loss of memory for how a fact came to be known (Schacter *et al.* 1984; Shimamura and Squire 1987), and memory for temporal order (Milner *et al.* 1985). Both of these latter abilities require meta-representation of the relationships between memories. Confabulation is a frequent occurrence in patients with frontal damage (Stuss *et al.* 1978). One interpretation of this disorder is that the patient loses the epi-representational label that enables him to distinguish between ideas and memories so that the first thought that comes to mind is recounted as a clear recollection producing 'delusional memory' (Kopelman 1987).

Patients with isolated retrograde amnesia are rare (Markowitsch *et al.* 1993) but this impairment may result from disruption to temporal–frontal interactions (Markowitsch 1995). Monkeys with frontal ablations may also exhibit isolated retrograde amnesia (Ridley *et al.* 1993). Stuss and Benson (1987) describe the milder effects seen in many patients with frontal lobe damage as 'forgetting to remember', i.e. failure to make use of memories. This is a defect of cognitive processing rather than of information storage.

In a classic paper, Mishkin (1964) described the consequence of frontal ablations in monkeys as the 'perseveration of central sets'. The deficits seen after frontal lesions still incorporate this flavour of behavioural and cognitive inflexibility, and an inability to perform conditional tasks (Petrides 1987). Impairment on these tasks would be predicted in an animal functioning in a 'single' mode only.

Primate studies have been used extensively to examine the localization of function within the frontal lobes. Much of this localization is dependent on the subject matter analysed rather than the nature of the processing carried out by different areas. For example, monkeys with ablations of the lateral premotor cortex have difficulty in learning to select an appropriate motor response but are unimpaired at learning to orientate towards an appropriate stimulus; the opposite effect is seen following lesions positioned a little more anteriorly (Halsband and Passingham 1985). Monkeys with lesions of the dorsal prefrontal cortex are unable to choose the location where they last saw the reward (Jacobsen 1935), although they can learn to choose the object under which the reward was hidden (Mishkin and Manning 1978). Impairment on this latter task is seen if the lesion is in a more ventral position within the prefrontal cortex (Mishkin and Manning 1978). A feature of almost all of the tasks that monkeys with frontal lesions find difficult is that they are conditional (Petrides 1987; Passingham 1993). Thus the frontal-lesioned monkey can learn an enormous number of tasks where one choice (of response or object) is invariably correct, but when reward depends on choosing objects or responses which are correct only under certain circumstances, or where reward can be obtained when a movement is made without it being 'cued' by an external event, then the monkey with frontal-lobe damage is seriously disadvantaged.

14.5 Meta-representation

14.5.1 Consciousness and self-awareness

Consciousness is a difficult topic for cognitive neuroscience because of a lack of consensus on definitions. We will adopt a working premise that humans and other mammals potentially have three levels of awareness: the unconsciousness of dreamless sleep, the normal consciousness of experience of the outside world, and the recursive self-awareness of 'knowing that one knows'. Hirst (1995) argues that 'any act of consciousness involves self-awareness as well as awareness of the world'. If this recursive view of consciousness were applied to animals one would be led to the conclusion that either monkeys are blundering about like invertebrates in a state of unconsciousness or they are engaging in perpetual introspection. Neither of these seems entirely likely; nor does it seem likely that consciousness and all its implications arose all in one go when man evolved from his recent predecessors. Monkeys, like humans, interact with and respond differently to the world when they are awake compared to when they are asleep, implying a similar transition between unconscious and normal conscious states. The central and peripheral visual systems of monkeys are similar to those of humans (with some anomalies in photoreceptor pigments in some species) so that it is likely that monkeys see shapes and colours in much the same way as we do. Since the perceptual images produced by our visual system enter into normal consciousness one must suppose that the percepts of monkeys also enter their consciousness. It would seem that monkeys are conscious (sentient) of the present, i.e. that they inhabit the present in the same explicit domain as humans. The important issue in most comparative neuropsychology is then to determine the extent to which the past and the future can also be brought into the explicit domain by the formation of secondary representations, i.e. to establish the extent to which animals can generate their own ideas and recollections. Analysis of recursive self-awareness only becomes important when meta-representation is critical for understanding behaviour, for example in the analysis of the social behaviour of the great apes (Premack and Woodruff 1978). Analysis of the social activity of monkeys provides little evidence that they are capable of meta-representation (Cheney and Seyfarth 1990).

14.5.2 Disorders of consciousness

Consciousness is of interest to the neuropsychologist when it is distorted by neurotrauma. Even when sensation is not lost, it may fail to influence perception, resulting in conditions of 'neglect'. Such conditions may be associated with damage to posterior neocortex and its associated white matter tracts and may include not only the loss of the primary representation of conscious percepts but also loss of the secondary representation of imagination and recollection of information (Bisiach and Luzzatti 1978). Neglect in humans often results from ischaemic damage following middle cerebral artery occlusion (stroke). In a primate model of this disorder, Marshall and Ridley (1996) found that marmosets also exhibited hemispatial neglect. This could be dissociated from motor impairments by the use of a specific test apparatus and occurred in the visual, tactual, and probably auditory modalities. Although it is difficult to be certain that this neglect was not due to a primary sensory loss, its occurrence in more than one modality, the absence of ischaemic damage in the primary visual cortex, and the freedom to move around within the test conditions (which would have enabled an animal with an hemianopia, but no neglect, to adjust its head position appropriately) argues in favour of a perceptual, representational impairment, which is therefore an impairment in consciousness.

Some patients also suffer from 'denial' or anosognosia, i.e. a failure to appreciate that they have a perceptual impairment (Bisiach and Geminiani 1991). A patient with recently acquired cortical blindness may deny being blind and explain away their behavioural difficulties with confabulatory stories about the lights being dim or their glasses having been stolen. This is the failure of a meta-representational system. Data relevant to this kind of meta-representational failure in monkeys is extremely limited but one experiment does suggest that they can be tricked into *not knowing that they know*. Rhesus monkeys can learn a number of simple two-choice discriminations such that the probability of making a correct choice on any trial, including the first trial in any test session, for that pair of stimuli exceeds 90 per cent, i.e. the task is well learnt. They can also form 'object learning sets' where they are presented with innumerable pairs of objects for a few trials each.

On the first-ever presentation of a pair they necessarily score 50 per cent correct, but if that pair is then presented again, their choices exceed 90 per cent correct (having learnt the rule that if reward is not under one object on the first trial it will be under the other one on all subsequent trials). However, if pairs of stimuli from previously well-learnt discriminations are then slipped into the sequence of novel pairs in the learning set, performance on the first presentation with these familiar objects drops to 50 per cent even though, when presented in isolation, performance on the first trial exceeds 90 per cent (Meyer 1971). This suggests that when the monkey is presented with familiar objects it *knows that it knows* where the reward is, but if the familiarity of these objects is obscured by surrounding them (temporally) with unfamiliar objects, the monkey fails to recognize them as objects that it knows something about. The monkey then *guesses* (with 50 per cent success) on the first trial and uses the outcome of that trial to score well on the second trial.

14.5.3 Psychosis

Autism is characterized by impairments in social competence as well as in perceptuo-motor integration (Kanner 1943). The ability to function at the level of meta-representation of the independent content of the minds of others is disproportionately impaired, relative to IQ, in autism (Baron-Cohen *et al.* 1985). This is described as the loss of a 'theory of mind'. But the disorder also includes a much more basic behavioural disturbance indicative of functioning in only a 'single' mode. Inability to appreciate the importance of the past and the future renders the patient largely incapable of independent living, and the 'insistence on sameness', overfocusing of interests, perseveration of ideas, and stereotypy of motor output are all suggestive of defective 'multi' processing. Against this background, the islands of exceptional achievement in the acquisition of restricted types of factual information, attention to detail, perceptual analysis, and repetitive arithmetical calculation which occur in some autistic individuals are indicative of an intact but isolated 'single' system. The supposition that 'multi' processing is defective in autism integrates the motor symptoms and the 'theory of mind' deficits which invariably co-exist in autism. The tendency for autistics to perform any task, from the perceptually very basic distinction of 'figure from ground' to the high-level appreciation of ironic context, at a level of analysis which fails to integrate relevant components, suggests that it is the mechanism of integration or appreciation of relationships (which requires 'multi' processing) which is faulty, rather than that the patient has a problem of functioning at a particular hierarchical level. The argument is, therefore, that 'social incompetence' is only one consequence of an 'across the board' dysfunction of data processing rather than that the patient suffers from a defect in a 'social functioning module' in the brain.

Frith (1992) has argued that schizophrenia can be understood as a disorder of meta- and epi-representation. At the highest level, a failure of meta-representation of the potential difference in the beliefs and intentions of other people and those one holds oneself, and of the relation of both of these to the outside world, will contribute to the special content of schizophrenic language. A failure of the recursive meta-representation of self-awareness and awareness of self-initiation of action will result in the experience of thought withdrawal and delusions of alien control. When epi-representational labels are weakened, imagination may be experienced as perception, resulting in hallucinations; hypothetical ideas may be experienced as factually based knowledge, resulting in delusional beliefs; thoughts lacking the quality of being self-generated may be experienced as 'thought insertion' or 'thought broadcast'. Negative symptoms, including poverty of speech production and content, and a loss of planned activity, will result from a weakening of the ability to form and use secondary representations. Thus this formulation accounts for most of the symptoms of psychosis except for the perseverative thought processes and motor stereotypy which are also seen in schizophrenia. But if failures of higher-order representation are seen as a consequence of the loss of 'multi' processing, such that the patient operates only in the 'single' mode, the features of perseveration, distractibility, stereotypy, and catatonia, which are seen in the severest form of the disease, can also be incorporated in the same theoretical framework. No other theory of schizophrenia is able to integrate the superficially very different social, cognitive, and behavioural aspects of the disorder.

This theory also offers particular hope for the development of an animal model of the cognitive defect underlying psychosis because, while it may be difficult to study symptoms of meta-representational deficits directly in animals, the study of underlying cognitive malfunctions may be more amenable to analysis in animals. Since amphetamine treatment (which increases dopamine release) exacerbates the symptoms of schizophrenia (Angrist *et al.* 1980) and may produce psychotic symptoms in otherwise healthy individuals (Griffiths *et al.* 1972), and since most antipsychotic drugs block dopamine, analysis of the role of dopamine in mental representation in primates has biochemical as well as cognitive validity.

Animal models of disease are often used when the aetiology and pathogenesis of a disease are at least crudely understood and a model is needed to test new treatments or to perform other analyses which would not be ethical in humans. The use of animal models to study a condition that is itself largely mysterious is much more problematic. Animal models of human neuropsychiatric disease could be based on anatomical, psychological, 'surface', aetiological, or pathogenetic validity. However, the anatomical basis of psychosis is poorly understood so that 'lesion' models are weak, and symptomological aspects of psychosis have usually been considered unsuitable for animal models because they are largely experiential and depend on verbal accounts by the patient. The surface behaviour of humans and monkeys is so different that comparison of overt symptoms across species is often crude. The problem is to go beyond the surface behaviours to the core cognitive deficits.

Ideally, the disparate symptoms of psychosis will be related to one 'basic' cognitive defect which, when reproduced in animals, results in a comparable set of disparate symptoms. High, acute or chronic, doses of amphetamine administered to primates induce stereotyped behaviours, social withdrawal, and behaviour compatible with visual and tactual hallucinations (Randrup and Munkvad 1974; Ellison *et al.* 1981; Ridley *et al.* 1983), but it is difficult to argue that this behaviour is more like the symptoms of schizophrenia than of toxic psychosis or delirium. Lower doses of amphetamine induce subtle effects on social interaction (Scraggs and Ridley 1978) and cognition. In particular, amphetamine induces perseveration of choice behaviour in the WGTA (Ridley *et al.* 1981*a*) which can be differentiated from motor stereotypy when choice of the same stimulus requires a different movement on different trials (Ridley *et al.* 1981*b*). This 'cognitive inflexibility' epitomizes the behaviour of an animal which is functioning only in a 'single' mode. One explanation for the involvement of dopamine in symptom expression in psychosis would be to suppose that in psychosis there is a defect in information processing in which higher-order representational processing is particularly weakened. There is evidence of functional 'hypofrontality' in schizophrenics (Andreasen *et al.* 1992). The behavioural response to amphetamine is enhanced in animals with frontal lesions (Iversen 1971), suggesting a mutually antagonistic role of ascending dopamine pathways (which project mainly to the basal ganglia) and descending influences from the frontal lobes (to the basal ganglia). Since there are arguments for the involvement of the frontal lobes in 'multi' processing (see above) it can be argued that increasing release of dopamine favours 'single' rather than 'multi' processing. Dopamine is released in response to conditions of high environmental demand and is required in normal functioning when immediate and simple responses may be life-saving (cf. *kinesia paradoxica* in Parkinson's disease). The speed and simplicity of these responses are best handled by a 'single' processor. But high levels of dopamine release in a brain that has difficulty functioning in a 'multi' mode may produce severe cognitive disability by biasing the brain even further towards the 'single' mode, resulting in the production of only limited, 'stimulus-bound' behaviour. Thus the study of the effects of low doses of amphetamine in animals not only has biochemical validity but may be able to illuminate cognitive aspects of psychosis in humans.

14.5.4 Meta-representation in monkeys and apes

While some people have been content to work on animal models of amnesia and psychosis without great regard to the level of mental representation at which they believe their model is operating, other investigators have addressed specifically the question of whether non-human primates are capable of higher levels of representation, especially meta-representation. Sometimes this work has been interpreted as providing (or destroying) an essential difference between humans and non-humans and has even been used in arguments over moral issues of the use and treatment of animals. This latter debate is deeply flawed since it is not necessary to show that a creature (human or animal) is like oneself in order to have due respect for its needs. On the other hand, it is important to know what an animal can understand and appreciate in order to provide it with an adequate environment. Almost all species, including invertebrates, use items in their environment (e.g. to make nests) and several species of mammals and birds use objects to obtain something else (e.g. using stones to break open food), although it is only amongst the primates that reports of using handy items as weapons or missiles, and sticks as pokers or levers, are frequent. Only capuchins and, more frequently, chimpanzees (there being little data on other apes) show the propensity to carry objects for long distances, or to modify objects, in order to use them as tools (reviewed by Passingham 1982). Thus tool use and tool-making have ceased to be regarded as the hallmark of being a human or being a primate. Similarly, attempts to teach sign or symbolic language to chimpanzees were sufficiently successful to indicate that 'word' use may be mastered by non-humans, but these attempts also fall so far short of complete success as to indicate that human language, in its full complexity, is uniquely human! But it may be reasonable to interpret many sounds and gestures made by monkeys and other species as being 'words', i.e. symbolic representations of events or items in the environment (Cheney and Seyfarth 1990).

The debate about whether monkeys and apes have a 'theory of mind' is subtle and sometimes confused. Cheney and Seyfarth (1990) maintain that vervet monkeys form 'alliances' on the basis of previous behavioural interactions (although whether this is dependent on remembering the interaction itself is not entirely clear) and are able to maintain these alliances by reciprocation of actions. They also argue that vervets know about the relationships between animals other than themselves and that these relationships must be represented in their minds. One of the factors in favour of this interpretation is that of parsimony. The permutations of interactions in social groups are too numerous to exist as separate learnt responses. Knowledge of the relationships between other animals could be regarded as a mental 'intervening variable' between social conditions and predicted behaviours. The evolution of mental representation is therefore seen as being driven by the complexity of social interactions (Whitten and Byrne 1988).

Many of the 'words' (calls which appear to inform other animals of various dangers) that vervets use appear to be intended to modify the *behaviour* of other vervets but not necessarily the *beliefs* of other monkeys, the latter being the requirement of a 'theory of mind'. Cheney and Seyfarth (1990) are careful to emphasize that they cannot know whether their vervets have a recursive awareness of their own representations. None of the 'words' which the vervets use refers to categories. Vervets have various 'danger' calls but no 'general danger' signal, suggesting that they have knowledge of dangerous events but no mental concept of danger.

14.6 Conclusions

Mental representations are the product, in consciousness, of unconscious brain information processing. Primary mental representations provide perceptual awareness of sensory input. That these can differ between people is evident, for example, from the consistently different descriptions that are given by people with various forms of anomalous colour vision. The close similarity in visual (and other sensory) peripheral and central neuroanatomy and neurophysiology between humans and other primates makes it reasonable to suppose that monkeys and humans form similar primary representations of percepts, except for the semantic background against which objects are identified. Secondary representations permit recollection of the past as an event, imagination of alternatives to the present, and apprehension of the future. These abilities emancipate the individual from current reality and their usefulness in directing individual behaviour, in providing the substrate of language, and as the basis of the development of a culture of shared knowledge provides a powerful explanation for the evolution of consciousness. The evolution of meta-representational abilities permits the development of a culture of unshared knowledge in which understanding that different people know different things allows for the development of collaboration as well as deception.

As a product of evolution, it must be supposed that consciousness differs subtly across species. Non-mammalian species are capable of responding in a fixed pattern to sensory information without it being necessary for us to suppose that they possess perceptual awareness. Behavioural responsiveness to the present, however intricate or subtle, is no proof of the existence of consciousness, though most mammals are likely to be conscious of the present because their neuroanatomical structures suggest that they are capable of perception. Behaviour which can only realistically be explained as resulting from a recollection of the past (rather than merely the modification of a behavioural repertoire as a consequence of experience), or from problem solving on the basis of hypothesis formation (rather than trial and error), or from the prediction of a probable future event, must depend on the formation of secondary representations, which would be evidence for the existence of an elaborated form of consciousness in another species. Proving that these mental events occur in another species may be as problematic as proving that another person's consciousness is, experientially, the same as one's own. While this difficulty should not be confused with assuming that other people experience less than oneself, it should not be forgotten that people with neural dysfunction may inhabit a very different world from one's own. When using animals to study cognition, it should be borne in mind that cognitive functions which, in humans, depend on particular levels of mental representation, can only be studied in species which also attain the same level of representational sophistication.

Acknowledgement

We would like to thank Professor Chris Frith for helpful comments on an earlier draft of this paper.

References

Aggleton, J. P. and Mishkin, M. (1983). Memory impairment following restricted medial thalamic lesions in monkeys. *Experimental Brain Research*, **52,** 199–209.

Aggleton, J. P. and Shaw, C. (1996). Amnesia and recognition memory: a re-analysis of psychometric data. *Neuropsychologia*, **34,** 51–62.

Andreasen, N. C., Rezai, K., Alliger, R., Swayze, V. W., Flaum, M., Kirchner, P. *et al.* (1992). Hypofrontality in neuroleptic-naive patients and in-patients with chronic schizophrenia. *Archives of General Psychiatry*, **49,** 943–58.

Angrist, B., Rotrosen, J., and Gershon, S. (1980). Differential effects of amphetamine and neuroleptics on negative versus positive symptoms in schizophrenia. *Psychopharmacology*, **72,** 17–19.

Bachevalier, J. and Mishkin, M. (1986). Visual recognition impairment follows ventromedial but not dorsolateral prefrontal lesions in monkeys. *Behavioural Brain Research*, **20,** 249–61.

Baddeley, A. D. and Hitch, G. (1974). Working memory. In *The Psychology of Learning and Motivation,* (ed. G. A. Bower), pp. 47–89. Academic Press, New York.

Baron–Cohen, S., Leslie, A. M., and Frith, U. (1985). Does the autisitic child have a 'theory of mind'? *Cognition*, **21,** 37–46.

Bartlett, F. C. (1932). *Remembering: an experimental and social study*. Cambridge University Press, Cambridge.

Bisiach, E. and Geminiani, G. (1991). Anosognosia related to hemiplegia and hemianopia. In *Awareness of deficit after brain injury*, (ed. G. P. Prigatano and D. L. Schacter), pp.17–39. Oxford University Press, New York.

Bisiach, E. and Luzzatti, C. (1978). Unilateral neglect of representational space. *Cortex*, **14,** 129–33.

Capaldi, E. J. (1971). Memory and learning: a sequential viewpoint. In *Animal memory*, (ed. W. K. Honig and P. H. R. James), pp. 115–54. Academic Press, New York.

Cheney, D. L. and Seyfarth, R. M. (1990). *How monkeys see the world.* University of Chicago, Chicago.

Cowey, A. and Gross, C. G. (1970). Effects of foveal prestriate and inferotemporal lesions on visual discrimination by rhesus monkeys. *Experimental Brain Research*, **11,** 128–44.

Davenport, R. K. and Rogers, C. M. (1971). Perception of photographs by apes. *Behaviour*, **39,** 318–20.

Dawkins, M. S. (1993). *Through our eyes only? The search for animal consciousness.* Freeman, Oxford.

Ellison, G. D., Nielson, E. B., and Lyon, M. (1981). Animal models of psychosis: hallucinatory behaviors in monkeys during the late stage of continuous amphetamine intoxication. *Journal of Psychiatric Research*, **16,** 13–22.

Eslinger, P. J. and Damasio, A. R. (1985). Severe disturbance of higher cognition after bilateral frontal lobe ablation: patient EVR. *Neurology*, **35,** 1731–41.

Frith, C. D. (1992). *The cognitive psychology of schizophrenia.* Erlbaum, Hove, UK.

Frith, C. D., Cahill, C., Ridley, R. M., and Baker, H. F. (1992). Memory for what it is and memory for what it means: a single case of Korsakoff's amnesia. *Cortex*, **28,** 53–67.

Frith, U. (1989). *Autism: understanding the enigma.* Blackwell, Oxford.

Funahashi, S., Bruce, C. J., and Goldman-Rakic, P. S. (1989). Mnemonic coding of visual space in the monkey's dorsolateral prefrontal cortex. *Journal of Neurophysiology*, **61,** 331–49.

Gaffan, D. (1974). Recognition impaired and association intact in the memory of monkeys after transection of the fornix. *Journal of Comparative and Physiological Psychology*, **86,** 1100–9.

Gaffan, D. (1992*a*). The role of the hippocampus–fornix–mammillary system in episodic memory. In *Neuropsychology of memory*, (ed. L. R. Squire and N. Butters), pp. 336–46. Guilford Press, New York.

Gaffan, D. (1992*b*). Amnesia for complex naturalistic scenes and for objects following fornix transection in the rhesus monkey. *European Journal of Neuroscience*, **4,** 381–8.

Gaffan, D. (1994). Scene-specific memory for objects: a model of episodic impairment in monkeys with fornix transection. *Journal of Cognitive Neuroscience*, **6,** 305–20.

Gaffan, D. and Harrison, S. (1988). Inferotemporal-frontal disconnection and fornix transection in visuomotor conditional learning by monkeys. *Behavioural Brain Research*, **31,** 149–63.

Gaffan, D. and Harrison, S. (1989). Place memory and scene memory: effects of fornix transection in the monkey. *Experimental Brain Research*, **74,** 202–12.

Gaffan, D. and Weiskrantz, L. (1980). Recency effects and lesion effects in delayed non-matching to randomly baited samples by monkeys. *Brain Research*, **196,** 373–86.

Gaffan, D., Gaffan, E. A., and Harrison, S. (1984*a*). Effects of fornix transection on spontaneous and trained non-matching by monkeys. *Quarterly Journal of Experimental Psychology*, **36B,** 285–303.

Gaffan, D., Saunders, R. C., Gaffan, E. A., Harrison, S., Shields, C., and Owen, M. J. (1984*b*). Effects of fornix transection upon associative learning in monkeys: role of the hippocampus in learned action. *Quarterly Journal of Experimental Psychology*, **36B,** 173–222.

Gaffan, D., Shields, C., and Harrison, S. (1984*c*). Delayed matching by fornix-transected monkeys: the sample, the push and the bait. *Quarterly Journal of Experimental Psychology*, **36B,** 305–17.

Gallup, G. G. (1975). Towards an operational definition of self-awareness. In *Socioecology and psychology of primates*, (ed. R. H. Tuttle), pp. 329–38. Mouton, The Hague.

Griffiths, J. D., Cavanaugh, J., Held, J., and Oates, J. A. (1972). Dextramphetamine —evaluation of psychomimetic properties in man. *Archives of General Psychiatry*, **26,** 97–100.

Haist, F., Shimamura, A. P., and Squire, L. R. (1992). On the relationship between recall and recognition memory. *Journal of Experimental Psychology (Learning, Memory and Cognition)*, **18,** 691–702.

Halsband, U. and Passingham, R. E. (1985). Premotor cortex and the conditions for movement in monkeys *(Macaca mulatta)*. *Behavioural Brain Research*, **18,** 269–76.

Harlow, H. F. (1949). The formation of learning sets. *Psychological Reviews*, **56,** 51–65.

Hayes, K. J. and Hayes, C. (1952). Imitation in a home-raised chimpanzee. *Journal of Comparative and Physiological Psychology*, **45,** 450–9.

Hirst, W. (1995). Cognitive aspects of consciousness. In *The cognitive neurosciences*, (ed. M. S. Gazzaniga), pp. 1307–19. MIT Press, Cambridge, MA.

Iversen, S. D. (1971). The effect of surgical lesions to frontal cortex and substantia nigra on amphetamine response in rats. *Brain Research*, **31,** 295–311.

Jacobsen, C. F. (1935). Functions of frontal association areas in primates. *Archives of Neurology and Psychiatry*, **33,** 558–69.

Jacoby, L. L. and Dallas, M. (1981). On the relationship between autobiographical memory and perceptual learning. *Journal of Experimental Psychology (General)*, **3,** 306–40.

Janowsky, J. S., Shimamura, A. P., Kritchevsky, M., and Squire, L. R. (1989*a*). Cognitive impairment following frontal lobe damage and its relevance to human amnesia. *Behavioral Neuroscience*, **103,** 548–68.

Janowsky, J. S., Shimamura, A. P., and Squire, L. R. (1989*b*). Memory and metamemory: comparison between patients with frontal lobe lesions and amnesic patients. *Psychobiology*, **17,** 3–11.

Kanner, L. (1943). Autistic disturbance of affective contact. *Nervous Child*, **2,** 217–50.

Kopelman, M. D. (1987). Amnesia: organic and psychogenic. *British Journal of Psychiatry*, **150,** 428–42.

Lhermitte, F. (1983). 'Utilization behaviour' and its relation to lesions of the frontal lobes. *Brain*, **106,** 237–55.

Leslie, A. M. (1987). Pretense and representation: the origins of 'theory of mind'. *Psychological Reviews*, **94,** 412–26.

Mahut, H. (1971). Spatial and object reversal learning in monkeys with partial temporal lobe ablations. *Neuropsychologia*, **9,** 409–24.

Malamut, B. L., Saunders, R. C., and Mishkin, M. (1984). Monkeys with combined amygdalo-hippocampal lesions succeed in object discrimination learning despite 24-hour intertrial intervals. *Behavioral Neuroscience*, **98,** 759–69.

Mandler, G. (1980). Recognising; the judgement of previous accounts. *Psychological Reviews*, **87,** 252–71.

Markowitsch, H. J. (1995). Anatomical basis of memory disorders. In *The cognitive neurosciences*, (ed. M. S. Gazzaniga), pp. 765–78. MIT Press, Cambridge, MA.

Markowitsch, H. J., Calabrese, P., Liess, M., Haupts, H. F., Durwen, H. F., and Gehlen, W. (1993). Retrograde amnesia after traumatic injury of the temporal–frontal cortex. *Journal of Neurology, Neurosurgery and Psychiatry*, **56,** 988–92.

Marshall, J. W. B. and Ridley, R. M. (1996). Assessment of functional impairment following permanent middle cerebral artery occlusion in a non-human primate species. *Neurodegeneration*, **5,** 275–86.

Meunier, M., Bachevalier, J., Mishkin, M., and Murray, E. A. (1993). Effects on visual recognition of combined and separate ablations of the entorhinal and perirhinal cortex in rhesus monkeys. *Journal of Neuroscience*, **13,** 5418–32.

Meyer, D. R. (1971). The habits and concepts of monkeys. In *Cognitive processes in non-human primates*, (ed. L. E. Jarrard), pp. 83–102. Academic Press, New York.

Milner, B. (1963). Effects of different brain lesions on card sorting. *Archives of Neurology*, **9,** 90–100.

Milner, B., Petrides, M., and Smith, M. L. (1985). Frontal lobes and the temporal organisation of memory. *Human Neurobiology*, **4,** 137–42.

Mishkin, M. (1954). Visual discrimination performance following partial ablations of the temporal lobe: II Ventral surface vs. hippocampus. *Journal of Comparative and Physiological Psychology*, **47,** 187–93.

Mishkin, M. (1964). Perseveration of central sets. In *The frontal granular cortex and behavior*, (ed. J. M. Warren and K. Akert), pp. 219–41. McGraw-Hill, New York.

Mishkin, M. (1972). Cortical visual areas and their interactions. In *The brain and human behavior*, (ed. A. G. Karczmar and J. C. Eccles), pp. 187–208. Springer, Berlin.

Mishkin, M. (1978). Memory severely impaired by combined but not by separate removal of amygdala and hippocampus. *Nature*, **273,** 297–8.
Mishkin, M. and Manning, F. J. (1978). Nonspatial memory after selective prefrontal lesions in monkeys. *Brain Research*, **143,** 313–23.
Mishkin, M., Malamut, B., and Bachevalier, J. (1984). Memories and habits: two neural systems. In *Neurobiology of learning and memory*, (ed. G. Lynch, J. L. McGough, and N. M. Weinberger), pp. 65–77. Guilford Press, New York.
Murray, E. A., Davidson, M., Gaffan, D., Olton, D. S., and Suomi, S. (1989). Effects of fornix transection and cingulate cortical ablation on spatial memory in rhesus monkeys. *Experimental Brain Research*, **74,** 173–86.
Nisbett, R. E. and Wilson, T. D. (1977). Telling more than we can know: verbal reports on mental processes. *Psychological Review*, **84,** 231–59.
Passingham, R. E. (1982). *The human primate*. Freeman, Oxford.
Passingham, R. E. (1993). *The frontal lobes and voluntary action*. Oxford University Press, Oxford.
Perner, J. (1993). *Understanding the representational mind.* MIT Press, Cambridge, Mass..
Petrides, M. (1987). Conditional learning and the primate frontal cortex. In *The frontal lobes revisited*, (ed. E. Perecman), pp. 91–108. IRBN Press, New York.
Premack, D. and Woodruff, G. (1978). Does the chimpanzee have a theory of mind? *Behavioral and Brain Sciences*, **1,** 516–26.
Pribram, K. H. and Mishkin, M. (1956). Analysis of the effects of frontal lesions in monkey. III. Object alternation. *Journal of Comparative and Physiological Psychology*, **45,** 565–75.
Prinz, W. (1992). Why don't we perceive our brain states? *European Journal of Cognitive Psychology*, **4,** 1–20.
Pylyshyn, Z. W. (1978). When is attribution of beliefs justified? *Behavioral and Brain Sciences*, **1,** 592–3.
Randrup, A. and Munkvad, I. (1974). Pharmacology and physiology of stereotyped behaviour. *Journal of Psychiatric Research*, **11,** 1–10.
Ridley, R. M. and Baker, H. F. (1991). A critical evaluation of monkey models of amnesia and dementia. *Brain Research—Brain Research Reviews*, **16,** 15–37.
Ridley, R. M. and Baker, H. F. (1997). Evidence for a specific information processing deficit in monkeys with lesions of the septo-hippocampal system. *Cortex*, **33**, 167–76.
Ridley, R. M., Haystead, T. A., and Baker, H. F. (1981*a*). An analysis of visual object reversal learning in the marmoset after amphetamine and haloperidol. *Pharmacology Biochemistry and Behaviour*, **14,** 345–51.
Ridley, R. M., Haystead, T. A., and Baker, H. F. (1981*b*). An involvement of dopamine in higher order choice mechanisms in the monkey. *Psychopharmacology*, **72,** 173–7.
Ridley, R. M., Baker, H. F., Owen, F., Cross, A. J., and Crow, T. J. (1983). Behavioural and biochemical effects of chronic treatment with amphetamine in the vervet monkey. *Neuropharmacology*, **22,** 551–4.
Ridley, R. M., Aitken, D. M., and Baker, H. F. (1989). Learning about rules but not about reward is impaired following lesions of the cholinergic projection to the hippocampus. *Brain Research*, **502,** 306–18.
Ridley, R. M., Durnford, L. J., Baker, J. A., and Baker, H. F. (1993). Cognitive inflexibility after archicortical and paleocortical prefrontal lesions in marmosets. *Brain Research*, **628,** 56–64.
Ridley, R. M., Pearson, C., Kershaw, T. R., Hodges, H., Maclean, C. J., Hoyle, C. *et al.* (1996). Learning impairment induced by lesion of the CA1 field of the primate

hippocampus: attempts to ameliorate the impairment by transplantation of fetal CA1 tissue. *Experimental Brain Research*, **115**, 83–94.

Rylander, G. (1939). Personality changes after operations on the frontal lobes. *Acta Psychiatrica et Neurologica Scandinavica*, Suppl. 20.

Schacter, D. L. (1987). Implicit memory: history and current status. *Journal of Experimental Psychology (Learning, Memory and Cognition)*, **13,** 501–18.

Schacter, D. L., Harbluk, J. L., and McLachlan, D. R. (1984). Retrieval without recollection: an experimental analysis of source memory. *Journal of Verbal Learning and Verbal Behavior*, **23,** 593–611.

Scraggs, P. R. and Ridley, R. M. (1978). Behavioural effects of amphetamine in a small primate: relative potencies of the d– and l–isomers. *Psychopharmacology*, **59,** 243–5.

Shallice, T. (1982). Specific impairments of planning. *Philosophical Transactions of the Royal Society (Series B)*, **298,** 199–209.

Shimamura, A. P. and Squire, L. R. (1987). A neuropsychological study of fact memory and source memory. *Journal of Experimental Psychology (Learning, Memory and Cognition)*, **13,** 464–73.

Smith, E. E. and Jonides, J. (1995). Working memory in humans: neuropsychological evidence. In *The cognitive neurosciences*, (ed. M. S. Gazzaniga), pp. 1009–20. MIT Press, Cambridge, MA.

Squire, L. R. (1986). Mechanisms of memory. *Science*, **232,** 1612–19.

Squire, L. R. (1992). Declarative and non-declarative memory: multiple brain systems supporting learning and memory. *Journal of Cognitive Neuroscience*, **99,** 195–231.

Squire, L. R. and McKee, R. D. (1993). Declarative and nondeclarative memory in opposition: when prior events influence amnesic patients more than normal subjects. *Memory and Cognition*, **21,** 424–30.

Squire, L. R., Shimamura, A., and Gray, P. (1985). Independence of recognition memory and priming effects. A neuropsychological analysis. *Journal of Experimental Psychology (Learning, Memory and Cognition)*, **11,** 34–44.

Stamm, J. S. (1964). Retardation and facilitation in learning by stimulation of frontal cortex in monkeys. In *The frontal granular cortex and behavior*, (ed. J. M. Warren and K. Akert), pp. 102–25. McGraw-Hill, New York.

Stuss, D. T. and Benson, D. F. (1987). The frontal lobes in control of cognition and memory. In *The frontal lobes revisited*, (ed. E. Perecman), pp. 141–58. IRBN Press, New York.

Stuss, D. T., Alexander, M. P., Lieberman, A., and LeVine, H. (1978). An extraordinary form of confabulation. *Neurology*, **28,** 1166–72.

Sugishita, M., Ettlinger, G., and Ridley, R. M. (1978). Disturbance of cage-finding in the monkey. *Cortex*, **14,** 431–8.

Tulving, E. (1985). Memory and consciousness. *Canadian Psychology*, **26,** 1–12.

Tulving, E. (1989). Memory: performance, knowledge and experience. *European Journal of Cognitive Psychology*, **1,** 3–26.

Volpe, B. T., Holtzman, J. D., and Hirst, W. (1986). Further characterization of patients with amnesia after cardiac arrest: preserved recognition memory. *Neurology*, **36,** 408–11.

Whitten, A. and Byrne, R. W. (1988). *Machiavellian intelligence: social expertise and the evolution of intellect in monkeys, apes, and humans*. Oxford University Press, Oxford.

Wilson, F. A. W., Scalaidhe, S. P., and Goldman-Rakic, P. S. (1993). Dissociation of object and spatial processing domains in primate prefrontal cortex. *Science*, **260,** 1955–8.

Winner, E. and Ettlinger, G. (1979). Do chimpanzees recognise photographs as representations of objects? *Neuropsychologia*, **17,** 413–20.

15

The specializations of the human neocortex

RICHARD E. PASSINGHAM

15.1 Introduction

In 1970, Drewe *et al.* compared the results of neuropsychological research on humans and monkeys. The paper grew out of discussions between George Ettlinger and a group of graduate students. It pointed to apparent differences in the results of neuropsychological studies carried out with human subjects and with monkeys, and suggested caution in generalizing from data on non-human primates to the human brain. This paper was followed in 1974 by another comparative paper (Passingham and Ettlinger 1974). This stressed possible differences in functional lateralization.

However, it occurred to Ettlinger that the conclusions of these reviews might be misleading, since they were based on comparisons between human subjects and monkeys rather than apes. So from 1974 to 1980 he carried out behavioural studies of six chimpanzees (Ettlinger 1983). For example, Muncer and Ettlinger (1981) tackled the crucial issue of whether a chimpanzee could be taught that in sign language the order of the signs was critical for meaning. They claimed preliminary evidence of competence in syntax, while stressing that the animal was unable to handle the negation of logical operators such as 'and' and 'or'. As always, Ettlinger was as interested in the differences between man and other primates as he was in the similarities.

The behavioural data reviewed in the comparative papers came mainly from the effects of brain lesions. The papers were written before the invention of positron emission tomography (PET) or functional magnetic resonance imaging (fMRI) for imaging the human brain at work. We now know much more about the functional organization of the human brain from imaging studies, and it is time for a reappraisal. This paper is the start of that enterprise.

15.1.1 Cytoarchitecture and anatomical connections

The study of living non-human primates is not the study of our ancestors. The hominid line diverged from that leading to the Old World monkeys 25 million years or more ago (Jones *et al.* 1992) and is thought to have diverged from the African apes some time between 5 and 8 million years ago (see also Chapter 13). Evidence on the evolution of the brain comes from the study of endocasts, but these provide only very limited information about the brains of our ancestors.

We can gain more clues from the detailed information that is available from comparisons of the human brain with that of our cousins, for example macaque monkeys or chimpanzees. These comparisons suggest the ways in which the human brain has become particularly specialized. Most comparisons have been with the macaque brain, because less is known of the brain of the chimpanzee. This is unfortunate because the chimpanzee has been shown by genetic studies to be our nearest relative (Jones *et al.* 1992). There is a danger, as foreseen by Ettlinger, that differences between the human and macaque brain be taken to reveal human specializations, when some of these characteristics are also apparent in the chimpanzee brain.

The present paper therefore cites anatomical data on the chimpanzee, where available. Figure 15.1 presents photographs of the left hemisphere of a rhesus monkey (*Macaca mulatta*), a chimpanzee (*Pan troglodytes*), and a human.

Comparisons rely on the identification of areas by their cytoarchitecture. Correspondence between areas in different species is judged by whether they have the same or similar cytoarchitecture. This procedure can, of course, be challenged, but it is one that has been widely adopted. Indeed, if it were not so, it would be difficult to interpret the results of studies of the human brain using functional brain imaging (PET, fMRI). These studies reveal distributed systems, and our knowledge of anatomical connections in the macaque brain is often helpful in suggesting anatomical connections between areas within these systems. Indirect evidence of this sort can only be used if a correspondence is assumed between areas in the human and macaque brain that have similar cytoarchitecture.

It would, of course, be better to have direct evidence on the anatomical connections of the human brain. However, it is not ethical or practical to use transport methods for tracing connections in human subjects. We have limited information from studies of retrograde degeneration (e.g. Meyer *et al.* 1947) and from the application of silver techniques to post-mortem material where brains can be found with discrete lesions (e.g. Clarke 1993). By comparison, we have a very detailed wiring diagram of the macaque neocortex (Felleman and van Essen 1991; Young 1993). Crick and Jones (1993) have commented on the 'backwardness of human neuroanatomy', and no doubt methods will be discovered in the future to remedy the situation. Until that time, however, the macaque model will be essential in interpreting the results.

Both degeneration studies and transport studies provide data that are unambiguous as to whether two areas are connected via a single synapse. It is for this reason that they supplanted the earlier technique of strychnine neuronography. In this technique, strychnine was applied to a small cortical area and electrophysiological recordings were taken elsewhere to detect spikes. The problem is that strychnine might fire cells trans-synaptically. Suppose that area A projects to area B, and area B to C; if strychnine is applied to area A, spikes might be recorded in area C. For this reason, little notice has been taken of the data obtained with this method for the macaque and chimpanzee brain (Bailey *et al.* 1950).

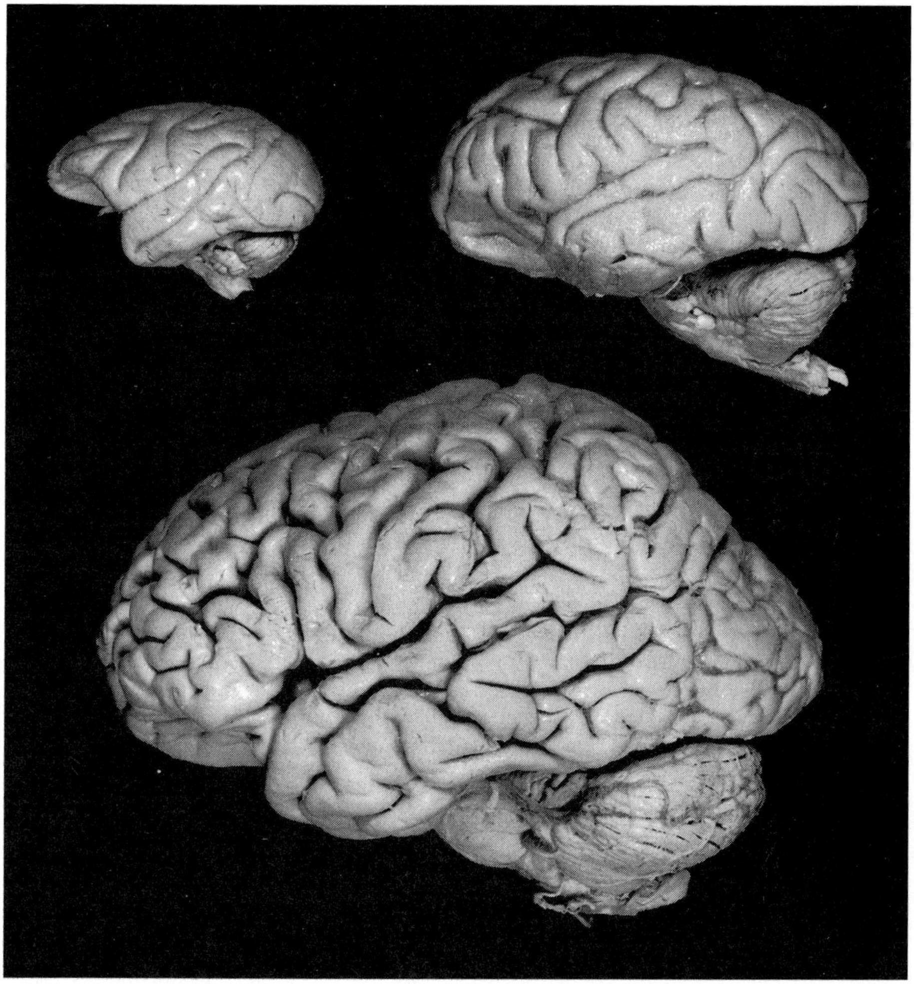

Fig. 15.1 Photographs of the brains of a rhesus monkey (*Macaca mulatta*) (top left), chimpanzee (*Pan troglodytes*) (top right), and human (bottom). The brains are shown in the correct relative sizes. George Ettlinger kindly gave me the chimpanzee brain.

The neglect may be unjustified. The connections shown for the macaque by Bailey *et al.* (1950, figure 293) can be compared with more recent charts obtained using transport methods (e.g. Young 1993). Many correspond. Consider, for example, the visual system. Bailey *et al.* (1950) give reciprocal projections between striate cortex (OC) and the cortex in the lunate sulcus (OB), where we now place V2 and V3 (Zeki 1993). Projections are given from this prestriate area to cortex anteriorly (OA) in which we now place V4 (Zeki 1993). Further projections are then described from here to infero-temporal cortex (TEO and TE). These projections have been confirmed in more detail using transport methods (Desimone and Ungerleider 1989; Young 1993). There is, however, a lack of detail in the account by Bailey *et al.* (1950) concerning the exact placement of the strychnine, and the map is clearly more coarse than that now available.

The *only* map of anatomical connections for the chimpanzee comes from the same authors, using the strychnine method (Bailey *et al.* 1950, figure 291). While accepting that results obtained with this method are not fully trustworthy, it would be foolish to ignore the chart provided. In this chapter, details of the connections claimed for the chimpanzee will be cited where the results are illuminating.

The following three sections discuss those areas that have been claimed to be unique to the human brain:

(1) Brodmann (1909) identified areas 39 and 40 in inferior parietal cortex in the human brain but not in the macaque brain.

(2) Wernicke's area is often assumed to be unique to the human brain; lesions in the left superior temporal cortex cause fluent dysphasia (Benson and Geschwind 1985), and electrical stimulation in this area interferes with language (Ojemann 1994).

(3) Finally, Brodmann (1909) identified area 44 (Broca's area) in the human but not the macaque brain.

15.2 Parietal cortex

15.2.1 The angular and supramarginal gyri

Brodmann (1909) identified areas 39 (angular gyrus) and 40 (supramarginal gyrus) below the intraparietal sulcus (IPS) in the human brain; and he identified areas 5 and 7 as lying above this sulcus (Fig. 15.2b). In the monkey (*Cercopithecus*) brain he identified only two areas: area 7 is shown as lying below the IPS, except for a small part of area 7 in the superior bank of the IPS at the back; area 5 is shown as lying superiorly to the IPS (Fig. 15.2a). However, Vogt and Vogt (1919) subdivided area 7 below the IPS into a posterior area 7a and an anterior 7b (Fig. 15.2a). Thus Brodmann's (1909) analysis of the human brain suggested two specialized areas, 39 and 40, below the intraparietal sulcus.

There are data that might be taken to support this view. In macaques, cells can be recorded in *inferior* parietal cortex which enhance their activity when the animal is required to attend covertly to visual stimuli (Bushnell *et al.* 1981). Yet when human subjects are required to attend covertly to visual stimuli, Corbetta *et al.* (1993) have reported that the peak activations lie in the *superior* rather than the inferior parietal cortex. Furthermore, when visual 'neglect' is measured by the extinction test, impairments have been reported after lesions of *inferior* parietal cortex in monkeys (Lynch and McLaren 1989), but after

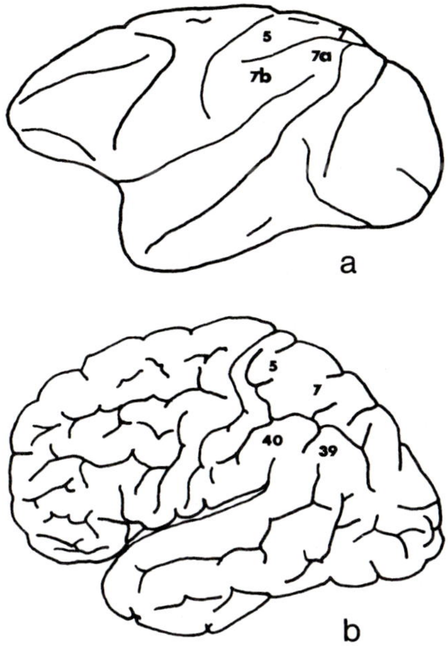

Fig. 15.2 Cytoarchitectural divisions of parietal cortex: (a) monkey (Brodmann 1909; Vogt and Vogt 1919); (b) human (Brodmann 1909).

lesions of *superior* parietal cortex in patients (Perenin and Vighetto 1988). Finally, misreaching to visual targets results from *inferior* parietal lesions in monkeys (Faugier-Grimaud *et al.* 1978; Lamotte and Acuña 1978; Rushworth *et al.* 1997) but misreaching (optic ataxia) has been claimed after *superior* parietal lesions in patients (Perenin and Vighetto 1988).

These studies could be taken to support the suggestion that there has been a fundamental reorganization of the parietal cortex in the human brain. It could then be argued that this reorganization occurred because of the development of language (Geschwind 1979). For example, Geschwind (1979) argued that when subjects read text, the information is routed to Wernicke's area via the left angular gyrus (area 39).

There is an inelegance in this story, though it is not fatal. It supposes that in evolution the homologous area shifted from one side of a sulcus to the other. It might be thought that this is not worthy of note. It is clear that in the evolution of the human brain there were 'shifts' in the location of particular areas. For example, it is agreed that there was a ventromedial shift in the visual areas. In the macaque brain, much of the primary visual cortex (area 17, V1), including the representation of the fovea, lies on the lateral surface, but in the human brain almost all of the primary visual cortex lies on the medial surface. Furthermore, PET studies suggest that the area V5 (MT) lies more ventrally in the human than in the macaque brain; whereas it lies in the fundus of the superior temporal sulcus (STS) in the macaque brain (Zeki 1993), it lies on the convexity below this sulcus in the human brain (Watson *et al.* 1993).

It could, of course, be argued that the 'intraparietal sulcus' in the human brain is not homologous with the IPS in the macaque brain. In the human brain, the 'intraparietal sulcus' often runs roughly horizontally whereas in the macaque brain it descends sharply as it runs anteriorly. Thus, it could be argued that the sulci are not the same. However, this solution is not tempting, since the IPS can run horizontally in the chimpanzee brain (Fig. 15.1).

There is, however, a solution which is more parsimonious. This directly relates the angular gyrus (39) and the supramarginal gyrus (40) in the inferior parietal cortex of the human brain to areas within the *inferior* parietal cortex in a macaque brain. The PET activations in 'superior parietal' cortex for covert attention are attributed to the visually responsive areas within and around the intraparietal sulcus. This re-analysis suggests that there may have been no fundamental change in the organization of parietal cortex.

15.2.2 Cytoarchitecture

The cytoarchitecture of the parietal cortex was re-analysed by von Economo (1929) and Eidelberg and Galaburda (1984). They used letters (PE, PF, PG) to distinguish the various areas of the human cortex. The advantage is that it is easy to label an area that is intermediate between two other areas: this can be done by combining the letters for each of the neighbouring areas. For example, below the IPS, Eidelberg and Galaburda (1984) label area 39 (angular gyrus) as PG, and area 40 (supramarginal gyrus) as PF, with an intermediate area PFG (Fig. 15.3c). Above the IPS, they identify a single area, PE. However, von Economo (1929) divided the superior cortex into an anterior PEm and a posterior PEp, and this division probably corresponds to Brodmann's 5 and 7 (Fig. 15.3c). Eidelberg and Galaburda (1984) also identified an area PEG in the ventral bank of the IPS; they believed this to be intermediate cortex between PE and PG (Fig. 15.3c).

In their analysis for the chimpanzee, Bailey *et al.* (1950) identified PG and PF below the IPS as in the human brain (Fig. 15.3b). However, they subdivided PE above the intraparietal sulcus into PEm anteriorly and PEp posteriorly. This layout corresponds to that proposed by von Economo (1929) for the human brain (Fig. 15.3c).

When von Bonin and Bailey (1947) analysed the cytoarchitecture of the rhesus monkey (*Macaca mulatta*), they identified areas PG and PF below the IPS sulcus and area PE above it (Fig. 15.3a). They therefore took PG and PF proposed by von Economo (1929) to correspond to 7a and 7b, respectively, in the macaque (Vogt and Vogt 1919). Pandya and Seltzer (1982) similarly identified PG and PF, but they also labelled an intermediate PFG, as in Eidelberg and Galaburda's chart for the human brain (Eidelberg and Galaburda 1984).

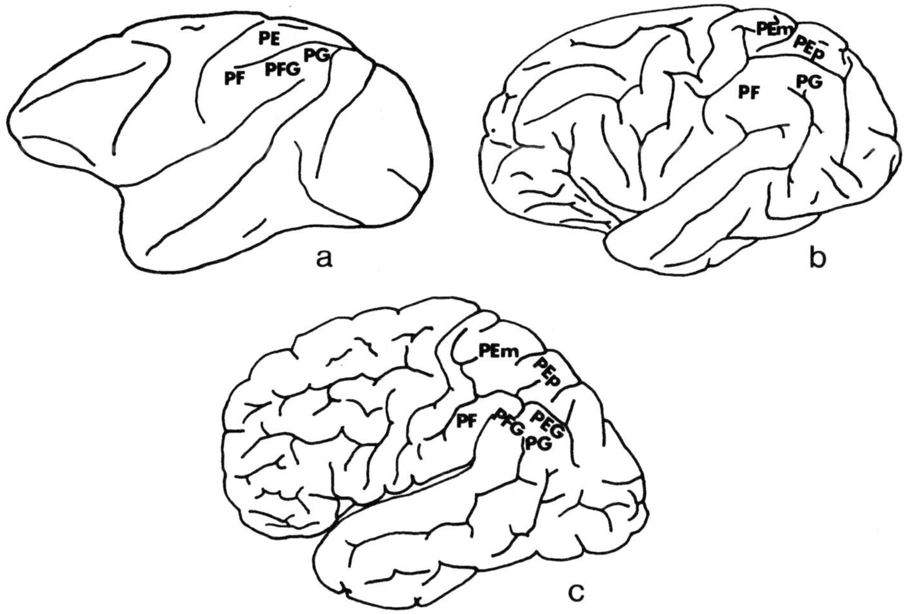

Fig. 15.3 Cytoarchitectural divisions of parietal cortex: (a) macaque (von Bonin and Bailey 1947; Pandya and Seltzer 1982); (b) chimpanzee (Bailey *et al.* 1950); and (c) human (von Economo 1929; Eidelberg and Galaburda 1984).

This re-analysis of the cytoarchitecture proposes that the areas of the inferior parietal cortex are similar in the macaque, chimpanzee, and human brain. A comparison of the numbering system in Fig. 15.2 and the letter system in Fig. 15.3 suggests that in the macaque brain PG corresponds to 7a, and PF to 7b. The intermediate area PFG corresponds to area 7ab in Fig. 15.4.

15.2.3 Behavioural functions

Attention

Many have argued that recent PET studies suggest a fundamental reorganization of the parietal lobe in the human brain. It is commonly stated that the *superior* parietal cortex is activated when subject attend covertly to visual stimuli (e.g. Corbetta *et al.* 1993). This is thought to be surprising because, in the macaque, area 7a lies *below* the IPS, and it is area 7a or more generally the 'PG complex' that receives a visual input (Desimone and Ungerleider 1989; Andersen *et al.* 1990). In the monkey, area 5 lies *above* the IPS (Brodmann 1909), and this area receives a somatic input (Pearson and Powell 1985).

However, the argument is not convincing. There are four other possibilities:

1. When the PET scans are co-registered with MRI scans, it is clear that the peak activation for covert attention to visual stimuli lies in the IPS (Nobre *et al.* 1997). Activation has also been reported in the IPS when subjects attend to the spatial aspects of a stimulus (Haxby *et al.* 1994). In the macaque brain, the area LIP is located in the *ventral* bank of the IPS (Fig. 15.4), and there are cells in this region that are active either when monkeys make overt eye movements (Andersen *et al.* 1990; Barash *et al.* 1991; Colby *et al.* 1996) or when they orient covertly (Robinson *et al.* 1995). In imaging studies of covert attention, no activation has been reported in the convexity cortex of the inferior parietal lobe. This might appear surprising, since Bushnell *et al.* (1981) reported that cells in inferior parietal cortex enhanced their rate of firing when monkeys covertly attended to visual stimuli. However, their paper makes it clear that many of these cells were in fact recorded in the ventral bank of the IPS and on the convexity nearby.

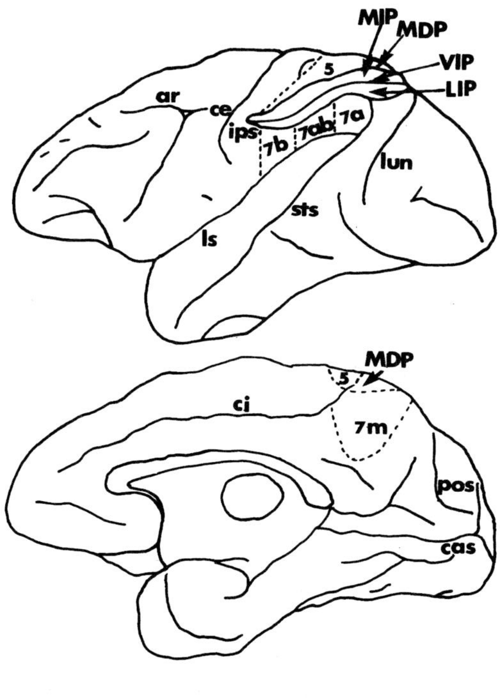

Fig. 15.4 Subareas of parietal cortex on lateral (above) and medial (below) surface of macaque brain (areas defined by Colby and Duhamel 1991). Ar, arcuate sulcus; ls, lateral sulcus; sts, superior temporal sulcus; lun, lunate sulcus; ips, intraparietal sulcus; ce, central sulcus; cas, calcarine sulcus; pos, parieto-occipital sulcus.

2. In the *superior* bank of the IPS there is area MIP in the macaque brain, which also receives a visual input (Colby and Duhamel 1991) (Fig. 15.4). Thus, visual activation in the intraparietal sulcus could also represent activation of MIP in the human brain.

3. There are also several visually receiving areas *at the back* of the IPS in the macaque brain. Even in the monkey (*Cercopithecus*) brain, Brodmann identified a small region which he labelled 7 in the superior bank of the IPS at the back. In more recent studies areas VIP, PIP, MDP, and PO have been described (Colby and Duhamel 1991). Some of these areas are shown in Fig. 15.4. Either MDP or MIP may correspond to the area labelled superior 7 by Brodmann (1909), and to the area labelled PEc by Pandya and Seltzer (1982). In the chimpanzee brain, Bailey *et al.* (1950) also claimed that there was a projection from prestriate cortex (OA) to the posterior part of the superior parietal lobule in the area that they labelled PEp.

4. Finally, in the macaque brain, area 7m (PGm) lies on the medial surface (Fig. 15.4). This area is connected with 7a (Andersen *et al.* 1990). In the chimpanzee brain, Bailey *et al.* (1950) identified PEp both on the medial surface and the lateral surface. It is possible that, in both the chimpanzee and human brains, area 7m has expanded on to the superior parietal surface.

Reaching

It has been shown that lesions of the *inferior* parietal cortex cause monkeys to misreach (Faugier-Grimaud *et al.* 1978; Lamotte and Acuña 1978; Rushworth *et al.* 1997). Yet, it has been claimed that in humans optic ataxia (misreaching) is caused by *superior* lesions. However, the lesions that cause optic ataxia lie in the vicinity of the intraparietal sulcus (Pierrot-Deseilligny *et al.* 1986; Perenin and Vighetto 1988), and lesions confined to the superior parietal lobe may not cause optic ataxia (Pause *et al.* 1989). There is no conflict. The lesions that were made in the monkeys included area LIP in the ventral bank of the intraparietal sulcus. It is clear that the lesions described by Perenin and Vighetto in patients included both banks of this sulcus. Furthermore, in a recent PET study Clower *et al.* (1996) found activation of the ventral bank of the IPS when subjects learned to reach under conditions in which they saw the targets through distorting prisms.

15.2.4 PET imaging of areas 39 and 40

In the macaque, the anterior and posterior divisions of inferior parietal cortex differ radically in their inputs and outputs. Area 7a receives visual projections (Andersen *et al.* 1990), and sends projections to dorsal prefrontal cortex (area 46) (Cavada and Goldman-Rakic 1989). Area 7b (PF) receives a projection from somatosensory cortex SI (Vogt and Pandya 1978; Pandya and Seltzer 1982), and sends projections to premotor cortex area 6 (Petrides and Pandya 1984; Matelli *et al.* 1986).

On the basis of strychnine neuronography, Bailey *et al.* (1950) claimed similar connections in the chimpanzee. They report that area PG (7a) receives an input from prestriate area OA, and that it sends a projection to the inferior frontal sulcus (area FD). In the human brain, this area lies in the dorsal prefrontal cortex; in a macaque it lies posteriorly within the principal sulcus in dorsal prefrontal cortex. They also report that area PF (7b) receives an input from somatosensory cortex PC, and sends a projection to the premotor cortex (areas FB, FC). We do not know the connections of these areas in the human brain, but given the similarity in the layout of the inferior parietal cortex in the human and chimpanzee brain (Fig. 15.3b,c), the most parsimonious assumption is that they are as described for the chimpanzee.

If so, it should be possible to demonstrate, using functional brain imaging, that the supramarginal gyrus (40, PF) is activated during motor tasks involving somatic information, and that the angular gyrus (39, PG) is activated during tasks involving visual information. This expectation is fulfilled. Area 40 (PF) is activated when subjects select between movements (Deiber *et al.* 1991; Jueptner *et al.* 1997*b*), decide when to make movements (Jahanshahi *et al.* 1995), prepare to make movements (Deiber *et al.* 1996, Krams *et al.* in press), or learn new sequences of movement (Jenkins *et al.* 1994; Jueptner *et al.* 1997*a*). The subjects performed with their eyes closed in some of these studies (Deiber *et al.* 1991; Jahanshahi *et al.* 1995; Jueptner *et al.* 1997*a,b*).

It is less easy to interpret PET studies in which activation is claimed in area 39 (PF). Unless the PET scans are co-registered with MRI scans, it is often difficult to tell whether the peak activation lies in the angular gyrus (area 39, PG) or in prestriate cortex (area 19) which lies directly behind it. For example, Kosslyn *et al.* (1994) reported activation of the angular gyrus when subjects have to identify objects from unusual views; but the coordinates are very close to area 19. Schwartz *et al.* (1995) claimed activation of the angular gyrus when subjects remembered abstract visual stimuli, and Paulesu *et al.* (1993) when subjects read and remembered Korean letters with which they were not familiar. However, without co-registering the PET scans to MRI scans, one cannot be certain that the activations lay in area 39 (PG) rather than in area 19. None the less, it remains a possibility that area 39 might be involved in the visuospatial processing of patterns, including letters.

In a recent study, Fink *et al.* (1997) required subjects to make a visuospatial judgement about a simple pattern. The subjects were presented with lines to the left or right of the fixation point, and were required to judge, without moving the eyes, on which end of a line a box was presented. In this study the PET data were co-registered with the MRI scans. There was activation which clearly lay within the angular gyrus, perhaps in area PFG.

The study by Fink *et al.* (1997) is important because the subjects were tested on their ability to *locate* an object with reference to a line. Mishkin *et al.* (1982) removed inferior parietal cortex, area 7, and showed that the animals were impaired when required to locate a foodwell with reference to a landmark. More studies are needed in which subjects are required to make allocentric spatial judgements. This is of especial importance since there are two studies in which it has been shown that lesions in the angular gyrus can cause visuospatial neglect in patients (Vallar and Perani 1986; Miklossy 1993).

15.2.5 Conclusion

According to this account, there has been no fundamental reorganization of the parietal cortex in the human brain. If this is so, there is a need to explain why neuropsychological studies have suggested a specialization of the left inferior parietal cortex for language (Geschwind 1979). The next section considers the language areas, and argues that the critical area is not the angular gyrus but the temporo-parietal area, Tpt.

15.3 Wernicke's area

In the present account, the term 'Wernicke's area' will be used to refer to the temporo-parietal cortex that can be shown to be involved directly in the analysis of spoken or written language. The borders of this area cannot be easily defined by analysing the effects of strokes: plotting the centre (Benson 1967) or the extent (Naeser 1994) of infarcts is a crude way of trying to delimit an area. However, Wernicke's area has been charted by the effects of electrical stimulation in disturbing speech (Penfield and Roberts 1959; Ojemann 1994). It will be seen from Fig. 15.5 that the sites include the superior temporal gyrus (area 22), the middle temporal gyrus (area 21), the temporo-parietal cortex round the back of the sylvian fissure (area Tpt), and inferior parietal perisylvian cortex. Figure 15.6c shows the location of these different cytoarchitectural areas in the human brain.

Functional brain imaging can also be used to chart the extent of Wernicke's area, and to distinguish the various specialized subareas within the larger region. This discussion will be restricted to differences that have been claimed between these areas in the human brain compared with the macaque or chimpanzee brain.

15.3.1 Area 22

The first of these is the functional asymmetry between the temporo-parietal cortex in the left and right hemisphere. Though the right (non-dominant) superior temporal cortex is activated when subjects process words, the activation on the left is very much more extensive when the activity for hearing sounds is subtracted (Demonet *et al.* 1992). It is widely believed that this dominance is unique to the human brain.

This belief is unfounded. Heffner and Heffner (1986) trained macaques (*Macaca fuscata*) to distinguish between different calls made by members of the same species. They then compared the effects of removing either the left or the

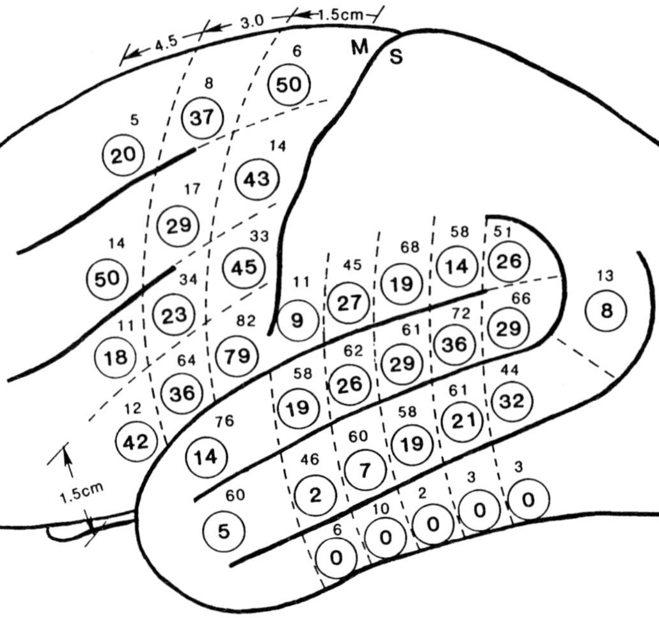

Fig. 15.5 Effects of stimulating temporal (and frontal) cortex in 117 patients. For each zone the upper number gives the number of subjects in which that zone was stimulated during naming. The lower number gives the percentage of patients with significant evoked errors in naming. (From Ojemann 1994.)

right superior temporal cortex (area 22) (Fig. 15.6a). The results were clearcut. Removal of the left area 22 resulted in a severe impairment in the ability to discriminate calls, whereas removal of the right was without effect.

It may, of course, be true that in the left area 22 of the human brain there are fine anatomical specializations which are not to be found in area 22 of either the macaque or chimpanzee brain. For example, Penhume *et al.* (1996) have reported that there is an asymmetry between the left and right auditory cortex in the human brain, and Seldon (1985) has claimed that the centre to centre distance between columns in the left auditory cortex is greater than in the right. Similarly, Galaburda *et al.* (1978) have reported an asymmetry in the temporo-parietal area, Tpt (Fig. 15.6c). It is, however, premature to assume that these asymmetries are unique to the human brain. In great apes the left sylvian fissure tends to be longer (Yeni-Komshian and Benson 1976) and to run lower (LeMay 1976) than the right; this is the same pattern as in the human brain (LeMay 1976; Rubens 1977). Witelson and Kigar (1992) have related the course of the sylvian fissure to handedness. Comparative studies are now needed of the fine architecture of the temporal and parietal cortex in the human brain and the ape brain.

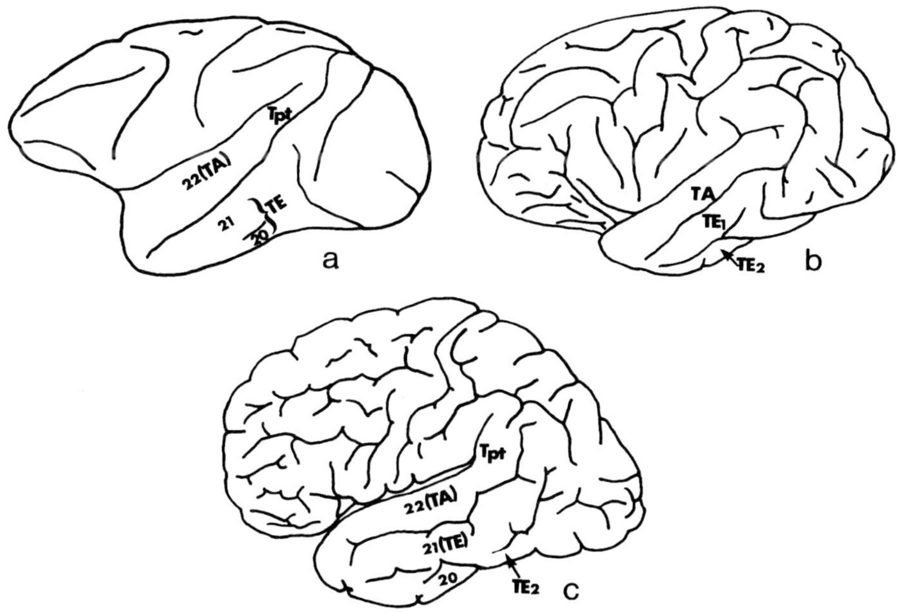

Fig. 15.6 Cytoarchitectural divisions of temporal cortex: (a) monkey (Brodmann 1909; von Bonin and Bailey 1947; Galaburda and Pandya 1983); (b) chimpanzee (Bailey *et al.* 1950); (c) human (Brodmann 1909; von Economo 1929; Galaburda *et al.* 1978).

15.3.2 Area 21

There is an apparent difference in the functions of area 21 in the human and monkey brain. This area forms the middle temporal gyrus in the human brain; that is, the convexity cortex between the superior and middle temporal sulci (STS and MTS) (Brodmann 1909; see Fig. 15.6c). It was labelled TE1 by von Economo (1929), with TE2 corresponding to area 20 which lies ventral to the MTS (Fig. 15.6c). In the chimpanzee, Bailey *et al.* (1950) distinguished TE1 between the STS and MTS, and TE2 ventromedially to the MTS as in the human brain (Fig. 15.6b). In the macaque brain, area 21 forms the ventral convexity of the temporal lobe, between the STS and MTS (Fig. 15.6a), though the latter is usually just a short furrow. Area 20 lies more medially, ventral to the MTS. The term TE is used to include both area 21 and 20 in the macaque brain (von Bonin and Bailey 1947).

In macaques, areas 21 and 20 (TE) act as *visual* association cortex. Lesions of areas 21 and 20 cause severe impairments in visual discrimination (Mishkin 1972), but an inferotemporal lesion has no effects on the ability to discriminate sounds (Dewson *et al.* 1969). Area 21 (TE) receives *visual* (Desimone and Ungerleider 1989) but not *auditory* (Pandya and Yeterian 1985) input, and single unit responses to visual stimuli can be recorded in area 21 (TE) (Miller and Desimone 1993, Tanaka 1993). Yet, there are PET studies in which it is claimed that the middle temporal gyrus (area 21, TE1) is activated—together with area 22—when human subjects repeat words that they hear (Howard *et al.* 1992), make judgements about adjective–noun pairs that they hear (Demonet *et al.* 1992), or generate verbs that are semantically related to nouns that they hear (Fiez *et al.* 1996). Furthermore, Creutzfeldt and Ojemann (1990) have recorded from single or multi-units during surgery on human patients, and they report that there are responses in the middle temporal gyrus when subjects respond to *spoken* words. Electrical stimulation of the middle temporal gyrus has also been reported to disturb the ability to produce spoken words (Penfield and Roberts 1959; Ojemann 1994) (Fig. 15.5).

It is easy to see how a visual association area could handle words that are presented visually. The problem is that in the human brain, but not in the macaque brain, the claim is that there are responses to words whether they are presented auditorily or visually (Howard *et al.* 1992; Fiez *et al.* 1996). One interpretation is that the development of language has led to a reorganization, such that the middle temporal gyrus handles words whether they are read or heard.

It is possible that there has been a shift in the location of certain areas. As mentioned before, there is evidence for a ventral shift in visual areas within the human temporal lobe. In the macaque brain the area V5 (MT) lies in the fundus of the STS, but PET studies locate V5 in the human brain on the middle temporal convexity (Watson *et al.* 1993). In the macaque brain, there are areas in the upper bank of the STS that are interconnected with the auditory association cortex (area 22) (Seltzer and Pandya 1991). It is possible that in the human brain these areas are to be found more ventrally, in the middle temporal gyrus.

However, there are two other ways of explaining the PET findings, each without supposing that there has been such a shift. The first is that the activations for words that are heard may lie in the STS, and not in the middle temporal gyrus. The PET studies by Howard *et al.* (1992) and Demonet *et al.* (1992) give coordinates for a group of subjects rather than for single subjects, and these studies locate the peaks of the activations by reference to an atlas (Talairach and Tournoux 1988) rather than by reference to the MRI scans of the individual patients. It is not possible from such studies to distinguish between activation of the middle temporal gyrus and activation of the upper bank of the STS. In group scans with considerable secondary filtering, activations show up as extensive swathes, whereas in individual scans with less secondary filtering they show as smaller peaks. When co-registered with the individual MRI scans it is possible to be much more accurate about the exact location of an activation.

A second possibility is that the activation *does* lie in the middle temporal gyrus, but that it is related not to the words as heard but to the *meaning* of the words. PET studies have shown that there is activation of widely distributed systems in the brain when subjects perform perceptual or cognitive tasks. For example, when subjects name pictures of tools, there is activation not only in visual areas but also in motor areas such as the premotor cortex and cerebellum (Martin *et al.* 1996). These motor areas are activated because the picture of the tool is associated with the use of the tool; it would clearly be wrong to conclude that the activation of these motor areas implies that they are involved in the visual analysis. Functional brain imaging shows the activation of the whole distributed network.

A similar argument can be used when considering the temporal lobe. Vandenberghe *et al.* (1996) have scanned subjects while they make semantic judgements. When presented with three words, the subjects had to decide which two words were most closely semantically related; subjects were required to judge that, for example, 'pliers' rather than 'saw' went with 'spanner'. The same task was also presented in pictorial form, with pictures of the relevant objects. The control task involved judging which of two objects was bigger than a third, and again the problems were set either by presenting the names of the objects or pictures of the objects. There was activation of the middle temporal gyrus (21, TE1) as well as in the inferior temporal gyrus (20, TE2) whether the semantic judgements were made in response to words or pictures.

The same experiment could be carried out with the difference that the semantic judgements had to be made on the basis of words that were *heard*. If area 21 was activated whether the words were read or heard, the suggestion would be that the activation was related to the semantic analysis of words, and that it represented the manipulation of knowledge about the objects to which the words referred. In monkeys, areas 21 and 20 form part of the 'object identification system' (Mishkin *et al.* 1983). This system is accessed when we make semantic judgements about words that refer to objects, and it may be amodal.

15.3.3 Tpt

When Brodmann (1909) studied the cytoarchitecture of the primate brain, he failed to note a distinctive area of temporo-parietal cortex. This is the area Tpt, described both for the rhesus monkey (Galaburda and Pandya 1983) and human brain (Galaburda and Sanides 1980). It is shown in Fig. 15.6. In the macaque brain it lies posteriorly in the superior temporal gyrus (Fig. 15.6a), but in the human brain it also extends round the back of the sylvian fissure and on to the ventral surface of the parietal cortex (Fig. 15.6c).

Unfortunately, in their description of the cytoarchitecture of the chimpanzee, Bailey *et al.* (1950) did not identify this area, and thus we do not know its extent. This is particularly unfortunate, because Galaburda *et al.* (1978) have shown that it is larger in the dominant than in the non-dominant hemisphere in the human brain, and until it is identified in the chimpanzee brain, we do not know whether there is a similar asymmetry in that species.

It is essential that the area Tpt be distinguished from the angular gyrus, area 39. Ojemann (1994) has reported that stimulation around the back of the sylvian fissure disrupts language (see Fig. 15.5), and this area corresponds to Tpt. Infarcts that involve the angular gyrus will usually include area Tpt as well. Thus the effects of such strokes on language and reading may result, not from damage to the angular gyrus (area 39), but to damage to area Tpt which lies directly in front. To distinguish the contribution of these areas, one needs to scan subjects while they perform language tasks.

Vandenberge *et al.* (1996) compared judgements made on the basis of written words or pictures. When they compared presentation in words or pictures, there was activation round the back of the sylvian fissure. In the atlas of Talairach and Tournoux (1988) the activation lies within the area that is labelled 39. However, it clearly corresponds to the location of area Tpt as described by Galaburda *et al.* (1978). Price *et al.* (1997) also report activation in this region when subjects name objects rather than colours.

15.3.4 Conclusion

It is reasonable to expect that the development of language is associated with specializations in the human temporal lobe. Apart from proportionate changes in the size of the different subregions, there may be finer architectural specializations and new anatomical connections. None the less, it has been argued that *the basic organization* of Wernicke's area is similar in the human and macaque brain. It is now important that detailed comparisons be made between the human and chimpanzee brain.

15.4 Broca's area

15.4.1 Cytoarchitecture

Broca's area is usually taken to be the inferior frontal areas *pars opercularis* and *pars triangularis*. These correspond to Brodmann's areas 44 and 45. Brodmann (1909) did not recognize either area in the brain of a *Cercopithecus* monkey. In his cytoarchitectural map of the human brain, von Economo (1929) labels *pars opercularis* as FCBm (Brodmann 44), and *pars triangularis* as FD (Brodmann 45) (Fig. 15.7c). Thus he classified *pars opercularis* as being part of premotor cortex (FB and FC), and *pars triangularis* as being part of the prefrontal cortex (FD).

In the chimpanzee, Bailey *et al.* (1950) identified area FCBm as lying in front of the 'anterior subcentral sulcus' (Fig. 15.7b). This sulcus appears to be a continuation of the sulcus that they label the 'inferior precentral sulcus'. Thus, this area can be regarded as being in the same general location as area 44 in the human brain.

When von Bonin and Bailey (1947) examined the brain of the rhesus monkey (*Macaca mulatta*), they identified the area FCBm as lying in the ventral premotor cortex, including the posterior bank of the inferior limb of the arcuate sulcus (Fig. 15.7a). They also identified an area FDγ in the anterior

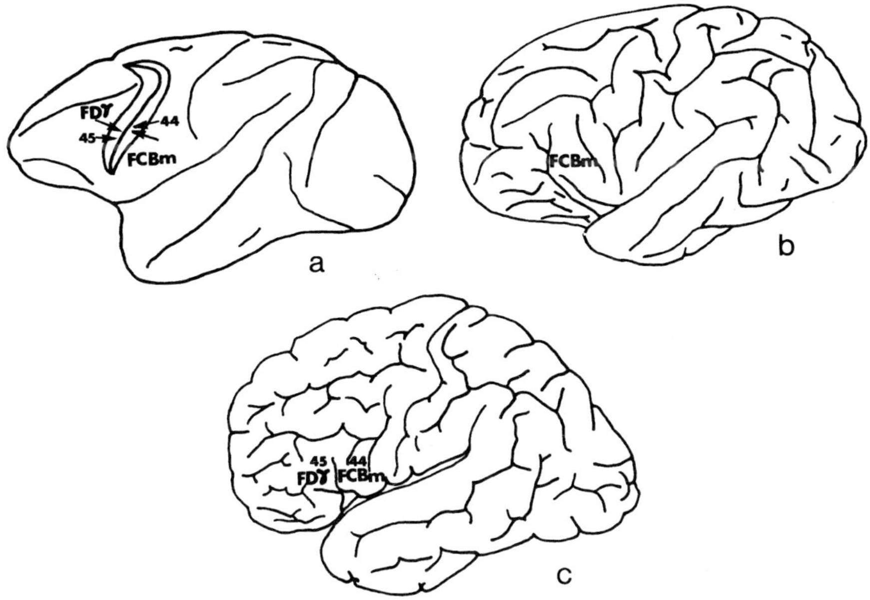

Fig. 15.7 Cytoarchitectural divisions of the inferior frontal cortex: (a) macaque (von Bonin and Bailey 1947; Matelli *et al.* 1986*b*; Petrides and Pandya 1995), b = chimpanzee (Bailey *et al.* 1950), c = human (Brodmann 1909; von Economo 1929; Petrides and Pandya 1995).

bank of the inferior limb of the arcuate sulcus. This roughly corresponds to Walker's (1940) area 45.

More recently, Petrides and Pandya (1995) have re-analysed the cytoarchitecture of the frontal lobe in man and macaque. Unlike Brodmann (1909), they suggest that area 44 can be identified in the macaque brain, and they place it in the posterior bank of the inferior limb of the arcuate sulcus (Fig. 15.7). Galaburda and Pandya (1982) made the same suggestion. The posterior bank of the limb of the arcuate sulcus is a part of the larger area FCBm, as identified by von Bonin and Bailey (1947). It also includes the area identified as F5 on the basis of staining with cytochrome oxidase (Matelli *et al.* 1985).

Like Walker (1940), Petrides and Pandya also identify area 45 in the macaque brain. However, both in the human and macaque brain, they divided it into 45B and 45A. In the macaque brain, 45B lies in the anterior bank of the inferior limb of the arcuate sulcus, and 45A lies more anteriorly on the inferior prefrontal convexity. In the human brain 45B is shown as lying in *pars triangularis*, and area 45A more anteriorly on the inferior prefrontal convexity.

15.4.2 Connections

It is often repeated in the literature that the arcuate fasciculus runs from Wernicke's area to Broca's area (e.g. Benson and Geschwind 1985). But the exact region of termination of the arcuate fasciculus has never been identified. As mentioned earlier, it would not be ethical to use the transport method for anatomical tracing in the human brain. It would be possible to use the silver method to identify terminal degeneration in a brain with a small lesion restricted to area Tpt, but this has not yet been attempted.

However, we do know the anatomical inputs of areas 44 and 45 as identified in the macaque brain. Area F5 (44?) receives an input from anterior inferior parietal cortex, including the area AIP in the ventral bank of the inferior parietal sulcus (Matelli *et al.* 1986; Pandya and Yeterian, 1996*a*). In both AIP and F5 there are cells that respond to visually presented objects that the monkey can reach and grasp (Rizzolatti *et al.* 1988; Sakata *et al.* 1995; Gallese *et al.* 1996). There are also cells that are responsive to touch. Using strychnine neuronography, Bailey *et al.* (1950) claimed that there was a projection from PF (anterior inferior parietal cortex) to FCBm in both macaque and chimpanzee.

Galaburda and Pandya (1982) claim that in the macaque there is an input from area Tpt to the posterior bank of the inferior limb of the arcuate sulcus (area 6, F5), but these data have never been published in full, and no other studies have reported this connection (e.g. Matelli *et al.* 1986). However, it is clear that there are auditory inputs to the inferior prefrontal convexity, and in particular to area 45A (Pandya and Yeterian 1996*a*). Mesulam (1990) claims that the superior temporal auditory association cortex sends projections to the *opercular* cortex lying ventral to the inferior limb of arcuate sulcus, and it is possible that it was this projection that was detected by Galaburda and Pandya (1982). There is clearly a need for further studies to clarify the exact region of termination of the fibres from the auditory association cortex.

15.4.3 Functional imaging

Macaque and man

PET can be used to test the hypothesis that the area F5 in the macaque brain corresponds to area 44 in the human brain. In the inferior limb of the arcuate sulcus (F5) there are cells with activity that is related to movements of the hand, mouth, or face (Gentilucci *et al.* 1988). Movements of the intrinsic laryngeal muscles can also be evoked by microstimulation in the sulcus and on the convexity below (Hast *et al.* 1974).

Two types of neurone are of especial interest. First, there are neurones that fire while monkeys view an object, reach to and then grasp it (Rizzolatti *et al.* 1988). For comparison, PET scans have therefore been taken while human subjects reach and grasp objects (Grafton *et al.* 1996). Though activation was reported in the dorsal premotor cortex, no activation was reported more ventrally. However, in monkeys the increase in activity often starts when the objects are presented and while the monkeys *prepare* to reach (Rizzolatti, personal communication). In a recent study, we have found activation in Broca's area 44 when subjects view a hand, and prepare to move a finger (Krams *et al.* in press). A finger was briefly marked, and the subjects waited for 3 seconds before moving that finger; the comparison condition was moving a finger as soon as it was marked. Activation also occurs in Broca's area when subjects imagine movements (Stephan *et al.* 1995).

The second type of neurone of interest are the 'mirror' neurones described by Gallese *et al.* (1996). These neurones fire when the monkey watches while the experimenter grasps and manipulates objects. An attempt has therefore been made using PET to identify the area corresponding to F5 by requiring subjects to watch while movements are made. In one study there was no activation in Broca's area (Decety *et al.* 1994); however, comparison was made, not with a resting condition, but with a condition in which the subjects inspected the object; and in that condition the subjects may have thought of the use of the objects. In another study, activation was found in the left area 45, but more anteriorly than expected (Rizzolatti *et al.* 1996*b*). However, in a recent fMRI study, activation of Broca's area has been reported when subjects copy movements (Erhard *et al.* 1996).

Unfortunately, no PET studies have been carried out to identify the premotor areas for the larynx. However, in the study mentioned above, Krams *et al.* (in press) also scanned subjects while they prepared to say letters. In one condition a letter appeared on the palm of a hand, and the subjects rehearsed that letter for 3 seconds before saying it; in the comparison condition they said the letter as soon as it appeared. Again there was activation in Broca's area 44. The peaks for preparing to move a finger and for preparing to say a letter appeared to have a similar location in *pars opercularis*. However, more studies are needed to map this area. Using fMRI, Erhard *et al.* (1996) have reported differences in localization for the tongue, toe, finger, and larynx.

If it can be shown that F5 in a macaque and area 44 in man are related, one can speculate about the evolution of this area. Rizzolatti *et al.* (1996*a*) have suggested that vocal communication evolved from facial gestures such as 'lip smacks'. An alternative is that the basic mechanism is one of repeating or copying. Old World primates repeat certain calls such as alarm calls. Gallese *et al.* (1996) have shown that there are 'mirror neurones' in F5, and these probably form the mechanism for the copying of actions that are viewed. If it can be confirmed that there are auditory projections to the underlying opercular cortex (Mesulam 1990), it is possible that the area provides the mechanism for producing sounds that match those that are heard. When human subjects make phonetic discriminations, there is activity in Broca's area (Zatorre *et al.* 1996), as would be predicted from the motor theory of speech perception (Liberman and Mattingly 1985).

Localization within Broca's area

In macaque monkeys, it is established that area 45 receives an auditory input from the superior temporal association cortex (Pandya and Yeterian 1996*a*). Fiez *et al.* (1995) have required subjects to detect tone triplets, consonant–vowel syllables, or three-letter words. They report activation in the left inferior frontal cortex, in a region they identify as area 45. This area was also activated when subjects discriminated whether words presented auditorily or visually had long vowels, but not when they discriminated whether the words had ascending letters (such as 'l'). These results implicate the area in phonological but not orthographic processing.

In the studies reported by Zatorre *et al.* (1996) the subjects discriminated between words that did or did not end in consonants, and in which the pitch of the second syllable was higher than the first. They found activations with a peak more posteriorly in Broca's area, and they suggest that they lie in area 44. The studies of Fiez *et al.* (1995) and Zatorre *et al.* (1996) differ in the control condition used. In the former it was fixation, and in the latter passive listening. This may matter, because Warburton *et al.* (1996) report activation anteriorly in Broca's area when subjects listen passively. Thus, in the studies reported by Zatorre *et al.* (1996), activation of area 45 may be subtracted out when a comparison is made with passive listening.

In none of these studies were the peaks of activation localized by co-registering the PET images with individual MRI scans. This means that, at the moment, it is a dubious procedure to try to allocate the peaks of activation to either area 44 or 45. To do so, one needs to visualize the sulcal pattern on MRI scans. Even when that is done, the results must be tentative, given the variation in cytoarchitecture of different brains.

15.5 Specializations

Brodmann (1909) identified specialized areas in the parietal and frontal lobe that he believed to be unique to the human brain. The literature is full of remarks that the human brain is specialized in this way and that. The present chapter has taken the areas for which these claims have most often been made; and the conclusion is that the *basic organization* of these areas may not differ from that found in the macaque or chimpanzee. By the term 'basic organization' I mean the general layout. For example, it has been argued here that there has been no functional shift from inferior to superior parietal cortex in the human brain.

However, this is not to say that there are no important *specializations* in the human brain. It would be very strange if there were none. When Preuss and Goldman-Rakic (1991) compared the brains of macaque monkey and bushbaby, they could distinguish areas 8A, 8B, and 45 in the bushbaby, but they could not identify a separate area 46. Area 46 in the macaque may have *differentiated* out of areas 8 and 8A or more medial cortex; it is similar in being involved in the selection of eye movements (Passingham 1993). In macaques, area 46 is *similar* to area 8 in having inputs from visual areas, but it differs in that these come from later stages of visual processing (Barbas and Pandya 1991). It would be strange if such specializations did not occur in the human brain.

The point is best illustrated by taking an example. It is claimed here that in Broca's area the regions 44 and 45 have *similarities* with the regions labelled 44 and 45 by Petrides and Pandya (1995) in the macaque brain. This claim is illuminating in three respects. First, it suggests that Broca's area includes two quite separate regions, a premotor area (44) and a prefrontal area (45). Secondly, it suggests that these two regions may differ in their inputs, from inferior parietal cortex to area 44, and from superior temporal cortex to area 45. Thirdly, there is a suggestion that, as in area F5 in the macaque brain, there is a representation in human area 44 of the hand and arm as well as the mouth and larynx.

The claim is, however, limited. It has been said that regions in the human and ape or macaque brain are *similar*. One might also say that they are *homologous*. Such a claim is a claim about evolutionary history, about the common origins of structures in two species. It is neither a claim about the relative *development* of the structures in the two species, nor a claim about *functional capacity*. Thus, it is illuminating to observe that the Wulst in birds and the neocortex in mammals may contain homologous regions to the dorsal ventricular ridge in reptiles (Benowitz 1980; Butler 1980), but this claim says nothing about the differentiation of the region in the different orders, nor about the efficiency with which the structures process information.

In the same way, it may be illuminating to say that the dorsal prefrontal cortex in macaque brains evolved as a late stage in an evolutionary trend for sequential architectonic differentiation that originates in archicortex (Sanides 1970; Pandya and Yeterian 1996*b*). But one should be wary of suggestions that, for example, the medial frontal cortex in a rat is the 'same' as the dorsal prefrontal cortex in a macaque. Although the dorsal frontal cortex may have evolved out of the more medial frontal cortex (Sanides 1970), it is not to be identified as 'the same as' the medial cortex of a rat (Preuss 1995). In macaques the dorsal prefrontal cortex has a different architecture and different connections, and the working memory of macaques is much superior to that of rats (Preuss 1995).

The claims made in this chapter only concern the *basic organization* of regions, and suggestions have been made as to possible homologies between regions in the human brain and regions in the brains of macaques or chimpanzees. But even if some of the suggestions are correct, no claims have been made concerning *functional capacity*. For example, human beings can pronounce consonants and speak grammatical sentences, but macaques and chimpanzees cannot. The implication is that there has been an elaboration of the mechanisms possessed by the common ancestors of humans, ape and monkey. The claim that area 44 can be detected in the macaque brain

(Petrides and Pandya 1995) is not a claim that the area is *identical* in cytoarchitecture to area 44 in the human brain; simply a claim that there are *similarities*. While Broca's area may be homologous, in that the area in man and monkey evolved out of an area shared by a common ancestor, it has without doubt become further differentiated. To say that area 44 is the same in humans and monkeys is probably as misleading as the claim that the medial frontal cortex in a rat is the same as dorsal prefrontal cortex in a macaque. The challenge is now to study the microstructure and the connections so as to reveal the specializations.

Acknowledgements

I am grateful to Matthew Rushworth with whom these ideas have been generated. David Milner and Amanda Parker made helpful comments on the manuscript.

References

Andersen, R. A., Asanuma, C., Essick, G., and Siegel, R. M. (1990). Corticocortical connections of anatomically and physiologically defined subdivisions within the inferior parietal lobule. *Journal of Comparative Neurology*, **296**, 65–113.

Bailey, P., von Bonin, G., and McCullogh, W. S. (1950). *The isocortex of the chimpanzee*. University of Illinois Press, Urbana.

Barash, S., Bracewell, R. M., Fogassi, L., Gnadt, J. W., and Andersen, R. A. (1991). Saccade-related activity in the lateral intraparietal area. I. Spatial properties. *Journal of Neurophysiology*, **66**, 1109–24.

Barbas, H. and Pandya, D. N. (1991). Pattern of connections of the prefrontal cortex in the rhesus monkey associated with cortical architecture. In *Frontal lobe function and dysfunction*, (ed. H. S. Levin, H. M. Eisenberg, and A. L. Benton), pp. 35–58. Oxford University Press, New York.

Benowitz, L. (1980). Functional organization of the avian telencephalon. In *Comparative Neurology of the Telencephalon*, (ed. S. O. E. Ebbeson), pp. 389–422. Plenum, New York.

Benson, D. F. (1967). Fluency in aphasia: correlation with radioactive scan localization. *Cortex*, **3**, 373–94.

Benson, D. F. and Geschwind, N. (1985). Aphasia and related disorders: a clinical approach. In *Principles of behavioral neurology*, (ed. M.-M. Mesulam), pp. 193–238. Davis, Philadelphia.

Brodmann, K. (1909). *Vergleichende Lokalisationlehre der Grosshirnrinde*. Barth, Leipzig.

Bushnell, M. C., Goldberg, M. E., and Robinson, D. L. (1981). Behavioral enhancement of visual responses in monkey cerebral cortex. I. Modulation in posterior parietal cortex related to selective visual attention. *Journal of Neurophysiology*, **46**, 755–72.

Butler, A. (1980). Cytoarchitecture and connectional organization of the Lacertilian telencephalon with comments on vertebrate forebrain evolution. In *Comparative neurology of the telencephalon*, (ed. S. O. E. Ebbesson), pp. 297–330. Plenum, New York.

Cavada, C. and Goldman-Rakic, P.S. (1989). Posterior parietal cortex in rhesus monkey: II. Evidence for segregated corticocortical networks linking sensory and limbic areas with the frontal lobe. *Journal of Comparative Neurology*, **287**, 422–45.

Clarke, S. (1993). Callosal connections and functional subdivision of the human occipital cortex. In *Functional organisation of the human visual cortex,* (ed. B. Gulyás, D. Ottoson, and P. E. Roland), pp. 138–49. Pergamon, Oxford.

Clower, D. M., Hoffman, J. M., Votaw, J. R., Faber, T. L., Woods, R. P., and Alexander, G. E. (1996). Role of posterior parietal cortex in the recalibration of visually guided reaching. *Nature*, **383**, 618–21.

Colby, C. L. and Duhamel, J.-R. (1991). Heterogeneity of extrastriate visual areas and multiple parietal areas in the macaque monkey. *Neuropsychologia*, **29**, 517–37.

Colby, C. L. Duhamel, J.-R., and Goldberg, M. E. (1996). Visual, presaccadic, and cognitive activation of single neurons in monkey lateral intraparietal area. *Journal of Neurophysiology*, **76**, 2841–51.

Corbetta, M., Miezin, F. M., Shulman, G. L., and Petersen, S. E. (1993). A PET study of visuospatial attention. *Journal of Neuroscience*, **13**, 1202–26.

Creutzfeldt, O. D. and Ojemann, G. (1990). Neuronal responses in the human temporal lobe. In *The principles of design and operations of the brain*, (ed. J. C. Eccles and O. Creutzfeldt), pp. 501–17. Vatican City, Rome.

Crick, F. and Jones, E. (1993) Backwardness of human neuroanatomy. *Nature*, **361**, 109–10.

Decety, J., Perani, D., Jeannerod, M., Bettinardi, V., Padary, B., Woods, R. *et al.* (1994). Mapping motor representations with positron emission tomography. *Nature*, **371**, 600–2.

Deiber, M.-P., Passingham, R. E., Colebatch, J. G., Friston, K. J., Nixon, P. D., and Frackowiak, R. S. J. (1991). Cortical areas and the selection of movement: a study with positron emission tomography. *Experimental Brain Research*, **84**, 393–402.

Deiber, M.-P., Ibanez, V., Sadato, N., and Hallett, M. (1996). The cerebral structures participating in motor preparation in humans: a positron emission tomography study. *Journal of Neurophysiology*, **75**, 233–47.

Demonet, J.-F., Chollet, F., Ramsay, S., Cardebat, D., Nespoulos, J.-L., and Wise, R. (1992). The anatomy of phonological and semantic processing in normal subjects. *Brain*, **115**, 1753–68.

Desimone, R. and Ungerleider, L. G. (1989). Neural mechanisms of visual processing in monkeys. In *Handbook of neuropsychology*, Vol. 2, (ed. F. Boller and J. Grafman), pp. 267–99. Elsevier, New York.

Dewson, J. H., Pribram, K. H., and Lynch, J. C. (1969). Effects of ablations of temporal cortex upon speech sound discrimination in the monkey. *Experimental Neurology*, **24**, 579–91.

Drewe, E. A., Ettlinger, G., Milner, A. D., and Passingham, R. E. (1970). A comparative review of the results of neuropsychological research on man and monkey. *Cortex*, **6**, 129–63.

Eidelberg, D. and Galaburda, A. M. (1984). Inferior parietal lobule: divergent architectonic asymmetries of the human brain. *Archives of Neurology*, **41**, 843–52.

Erhard, P., Kato, T., Strupp, J. P., Andersen, P., Adriany, G., Strick, P. L. *et al.* (1996). Functional mapping of motor cortex in and near Broca's area. *Neuroimage*, **3**, S367.

Ettlinger, G. (1983) A comparative evaluation of the cognitive skills of the chimpanzee and monkey. *International Journal of Neuroscience*, **22**, 7–19.

Faugier-Grimaud, S., Frenois, C., and Stein, D. G. (1978). Effect of posterior parietal lesions on visually guided behavior in monkeys. *Neuropsychologia,* **16**, 151–68.

Felleman, D. J. and van Essen, D. C. (1991). Distributed hierachical processing in the primate cerebral cortex. *Cerebral Cortex*, **1**, 1–47.

Fiez, J. A., Raichle, M. E., Miezin, F. M., and Petersen, S. E. (1995). PET studies of auditory and phonological processing: effects of stimulus characteristics and task demands. *Journal of Cognitive Neuroscience*, **7**, 357–75.

Fiez, J. A., Raichle, M. E., Balota, D. A., Tallal, P., and Petersen, S. E. (1996). PET activation of posterior temporal regions during auditory word presentation and verb generation. *Cerebral Cortex*, **6**, 1–10.

Fink, G. R., Dolan, R. J., Halligan, P. W., Marshall, J. C., and Frith, C. D. (1997). Space-based and object-based visual attention: shape and specific neural domains. *Brain*, **120**, 2013–28.

Galaburda, A. M. and Pandya, D. N. (1982). Role of architectonics and connections in the study of primate brain evolution. In *Primate brain evolution*, (ed. E. Armstrong and D. Falk), pp. 203–16. Plenum, New York.

Galaburda, A. M. and Pandya, D. M. (1983). The intrinsic architectonic and connectional organization of the superior temporal region of the rhesus monkey. *Journal of Comparative Neurology*, **221**, 169–84.

Galaburda, A. and Sanides, F. (1980). Cytoarchitectonic organization of the human auditory cortex. *Journal of Comparative Neurology*, **190**, 597–610.

Galaburda, A. M., Sanides, F., and Geshwind, N. (1978). Human brain: cytoarchitectonic left-right asymmetries in the temporal speech region. *Archives of Neurology*, **35**, 812–17.

Gallese, V., Fadiga, L., Fogassi, L., and Rizzolatti, G. (1996) Action recognition in the premotor cortex. *Brain,* **119**, 593–610.

Gentilucci, M., Fogassi, L., Luppino, G., Matelli, M., Camarda, R., and Rizzolatti, G. (1988). Functional organization of inferior area 6 in the macaque monkey. I. Somatotopy and the control of proximal movements. *Experimental Brain Research*, **71**, 475–90.

Geschwind, N. (1979). Specializations of the human brain. *Scientific American*, **241**, 180–99.

Grafton, S. T., Fagg, A. H., Woods, R. P., and Arbib, M. A. (1996). Functional anatomy of pointing and grasping in humans. *Cerebral Cortex*, **6**, 226–37.

Hast, M. H., Fischer, J. M., Wetzela, B., and Thompson,V. E. (1974). Cortical motor representation of they laryngeal muscles in *Macaca mulatta. Brain Research*, **73**, 229–40.

Haxby, J. V., Horwitz, B., Ungerleider, L. G., Maisog, J. M., Pietrini, P., and Grady, C. L. (1994). The functional organization of human extrastriate cortex: a PET-rCBF study of selection attention to faces and locations. *Journal of Neuroscience*, **14**, 6336–53.

Heffner, H. and Heffner, S. (1986). Effect of unilateral and bilateral auditory cortex lesions on the discrimination of vocalizations by Japanese macaques. *Journal of Neurophysiology*, **56**, 683–90.

Howard, D., Patterson, K., Wise, R., Brown, W. D., Friston, K., Weiller, C. *et al.* (1992). The cortical localization of the lexicons. *Brain,* **115**, 1769–82.

Jahanshahi, M., Jenkins, I. H., Brown, R. G., Marsden, C. D., Passingham, R. E., and Brooks, D. J. (1995). Self-initiated versus externally triggered movements. *Brain*, **118**, 913–33.

Jenkins, I. H., Brooks, D. J., Nixon, P. D., Frackowiak, R. S. J., and Passingham, R. E. (1994). Motor sequence learning: a study with positron emission tomography. *Journal of Neuroscience*, **14**, 3775–90.

Jones, S., Martin, R., and Pilbeam, D. (1992). *The Cambridge encyclopedia of human evolution*. Cambridge University Press, Cambridge.

Jueptner, M., Frith, C. D., Brooks, D. J., Frackowiak, R. S. J., and Passingham, R. E. (1997*a*). Anatomy of motor learning. II. Subcortical structures and learning by trial and error. *Journal of Neurophysiology*, **77**, 1313–24.

Jueptner, M., Stephan, K. M., Frith, C. D., Brooks, D. J., Frackowiak, R. S. J., and Passingham, R. E. (1997*b*). Anatomy of motor learning. I. Frontal cortex and attention to action. *Journal of Neurophysiology*, **77**, 1325–37.

Kosslyn, S. M., Alpert, N. M., Thompson, W. L., Chabris, C. F., Fauch, S. L., and Anderson, A. K. (1994). Identifying objects seen from different viewpoints: a PET investigation. *Brain*, **117**, 1055–71.

Krams, M., Rushworth, M., Deiber, M.-P., Frackowiak, R. S. J. and Passingham, R. E. (in press). The preparation, execution and suppression of copied movements in the human brain. *Experimental Brain Research*.

Lamotte, R. H. and Acuña, C. (1978). Deficits in accuracy of reaching after removal of posterior parietal cortex in monkeys. *Brain Research*, **139**, 309–26.

LeMay, M. (1976). Morphological cerebral asymmetries of modern man, fossil man, and non-human primates. *Annals of the New York Academy of Sciences*, **280**, 349–66.

Liberman, A. M. and Mattingly, I. G. (1985). The motor theory of speech perception revisited. *Cognition*, **21**, 1–36.

Lynch, J. C. and McLaren, J. W. (1989). Deficits of visual attention and saccadic eye movements after lesions of parietooccipital cortex in monkeys. *Journal of Neurophysiology*, **61**, 74–90.

Martin, A., Wiggs, C. L., Ungerleider, L. G., and Haxby, J. V. (1996). Neural correlates of category-specific knowledge. *Nature*, **379**, 649–52.

Matelli, M., Luppino, G., and Rizzolatti, G. (1985). Pattern of cytochrome oxidase activity in frontal agranular cortex of the macaque monkey. *Behavioural Brain Research*, **18**, 125–36.

Matelli, M., Camarda, M., Glickstein, M., and Rizzolatti, G. (1986). Afferent and efferent projections of the inferior area 6 in the macaque monkey. *Journal of Comparative Neurology*, **251**, 281–98.

Mesulam, M.-M. (1990). Large-scale neurocognitive networks and distributed processing for attention, language, and memory. *Annals of Neurology*, **28**, 597–613.

Meyer, A., Beck, E., and McLardy, T. (1947). Prefrontal leucotomy: a neuroanatomical input. *Brain*, **70**, 18–49.

Miklossy, J. (1993). The geniculocalcarine pathway in man, and some putative rostral visual areas involved in visuo-spatial attention. In *Functional organisation of the human visual cortex*, (ed. B. Gulyás, D. Ottoson, and P. E. Roland), pp. 123–36. Pergamon, Oxford.

Miller, E. K. and Desimone, R. (1993). Activity of neurons in anterior inferior temporal cortex during a short-term memory task. *Journal of Neuroscience*, **13**, 1460–78.

Mishkin, M. (1972). Cortical visual areas and their interactions. In *The brain and human behavior*, (ed. A. G. Karczmar and J. C. Eccles), pp. 187–208. Springer-Verlag, Berlin.

Mishkin, M., Lewis, M. E., and Ungerleider, L. G. (1982). Equivalence of parieto-preoccipital subareas for visuospatial ability in monkeys. *Behavioural Brain Research*, **6**, 41–55.

Mishkin, M., Ungerleider, L. G., and Macko, K. A. (1983). Object vision and spatial vision: two cortical pathways. *Trends in Neurosciences*, **6**, 414–17.

Muncer, S. J. and Ettlinger, G. (1981). Communication by a chimpanzee: first-trial mastery of word order that is critical for meaning. *Neuropsychologia*, **19**, 73–8.

Naeser, M. A. (1994). Neuroimaging and recovery of auditory comprehension and spontaneous speech in aphasia with some implications for treatment in severe aphasia. In *Localization and neuroimaging in psychology*, (ed. A. Kertesz), pp. 35–56. Academic Press, New York.
Nobre, A. C., Sebestyen, G. N., Gitelman, D. R., Mesulam, M.-M., and Frackowiak, R. S. J. (1997). Functional localisation of the neural network for visual spatial attention by positron emission tomography. *Brain*, **120**, 515–33.
Ojemann, G. A. (1994). Cortical stimulation and recording in language. In *Localization and neuroimaging in psychology*, (ed. A. Kertesz), pp. 245–96. Academic Press, New York.
Pandya, D. N. and Seltzer, B. (1982). Intrinsic connections and architectonics of posterior parietal cortex in the rhesus monkey. *Journal of Comparative Neurology*, **204**, 196–210.
Pandya, D. N. and Yeterian, E. H. (1985). Architecture and connections of cortical association areas. In *Cerebral cortex*, Vol. 4, (ed. A. Peters and E. G. Jones), pp. 3–61. Plenum, New York.
Pandya, D. N. and Yeterian, E. H. (1996*a*). Comparison of prefrontal architecture and connections. *Philosophical Transactions of the Royal Society of London, B*, **351**, 1423–33.
Pandya, D. N. and Yeterian, E. H. (1996*b*). Morphological correlations of human and monkey frontal lobe. In *Neurobiology of decision-making*, (ed. A. R. Damasio, H. Damasio, and Y. Christen), pp. 13–46. Springer, Berlin.
Passingham, R. E. (1993). *The frontal lobes and voluntary action.* Oxford University Press, Oxford.
Passingham, R. E. and Ettlinger, G. E. (1974). A comparison of cortical functions in man and other primates. *International Review of Neurobiology*, **16**, 233–99.
Paulesu, E., Bottini, G., Bench, C. J., Grasby, P. M., Frith, C. D., and Frackowiak, R. S. J. (1993). The double anatomical dissociation of verbal and visual short-term memory. *Society for Neuroscience Abstracts*, **19**, 413.
Pause, M., Kunesch, E., Binkofski, F., and Freund, H.-J. (1989). Sensorimotor disturbances in patients with lesions of the parietal cortex. *Brain*, **112**, 1599–625.
Pearson, R. C. A. and Powell, T. P. S. (1985). The projection of the primary somatic sensory cortex upon area 5 in the monkey. *Brain Research Reviews*, **9**, 89–107.
Penfield, W. and Roberts, L. (1959). *Speech and brain mechanisms.* Princeton University Press, Princeton.
Penhume, V. B., Zatorre, R. J., MacDonald, J. D., and Evans, A. C. (1996). Interhemispheric anatomical differences in human primary auditory cortex: probabilistic mapping and volume measurement from magnetic resonance imaging. *Cerebral Cortex*, **6**, 661–72.
Perenin, M.-T. and Vighetto, A. (1988). Optic ataxia: a specific disruption in visuomotor mechanisms. I. Different aspects of the deficit in reaching for objects. *Brain*, **111**, 643–74.
Petrides, M. and Pandya, D. N. (1984). Projections to the frontal lobe from the posterior-parietal region in the rhesus monkey. *Journal of Comparative Neurology*, **228**, 105–16.
Petrides, M. and Pandya, D. N. (1995). Comparative architectonic analysis of the human and macaque frontal cortex. In *Handbook of neuropsychology*, Vol. 9, (ed. F. Boller and J. Grafman), pp. 17–58. Elsevier, Amsterdam.
Pierrot-Deseilligny, C., Gray, F., and Brunet, P. (1986). Infarcts of both inferior parietal lobules with impairment of visually guided eye movements, peripheral visual inattention and optic ataxia. *Brain*, **109**, 81–97.

Preuss, T. M. (1995). Do rats have prefrontal cortex? The Rose–Woolsey–Akert program reconsidered. *Journal of Cognitive Neuroscience*, **7**, 1–24.

Preuss, T. M. and Goldman-Rakic, P. S. (1991). Myelo- and cyto-architecture of the granular frontal cortex and surrounding regions in the strepsirhine primate *Galago* and the anthropoid primate *Macaca*. *Journal of Comparative Neurology*, **310**, 429–74.

Price, C. J. I., Moore, C. J., Humphreys, G. W., Frackowiak, R. S. J., and Friston, K. J. (1997). The regions sustaining object and colour naming. *Proceedings of the Royal Society of London, B*, **263**, 1501–7.

Rizzolatti, G., Camarda, R., Fogassi, L., Gentilucci, M., Luppino, G., and Matelli, M. (1988). Functional organization of inferior area 6 in the macaque monkey: II. Area F5 and the control of distal movements. *Experimental Brain Research*, **71**, 491–507.

Rizzolatti, G., Fadiga, L., Gallese, V., and Fogassi, L. (1996*a*). Premotor cortex and the recognition of motor actions. *Cognitive Brain Research*, **3**, 131–42.

Rizzolatti, G., Fadiga, L. Matelli, M., Bettinardi, V., Paulesu, E., Perani, D., and Fazio, F. (1996*b*). Localization of grasp representations in humans by PET. 1 Observation versus execution. *Experimental Brain Research*, **111**, 246–52.

Robinson, D. L., Bowman, E. M., and Kertzman, C. (1995). Covert orienting of attention in macaques. II. Contribution of parietal cortex. *Journal of Neurophysiology*, **74**, 698–712.

Rubens, A. B. (1977). Anatomical asymmetries of the human cerebral cortex. In *Lateralization in the nervous system*, (ed. S. Harnad, R. W. Doty, L. Goldstein, J. Jaynes, and G. Krauthamer), pp. 503–16. Academic Press, New York.

Rushworth, M., Nixon, P. D., and Passingham, R. E. (1997). Parietal cortex and movement. I. Movement selection and reaching. *Experimental Brain Research*, **117**, 292–310.

Sakata, H., Taira, M., Murata, A., and Mine, S. (1995). Neural mechanisms of visual guidance of hand action in the parietal cortex of the monkey. *Cerebral Cortex*, **5**, 429–38.

Sanides, G. A. (1970). Functional architecture of motor and sensory cortices in primates in the light of a new concept of neocortex evolution. In *The primate brain*, (ed. C. R. Noback and W. Montagna) , pp. 137–208. Appleton-Century-Crofts, New York.

Schwartz, B. E., Halgren, E., Fuster, J. M., Simkins, F., Gee, M., and Mandelkern, M. (1995). Cortical metabolic activation in humans during a visual memory task. *Cerebral Cortex*, **5**, 205–14.

Seldon, H. L. (1985). The anatomy of speech perception: human auditory cortex. In *Cerebral cortex*, Vol. 4, (ed. A. Peters and E. G. Jones), pp. 273–328. Plenum, New York.

Seltzer, B. and Pandya, D. N. (1991). Post-rolandic cortical projections of the superior temporal sulcus in the rhesus monkey. *Journal of Comparative Neurology*, **312**, 625–40.

Stephan, K. M., Fink, G. R., Passingham, R. E., Silbersweig, D., Ceballos-Baumann, A., Frith, C. D. *et al.* (1995). Imagining the execution of movements: functional anatomy of the mental representation of upper extremity movements in healthy subjects. *Journal of Neurophysiology*, **73**, 373–86.

Talairach, J. and Tournoux, P. (1988). *Co-planar stereotaxic atlas of the human brain*. Thième, Stuttgart.

Tanaka, K. (1993). Neuronal mechanisms of object recognition. *Science*, **262**, 685–8.

Vallar, G. and Perani, D. (1986). The anatomy of unilateral neglect after right-hemisphere stroke lesions. A clinical / CT-scan correlation study in man. *Neuropsychologia*, **24**, 609–22.

Vandenberghe, R., Price, C., Wise, R., Josephs, O., and Frackowiak, R. S. J. (1996). Functional anatomy of a common semantic system for words and pictures. *Nature*, **383**, 254–6.

Vogt, B. A. and Pandya, D. N. (1978). Cortico-cortical connections of somatic sensory cortex (areas 3, 1 and 2) in the rhesus monkey. *Journal of Comparative Neurology*, **177**, 179–92.

Vogt, C. and Vogt, O. (1919). Allgemeine Ergebnisse unserer Hirnforschung. *Journal of Psychology and Neurology*, **25**, 279–462.

von Bonin, G. and Bailey, P. (1947). *The neocortex of* Macaca mulatta. University of Illinois Press, Urbana.

von Economo, C. (1929). *The cytoarchitectonics of the human cerebral cortex*. Oxford University Press, London.

Walker, A. E. (1940). A cytoarchitectural study of the prefrontal areas of the macaque monkey. *Journal of Comparative Neurology*, **73**, 59–86.

Warburton, E., Wise, R. J. S., Price, C. J., Weiller, C., Hadar, U., Ramsay, S. *et al.* (1996). Noun and verb retrieval by normal subjects: studies with positron emission tomography. *Brain*, **119**, 159–79.

Watson, J. D. G., Myers, R., Frackowiak, R. S. J., Hajnal, J.V., Woods, R. P., Mazziotta, J. C. *et al.* (1993). Area V5 of the human brain: evidence from a combined study using positron emission tomography and magnetic resonance imaging. *Cerebral Cortex*, **3**, 79–94

Witelson, S. F. and Kigar, D. L. (1992). Sylvian fissure morphology and asymmetry in men and women. Bilateral differences in relation to handedness in men. *Journal of Comparative Neurology*, **323**, 326–40.

Yeni-Komshian, G. H. and Benson, D. A. (1976). Anatomical study of cerebral asymmetry in the temporal lobe of humans, chimpanzees and rhesus monkeys. *Science*, **192**, 387–9.

Young, M. P. (1993). The organization of neural systems in the primate cerebral cortex. *Proceedings of the Royal Society of London, B*, **252**, 13–18.

Zatorre, R. J., Meyer, E., Cjedde, A., and Evans, A. C. (1996). PET studies of phonetic processing of speech: review, replication and reanalysis. *Cerebral Cortex*, **6**, 21–30.

Zeki, S. (1993). *A vision of the brain*. Blackwell, Oxford.

Index

achromatopsia 26, 45
agnosia
  apperceptive 40–1, 48
  associative 15, 30–2, 41, 48
AIP 73, 77, 80, 288
allocentric (coding) 113, 255, 280
amnesia 97–8, 109–12, 248, 253, 255–6, 258, 263
amygdala 57–9, 61–2, 95, 97, 99–100, 113
anterior commissure, *see* commissures
apperceptive agnosia 40–1, 48
apraxia 3, 184–91, 204
area 6, *see* premotor cortex
area 7a 74, 79, 86, 274, 277, 279
area 8, *see* frontal eye fields
area 46 279, 290–1
associative agnosia 15, 30–2, 41, 48
asymmetry, cerebral 167, 191, 281–2, 285
auditory cortex 282
auditory perception 51, 59–60, 62, 65-6, 122, 160, 172, 189, 218, 260, 282–4, 288–90
autism 261
awareness, *see* consciousness

basal ganglia 176, 199, 222, 263

caudate nucleus, *see* basal ganglia 56
cerebellum (and cerebellar) 73, 194, 199, 285
colliculus 73, 148, 157
commissures
  anterior 64, 127, 129–38, 144–9, 153, 156–7, 159, 161–2
  hippocampal 153, 158–9
  posterior 148, 161
  see also corpus callosum
consciousness 77, 148, 220, 246, 249–50, 255, 257, 259–60, 262, 264–5
constructional apraxia 187–8
corpus callosum 2, 3, 79, 115, 127–38, 143, 145–9, 155–61, 189
  agenesis of 129, 149, 156
corpus striatum, *see* basal ganglia
cortical blindness 131, 213, 215, 260
cross-modal integration 2, 51–66

directional hypokinesia 217

emotion 175, 249
enhancement 120–1, 199, 221
episodic memory, *see* memory
Ettlinger, G. 1, 2, 16–18, 23, 26–7, 30–2, 45, 48, 52–6, 58, 66, 70–3, 79, 82–6, 88, 95–6, 100, 103, 105, 129, 133, 143, 148, 167–8, 185, 187, 190, 203, 214–16, 218, 220, 222–3, 247, 271–2
eye movements 73, 85, 223
  pursuit 75, 87–8, 191
  saccadic 75–6, 82–3, 87, 221, 223
extinction 84, 216, 220–3, 229, 274

face perception 18–19, 21–2
fMRI 97, 271–2, 289
frontal eye fields 75, 222, 291
functional MRI 97, 271–2, 289
FST 73

grasping 77–80, 87, 168, 175

hand preferences 168–9, 173–7
hemianopia, *see* cortical blindness
hemispatial neglect, *see* neglect
hippocampal commissure, *see* commissures
hippocampus 59, 61, 95, 97–8, 100–5, 109, 113, 115, 153, 156, 158–9, 252–3, 256–7

imagery
  visual 254
  motor 199
inattention, *see* neglect
inferior temporal cortex 2, 30, 32, 38, 41, 45, 56, 58, 60, 64–5, 70, 73–4, 80–1, 122, 129, 274, 283
inferotemporal cortex, *see* inferior temporal cortex
insula 58, 65
intraparietal sulcus 74, 77–8, 86–7, 204, 221, 274, 276, 279

Korsakoff 257

lateral geniculate nucleus, *see* thalamic nuclei
laterality 3, 101–2, 170, 214, 222, 237
lateralization 131, 136, 169–70, 271
left hemisphere 19, 22, 130, 138, 152, 162, 167–78, 190–1, 215, 217, 272
LGN, *see* thalamic nuclei
LIP 73–6

magnetic resonance imaging 100, 101–2, 145, 149, 156, 271, 278, 280, 284, 290
memory
  episodic 109–10, 112–14, 116, 122, 250–1, 254
  implicit 249–50, 253
  semantic 66, 109–10, 113–14, 116
mental representation 216, 236, 238, 245–8, 250, 262–5
  see also imagery
misreaching 71–2, 79, 84–6, 275, 279
motor control 160, 170, 176, 178, 191, 201
MRI 100, 101–2, 145, 149, 156, 271, 280, 284, 290
MST 278–9
MT 73, 75, 88, 275, 284

neglect 86, 213–23, 260
  object-based 223

object-based coding 157
oculomotor, *see* eye movements
optic ataxia 85–7, 221, 285, 279

parietal lobe, inferior (human) 186, 190, 223, 278
parietal lobe, superior (human) 279
Parkinson's disease 176, 263
parvocellular channel 31
PET 97, 195, 254, 271–2, 275–80, 287–90
planning 184, 186, 188, 199, 201
PO 234, 257
pontine nuclei 73
positron emission tomography 97, 195, 254, 271–2, 275–80, 287–90
posterior commissure 148, 161
posterior parietal cortex (monkey) 70, 73, 75, 77, 80, 82, 85, 221
prefrontal cortex 56–7, 128, 189, 192, 194, 199, 259, 279–80, 286–8, 291–2
prehension 77–80, 87, 168, 175
premotor cortex 56, 75–7, 187, 189, 192, 195, 197, 201, 204, 259, 279–80, 285–6, 288–9
primary visual cortex, *see* V1
prosopagnosia 23
pulvinar nucleus, *see* thalamic nuclei
putamen, *see* basal ganglia

representation, *see* mental representation
right hemisphere 19, 21–2, 63, 130, 132, 138, 148, 152–3, 162, 168, 170–8, 190–1, 214–15, 217, 281

saccades, *see* eye movements
schizophrenia 261–3
scotoma, *see* cortical blindness
semantic memory 66, 109–10, 113–14, 116
sensory deficits 26, 214
SI, *see* somatosensory cortex
SII, *see* somatosensory cortex
somatosensory cortex 117, 189, 194, 279–80
somatosensory discrimination, *see* tactile
spatial attention 217
spatial neglect, *see* neglect
spatial perception 70, 78–9, 83, 86, 148, 187
speech 146, 169, 188, 191, 254, 262, 281, 289
stereopsis 130, 157, 160
stereotypy 261–3
striate cortex 32, 45, 273
sulcus principalis, *see* area 46
superior colliculus 73, 148, 156
superior temporal 56, 73, 129, 274, 276, 281–2, 285, 288, 290–1
supplementary motor 187, 192, 199, 204

tactile discrimination 53–9, 61–6, 70, 80, 117, 122, 132–5, 141, 189, 218, 260, 263, 279–80
TE, *see* inferior temporal cortex
TEO 32–3, 274
thalamic nuclei 112–13, 115
  pulvinar nucleus 73
  anterior thalamus 111–13, 115

visual areas
  AIP 73, 77, 80, 288
  FST 73
  LIP 73–6
  MST 278–9
  MT 73, 75, 88, 275, 284
  PO 234, 257
  TEO 32–3, 274
  V1 72–4, 79, 82, 260, 275
  V2 32, 74, 273
  V3 74, 273
  V3A 73, 75
  V4 32–3, 45, 80, 273
visual form agnosia, *see* agnosia, apperceptive
visuomotor integration 73–4, 76–80, 84–6, 88, 201, 222–3
visuomotor disorders, *see* optic ataxia
visuospatial neglect, *see* neglect
V1 72–4, 79, 82, 260, 275
V2 32, 74, 273
V3 74, 273
V3A 73, 75
V4 32–3, 45, 80, 273
V5, *see* visual areas, MT